DR. AMANDA ARCHULETA

Wired For Balance

Acupuncture, the Nervous System, and the Secrets of Longevity

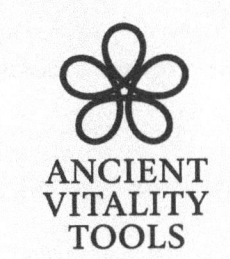

ANCIENT
VITALITY
TOOLS

First published by Ancient Vitaltiy Tools Press 2025

Copyright © 2025 by Dr. Amanda Archuleta

All rights reserved. No part of this publication may be reproduced, stored or transmitted in any form or by any means, electronic, mechanical, photocopying, recording, scanning, or otherwise without written permission from the publisher. It is illegal to copy this book, post it to a website, or distribute it by any other means without permission.

Dr. Amanda Archuleta asserts the moral right to be identified as the author of this work.

Dr. Amanda Archuleta has no responsibility for the persistence or accuracy of URLs for external or third-party Internet Websites referred to in this publication and does not guarantee that any content on such Websites is, or will remain, accurate or appropriate.

This book is intended for educational and informational purposes only. It is not a substitute for professional medical advice, diagnosis, or treatment. Always seek the advice of your physician or other qualified health provider with any questions you may have regarding a medical condition. Never disregard professional medical advice or delay seeking it because of something you have read in this book.

The case studies and stories in this book are composite accounts inspired by real clinical experiences. They are for educational purposes only and do not depict actual patients. These examples are not meant to diagnose, treat, or prescribe.
Readers should always consult a qualified healthcare provider for personalized care. This content is not a substitute for medical advice and does not establish a provider-patient relationship.

The author and publisher disclaim any liability for any adverse effects or consequences from the use of any suggestions, preparations, or procedures discussed in this book.

Acknowledgment of Previously Published Material

Certain sections of this book were originally published in Acupuncture Today. They are republished here with permission from Acupuncture Today.

First edition

ISBN: 979-8-9933130-1-6

This book was professionally typeset on Reedsy.
Find out more at reedsy.com

Dedication
To all the patients who have trusted me with their healing,
To my family and friends who have walked beside me,
To the teachers, mentors, and communities that have shaped me,
And to the world—
May we all find our way back to rhythm, balance, and vitality.

"I've heard that in the days of old everyone lived one hundred years without showing the usual signs of aging. In our time, however people age prematurely, living only fifty years. Is this due to a change in the environment, or is it because people have lost the correct way of life"

— Huang Di

Contents

Preface   iv
Acknowledgments   vi
Authors Note   vii
Introduction   1

I   Foundations of Acupuncture and the Nervous System

  1   Homeostasis & the Healing Body   7
  2   The Body's Electrical Language - How the Nervous System...   11
  3   The Autonomic Nervous System - The Hidden Healer   18
  4   The Vagus Nerve - The Body's Healing Superhighway   23

II   When Survival Becomes the Pattern

  5   Yin and Yang in the Nervous System - Ancient Insights,...   31
  6   Trauma and the ANS - Rewiring the Survival Response   36
  7   The Liver, the Mind, and the Movement of Qi   40

III   The Channels of Regulation

  8   Channels and Nerves - Where Ancient Pathways Meet...   49
  9   Spinal Pathways and the Energetics of Organ Regulation   57
  10   Spinal Gateways - The Ling Shu and the ANS   60

IV The Emotional Body

11 When Emotions Take Shape - The Psychosomatic Roots of... — 67
12 Quieting the Storm - Acupuncture, Autonomic Balance, and... — 71
13 The Spirit and the Shen – Emotional Regulation in Classical... — 82
14 Trauma and the Po – Grief, the Lungs, and Somatic Release — 90
15 Digesting Life -The Spleen, the Yi, and the Nervous System — 102
16 The Wellspring Within - The Kidneys, Zhi, and the Blueprint... — 128
17 The Ethereal Soul - Honoring the Hun for Vision, Flow, and... — 150
18 Emotional Harmony and the Nervous System - A Lifelong Key to... — 174
19 Integration – The Healing Rhythm of Balance — 181

V Tracing the Currents of Balance

20 How Modern Science Validates Acupuncture's Ancient Wisdom — 189
21 The Science of Balance - What Research Reveals About... — 192
22 From Systemic Balance to the Wandering Nerve — 199
23 When Pain Signals a System Out of Balance — 207
24 The Heart Remembers - Acupuncture, Autonomic Rhythm, and the... — 215
25 Regulating the Gut - Acupuncture, Autonomic Balance, and... — 222
26 Breath and Balance - Acupuncture's Autonomic Influence on... — 233
27 Final Reflections - A Unified Path of Healing — 241

VI From Regulation to Renewal

28 Acupuncture and Longevity - Restoring the Rhythms of Vital...	245
29 Key Research on Acupuncture, the ANS, and Longevity	247
30 The Pulse of Longevity - How Vessels Carry Time	254
31 Inflammaging and Lingering Heat - The Slow Fire of Aging	262
32 Acupuncture and Cellular Health	269
33 Essence Woven in Time - Telomeres and the Sentinels of...	277

VII Rhythms of Renewal

34 Living in Rhythm - Daily Tools for Autonomic Balance	291
35 Morning Grounding Practices - Waking the Body with Rhythm...	293
36 Breathwork for Vagal Stimulation - Returning to Calm, One...	296
37 Nourishment as Regulation - Eating in Rhythm with the...	306
38 The Night Gate - Calming Rituals for the Shen and Vagal Tone	313
39 Restoring Rhythm - Touch as Medicine for Emotion and...	321
40 The Rhythm of Return - Acupuncture, Autonomic Healing, and...	336

Notes	342
Appendix A. Epigraph Sources	401
About the Author	404
Stay Connected	406
Share Your Experience	407

Preface

My journey into acupuncture began with pain of my own. For years I carried discomfort that no amount of doctor visits or therapies seemed to resolve. It wasn't until a friend suggested acupuncture that something shifted. Skeptical but curious, I booked a session. After just a few treatments, the pain that had weighed on me began to melt away. But something deeper changed as well. I felt like myself again. That experience planted a seed.

Physical activity slowly became easier, and with that came a sense of freedom in my body I hadn't felt in years. That spark grew into a passion for movement, which eventually led me to train as a fitness instructor. From there, I went on to study exercise science and began teaching fitness classes, helping others discover the same strength and vitality I had found.

The memory of acupuncture's profound effect stayed with me. In 2008, I decided to devote my life to the medicine that gave me mine back. I earned my Master of Science in Oriental Medicine from Southwest Acupuncture College in Santa Fe, New Mexico. A few years later received my Doctorate in Acupuncture and Oriental Medicine from Five Branches University in San Jose, California. During my studies, I also had the honor of interning at Heilongjiang University in Harbin, China, where I witnessed firsthand the integration of acupuncture into hospital-based care.

After graduation, I took my skills to the sea. I traveled the world as an acupuncturist aboard cruise ships, treating thousands of patients from every walk of life. From the Mediterranean to Southeast Asia, I saw how universal the need for balance was, and how deeply acupuncture could meet that need.

Wired for Balance began as a doctoral capstone. But the more I studied, practiced, and reflected, the more I realized this wasn't just a project, it was a calling. I wanted to understand, and more importantly, share how acupuncture influences the Autonomic Nervous System (ANS), the master regulator of our internal balance. What I found confirmed what many practitioners have long observed, acupuncture doesn't just treat symptoms. It rewires our ability to heal.

Blending the wisdom of TCM with modern science and clinical insight, this book explores how acupuncture restores balance by regulating the ANS. It is written for practitioners, students, and anyone who wants to understand how a needle can calm anxiety, ease pain, improve sleep, and bring the body back into its natural rhythm.

We live in an age of over stimulation. Chronic stress has become a baseline, and many of us are disconnected from the body's wisdom. Acupuncture invites us back to slowness, to breath, to balance. It is both art and science, both ancient and urgently modern.

Thank you for walking this path with me. I hope this book serves as a bridge between worlds and a reminder that healing is not just possible. It is our nature.

With warmth and gratitude,
Dr. Amanda Archuleta

Acknowledgments

Acknowledgments

This book would not be possible without the love, counsel, and support of many people who have walked with me on my journey of healing and discovery.

I want to express my gratitude to my family for their consistent support and patience during the long writing sessions, and faith in my vision. Your presence has consistently given me courage and motivation.

Thank you to my teachers and deans at Southwest Acupuncture College and Five Branches University for sharing your knowledge and allowing me to grow as a student and healer. The instruction I got in your classrooms provided the groundwork for all this book represents.

A special acknowledgment to Dr. Maya Yu, my teacher, mentor, dean, and employer. Your instruction has been grounding, thoughtful, and supportive. Your dedication to this medicine inspires me every day. Thank you for supporting me, encouraging me, and believing in my abilities.

To the patients I have had the honor to treat. You are my greatest teacher. It is through your healing journeys that I have learned the depth of this medicine.

And to every reader picking up this book, thank you for being part of the ongoing story. May this work support you, ground you, and help you reconnect with balance.

With heartfelt gratitude,
Dr. Amanda Archuleta

Authors Note

Longevity is more than the number of years you live. It is the quality of those years. It is your body's ability to move with strength, think with clarity, and meet each day with energy and purpose.

This book is one branch of the larger tree that is longevity. A vibrant, healthy life grows from many interconnected roots. It is nourished by regular movement, wholesome food, deep and restorative sleep, emotional balance, meaningful relationships, and, when needed, carefully chosen supplements under the guidance of a qualified practitioner. Breath practices, mindfulness, and other tools for calming the mind are among the most powerful of these roots, helping the body return to balance and repair. No single branch stands alone. Together, they create the living system that sustains vitality across a lifetime.

In this book, longevity focuses on a science-based framework for supporting the body's natural repair systems, emotional resilience, and physiological balance. These are part of the foundations of living not just longer, but well.

For over two thousand years, Chinese medicine has viewed longevity as the art of nourishing life. The *Huang Di Nei Jing* taught that those who live in harmony with the seasons, regulate their emotions, and care for their vital energy could reach one hundred years. Today, modern research echoes this wisdom. Studies show that the state of your ANS, the delicate balance between sympathetic and parasympathetic function, shapes inflammation, immune health, hormonal balance, and even how your cells age.

In *Wired for Balance*, we bring these worlds together. Through acupuncture, breath, mindfulness, and lifestyle strategies, you will learn how to regulate your nervous system and activate the body's innate capacity for repair. Each chapter blends evidence from peer-reviewed research with timeless longevity practices from Chinese medicine, creating a blueprint that is both ancient in its roots and modern in its application.

If you would like to continue exploring these practices beyond the book, I invite you to join me for seasonal, self care rituals, wellness reflections, foods, and guided meditations, at ancient-vitality-tools.com.

Introduction

Have you ever wondered why acupuncture can feel so deeply relaxing? Or why does it help with pain, sleep, and even digestion? At the heart of this ancient therapy is its ability to influence the body's Autonomic Nervous System (ANS), the part of our physiology that quietly regulates everything from our heartbeat to our stress response.

In this book, we will explore how acupuncture influences the ANS. We will explore why this understanding matters not only for healthy aging and longevity, but also how it helps with emotional health, chronic pain and disease. At the same time, we will see how these modern insights echo the ancient wisdom of yin and yang and the meridian systems of Chinese medicine.

By integrating scientific research with the wisdom of Traditional Chinese Medicine (TCM), we begin to see how these two frameworks converge on the same truth. Acupuncture emerges as a profound tool for cultivating longevity, restoring the body's physiological rhythms, and replenishing the deeper currents of energy that sustain life.

Introduction to Acupuncture and Chinese Medicine

For over 3,000 years, Traditional Chinese Medicine (TCM) has offered a holistic view of health. One that sees the body not as separate parts, but as an interconnected whole. Rooted in observation, rhythm, and balance, TCM has long recognized patterns of disharmony behind pain and disease.[1] Among its most widely practiced modalities is acupuncture, a technique that uses fine needles to stimulate specific points along the body's meridians, channels through which vital energy, or qi, flows.

Today, acupuncture is increasingly recognized as both primary and complementary therapy for treating chronic conditions.[2] The purpose is simple yet profound. To restore balance and awaken the body's natural healing intelligence. In Western terms, this means activating key regulatory systems, especially the ANS, to shift the body out of survival mode and into a state of healing and repair.[3]

Ancient practitioners worked with sharpened stones, bones, or bronze tools to move qi through the twelve primary meridians. Today's acupuncturists use ultra-fine, sterile needles to gently stimulate the same points, often eliciting a feeling known as *da qi*, a dull, heavy, or spreading sensation that signifies the body is responding.[4] Across both ancient and modern approaches, the goal remains the same. To restore flow, release stagnation, and return the body to balance.

To understand how this healing process works, we must first explore the concept of homeostasis. This is the body's natural ability to maintain internal stability. It relies on a set of sophisticated systems that constantly work to keep us well

Acupuncture, ANS, and Longevity

Modern research increasingly shows that the key to a longer, healthier life is not just genetics, it's how well our body adapts to stress. The ANS plays a vital role in this adaptability. It regulates our heart rate, breath, digestion, sleep, inflammation, and even our immune response. These are all critical for long-term health and vitality. When the ANS is imbalanced, the body stays stuck in survival mode, contributing to chronic conditions like hypertension, insomnia, digestive issues, and systemic inflammation.[5] Acupuncture appears to restore balance within the ANS, guiding the body toward rest, recovery, and resilience..[6]

From a Chinese medicine perspective, this makes intuitive sense. Acupuncture moves qi and restores harmony. These concepts mirror the body's internal regulation. By supporting nervous system balance, acupuncture does more than relieve symptoms. It supports the body's ability to heal, adapt, and thrive, which are key elements of what we now understand as the foundations of healthy aging and longevity.

Yin, Yang & the Nervous System

INTRODUCTION

In Chinese medicine, the concept of balance is rooted in the dynamic interplay of yin and yang, opposing yet complementary forces that govern all aspects of life and physiology. Yin represents stillness, nourishment, rest, and cooling qualities. Yang embodies movement, heat, activity, and stimulation. For thousands of years, this framework has guided practitioners in understanding health, disease, and the nature of vitality.[7]

What is remarkable is how closely this ancient model aligns with modern understandings of the ANS. The parasympathetic branch, which governs rest, digestion, and regeneration, is distinctly yin in nature. It slows the heart, calms the mind, and supports long-term healing. The sympathetic branch, which primes us for action and alertness, is yang. Yang is energizing, activating, and protective. Health arises not from suppressing one or the other, but from maintaining their dynamic balance. Just as too much yang leads to burnout, excess yin can result in stagnation and depletion.[8]

Acupuncture helps regulate this yin-yang relationship by influencing the body's bioelectrical and neurochemical systems. Through specific point combinations, practitioners can tonify yin, subdue excess yang, or restore flow between the two. This ability to modulate nervous system tone through the lens of yin and yang is what makes acupuncture such a powerful tool for modern chronic disease. Imbalance, rather than a single pathogen, is often the root cause.[9]

Meridian Theory & the Body's Internal Wiring

Chinese medicine describes a network of meridians. Meridians are energetic pathways through which qi (vital energy) flows to nourish the body's organs, tissues, and spirit. For centuries, these pathways have been mapped, palpated, and treated to restore balance and health. While qi and meridians may sound abstract through a Western lens, scientists now believe they closely mirror the body's internal communication systems, especially the nervous system and fascia network.[10]

Meridians are not anatomical structures in the traditional sense. They follow patterns that correlate with major nerve pathways, blood vessels, and connective tissue planes.[11] Studies using imaging, electrical conductance, and ultrasound have shown that acupuncture points often lie at sites of high electrical conductivity, nerve bundles, or intermuscular fascia junctions, suggesting a physical basis for their energetic descriptions.[12]

Just as nerves transmit electrical signals to regulate organ function and perception, meridians carry vital information that helps the body adapt, heal, and maintain equilibrium. When we place a needle along a meridian, we interact with the energy of the nervous system. We are initiating a response for the body to break feedback loops that are causing blockages. This stimulation is what promotes blood flow and circulation to an area that needs it.[13]

In the chapters ahead, we will dive deeper into how acupuncture awakens the body's healing intelligence through both the lens of modern science and the wisdom of Chinese medicine. You will discover how meridians mirror the body's internal wiring, how yin and yang reflect autonomic rhythms, and how restoring balance within your nervous system can lead to real, lasting change in your physical, emotional, and energetic well-being.

This is more than a book about acupuncture. It's a map of the body's deeper intelligence. Whether you're a practitioner, a patient, or simply someone searching for healing and clarity, *Wired for Balance* invites you to reimagine wellness not as a destination, but as a state of dynamic harmony. One needle at a time, one breath at a time, we begin the journey toward restoring balance, vitality, and the ancient rhythm of health that still lives within us all.

I

Foundations of Acupuncture and the Nervous System

The Healing Blueprint Within

"The law of yin and yang is the natural order of the universe, the foundation of all things, mother of all changes, the root of life and death. In healing, one must grasp the root of the disharmony, which is always subject to the law of yin and yang"
— Huang Di

"The people of high antiquity, those who knew the Way, they modeled [their behavior] on yin and yang."
— Huang Di

1

Homeostasis & the Healing Body

Your body is always in motion. It gently adjusts, responds, and finds its way back to balance as it works quietly to keep you safe, alive, and well. This remarkable process is called homeostasis. Homeostasis is a state of balance that keeps your internal environment stable, even when the world around you changes.[1] Whether it's regulating temperature, fluid levels, or nutrient delivery, your body is always working behind the scenes to ensure every cell has what it needs to function.

The Architecture of Balance

To maintain this internal harmony, the body relies on essentials: oxygen, hydration, nutrients, and warmth.[2] When these are in balance, blood flows freely throughout the body. This supports tissue repair and makes energy available for healing and restoration. Yet life brings many disruptions. Stress, trauma, inflammation, poor sleep, and chronic pain can easily throw this system off course. Fortunately, the body is equipped with complex feedback systems that constantly monitor for imbalances and activate real-time adjustments to restore balance.[3]

The ability to restore balance is what makes healing possible. When feedback systems become overwhelmed or stuck, stress becomes chronic, and inflammation can persist. As a result, core systems may begin to shut down, and disease can take root. According to both Western physiology and Chinese medicine, chronic illness is often the result of homeostatic imbalance.[4]

As we will soon explore, acupuncture is a tool that helps the body restore its natural balance by engaging the very systems that support homeostasis.

Yin, Yang, and the Stress Response

In TCM, homeostasis arises from the ever-shifting dance of yin and yang. These two forces are in constant dialogue within us. This balance is also maintained from the harmonious interplay of the five elements that shape our inner world.[5]

Each element is linked to an organ system, which is further divided into yin and yang organ pairs. These aren't just anatomical references, they represent energetic functions, emotional tendencies, and physiological responses.

Among these, the liver plays a central role. According to Chinese medicine, the liver stores blood, regulates qi, and governs the smooth flow of energy throughout the body. Its influence goes even deeper. The liver acts as the body's first responder to stress, whether emotional or physical.[6] When we face pressure, the liver's yang aspect helps the nervous system respond. It promotes circulation, and directs blood and energy to where they're needed most. In this way, the liver helps the body rise to the occasion and restore internal order.[7]

From a Western perspective, this mirrors how the ANS responds to stress. When triggered, it shifts us into high alert to protect the body. Prolonged activation can create an imbalance. If the body cannot return to homeostasis after stress or trauma, dysfunction sets in. Over time, this unresolved stress response contributes to chronic conditions, something both Eastern and Western medicine acknowledge.[8]

Feedback Loops & the Roots of Imbalance

In Western medicine, the body maintains homeostasis through a series of feedback mechanisms. These feedback mechanisms are internal communication loops that regulate various functions, including temperature, hormone levels, and immune responses.[9] The most common of these are negative feedback loops. They act to correct changes and restore balance. For example, if your body temperature rises, these loops trigger sweating to cool you down. It's a constant, intelligent dance of adjustment.[10]

When the system is overwhelmed by chronic stress, unresolved trauma, or physical injury, the body's negative feedback loops can fail to restore balance. In their place, positive feedback loops may begin to dominate. Unlike negative feedback, positive feedback amplifies a response instead of calming it. It's meant to be temporary, like in childbirth or blood clotting. However, when it persists unnecessarily, it can lead to dysfunction.[11]

A common example of positive feedback is muscle spasms. The initial spasm might protect an injured area, but ongoing pain can trigger more spasms. This response causes more pain, creating a loop that won't stop until something breaks the cycle.[12] These unchecked loops often underlie chronic pain and inflammatory conditions.

At the center of these loops is the nervous system, the body's primary communication network. It gathers information, makes decisions, and directs responses throughout the entire body.[13] To understand how acupuncture supports regulation, we must first examine the central and peripheral nervous systems and their roles in homeostasis and disease

Acupuncture, Homeostasis & the Path to Longevity

Acupuncture helps restore homeostasis by modulating the body's core regulatory systems, such as the ANS, the endocrine system, and the immune system. When the body is under chronic stress or disease, its natural feedback mechanisms often become impaired. Acupuncture helps reestablish communication between these systems by stimulating sensory nerves, activating brain centers like the hypothalamus, and modulating hormonal and immune responses.[14]

By activating specific points along the meridians, acupuncture sends signals to the central nervous system. This triggers the release of endorphins, serotonin, and hormones that regulate cortisol. Together, these shifts help the body move from a state of overdrive, known as sympathetic dominance, into a state of repair and regulation through parasympathetic activation.[15] This shift is crucial for homeostasis. In effect, acupuncture reminds the body how to reset itself.

The importance of homeostasis goes far beyond symptom relief.

Longevity science shows that people who maintain greater physiological adaptability live longer and healthier lives. This adaptability reflects the body's ability to return to balance after experiencing stress. [16]

In TCM, longevity is seen as the result of harmony. This is seen as a balanced flow of qi, blood, and spirit. By supporting the body's natural rhythms and restoring balance, acupuncture offers not just symptom relief, but a path toward deeper vitality and extended health span. It doesn't force healing; it reawakens it.

2

The Body's Electrical Language - How the Nervous System Communicates

Deep within us, countless signals move in conversation. Every second, they gather information, interpret messages, and send instructions. This intelligent network adjusts everything from heart rate to immune activity. Together, the nervous and endocrine systems regulate the body's internal environment, transmitting messages through electrical impulses along nerves and chemical messengers in the blood known as hormones.[1]

Sensory information travels through afferent and efferent pathways. These pathways define the direction of communication within the nervous system. Afferent signals carry messages *toward* the brain or spinal cord, helping the body notice what is happening within and around it. Efferent signals carry instructions *away* from the brain and spinal cord, guiding the body in how to respond.[2] For example, if you touch something hot, an afferent signal races to your brain, and an efferent signal immediately tells your hand to pull away.

This two-way communication allows the body to stay balanced through built-in feedback loops. When something shifts, like a change in temperature or a rise in stress hormones, the nervous system notices. It sends signals to help the body return to balance.[3] These rapid adjustments are essential to homeostasis, and they depend entirely on the integrity of the central and peripheral nervous systems.

Feedback Loops - The Body's Balancing Act

To maintain internal balance, the body relies on mechanisms called feedback loops. These mechanisms either suppress or amplify a response depending on what's needed. These loops are vital to homeostasis. They help keep blood pressure steady, hormones in check, and stress responses appropriate.[4]

There are two primary types of feedback: negative and positive. Negative feedback loops are protective and stabilizing. They detect a change and trigger a response that reverses it. This response helps to bring the body back to equilibrium. For instance, if your body temperature rises, you begin to sweat; if it drops, you start to shiver. These loops help prevent sudden or extreme shifts in the body's internal environment[5].

Positive feedback loops, on the other hand, amplify change. They push the body further away from its baseline. This usually happens for short-term and necessary functions, such as blood clotting or childbirth. When these loops persist without interruption, they can contribute to dysfunction. For example, chronic pain triggers muscle tension. The increased tension amplifies pain signals. In turn, heightened pain leads to further tension. This cycle reinforces itself and often requires intervention to restore balance.[6]

When negative feedback systems become overwhelmed, positive feedback can dominate, leading to a breakdown in homeostasis. Many diseases arise when these regulatory systems fail to recalibrate. In this way, imbalance in the body's internal messaging system does not simply cause discomfort. It can also create conditions that lead to chronic illness.

Understanding how these feedback loops function is essential to understanding how acupuncture supports healing. Acupuncture helps interrupt harmful cycles and restore healthy communication within the nervous system. As this communication is restored, the body can regulate itself more effectively.[7]

The Central Nervous System - The Body's Command Center

At the core of the body's regulatory system is the Central Nervous

System (CNS). It consists of the brain and spinal cord. It acts as the body's command center, processing sensory input and issuing instructions to maintain stability. Every thought, movement, hormone release, immune defense, and pain response begins here. In terms of homeostasis, the CNS constantly monitors the internal environment and determines the appropriate response to keep the body within optimal range.[8]

When the CNS detects stress, injury, or imbalance, it orchestrates a coordinated reaction through nerve signaling, hormonal messengers, and motor responses. If the stress is acute, this reaction is protective. When the CNS stays activated for too long, it starts to form unhealthy patterns. Long periods of anxiety or trauma can lead to chronic pain. Muscles may stay tense. Sleep may become disturbed. Hormones may shift out of balance.

This is where acupuncture comes in as a modulator of CNS activity. Neuroimaging studies show that acupuncture stimulation affects multiple areas of the brain, including the hypothalamus, brainstem, amygdala, and anterior cingulate cortex. All of these regions are involved in autonomic regulation, emotional processing, and pain perception.[9] Acupuncture quiets overactive neural circuits, helping shift the brain from hypervigilance to restoration.

From the perspective of TCM, this mirrors the process of calming liver yang, anchoring the Shen (spirit), and opening flow through the Governing Vessel, which runs along the spine and connects to the brain.[10] Ancient texts recognized that when one's spirit and brain were disturbed, the body could not maintain harmony. Today, neuroscience is confirming this same principle. A regulated brain supports a regulated body.

By calming the CNS, acupuncture initiates a ripple effect across all systems. This effect lowers blood pressure, enhances digestion, reduces inflammation, and improves sleep. This brain-body connection is central to restoring homeostasis and promoting long-term vitality.[11]

The Peripheral Nervous System - Extending the Brain's Reach

Every thought, movement, and emotion involves the nervous system. It coordinates each function, allowing your body and mind to respond to the world around you. It's the body's master communication network, and is working nonstop to process what's happening both inside and around you.[12] Millions of sensory receptors constantly monitor your internal state and your environment, sending signals to your brain and spinal cord to determine how you should respond.[13]

The nervous system has two main branches. The Central Nervous System (CNS) includes the brain and spinal cord. The Peripheral Nervous System (PNS) consists of all the nerves that branch out from the center and extend throughout the body.[14] While the CNS serves as the control center, the PNS functions like a vast information highway. It carries signals between the brain and the rest of the body.[15]

Anatomically, the PNS includes 12 pairs of cranial nerves and 33 pairs of spinal nerves.[16] These nerves are made up of two major types of cells: sensory (afferent) neurons, which carry information *to* the brain, and motor (efferent) neurons, which carry instructions *away* from it.[17] This flow of input and output allows your body to respond to everything from a change in temperature to a moment of danger, or to the calming touch of an acupuncture needle.

The fundamental building block of this system is the neuron. Often called the "signal unit" of the nervous system, it transmits messages using electrical impulses and chemical messengers.[18] Acupuncture interacts with these neurons at key points along the body, altering their signaling to regulate pain, tension, and physiological stress responses.[19]

In essence, the Peripheral Nervous System is an extension of your brain. It reaches out to connect every organ, tissue, and cell. When it's out of sync, your body can't respond to stress effectively or heal properly. When it's balanced, the entire system functions with greater intelligence, adaptability, and vitality.

Acupuncture & the Nervous System - Rewiring the Loop

Acupuncture has a unique ability to influence the nervous system in ways that restore balance and interrupt harmful feedback loops. Acupuncture stimulates specific points on the body. Many of these points are located near nerve bundles or connective tissue junctions. The stimulation sends signals to the brain and spinal cord. This activates a cascade of physiological responses that support regulation.[20]

These signals can modulate activity in the ANS, shifting the body out of a sympathetic "fight-or-flight" state and into parasympathetic "rest-and-digest" mode. This is where healing occurs. Recent observations shows that acupuncture promotes the release of endorphins, serotonin, and oxytocin. These neurochemicals calm the mind, reduce pain, and regulate stress hormones such as cortisol.[21] These changes help reverse the very loops that contribute to chronic pain, inflammation, insomnia, and anxiety.

In practical terms, acupuncture serves as an external signal that helps the body recalibrate. If a feedback loop becomes destructive, such as chronic muscle tension from stress or an ongoing inflammatory response, acupuncture can act as a reset button. It interrupts the pattern and allows the body to return to homeostasis.[22]

TCM describes this in energetic terms. When qi is stuck or chaotic, symptoms arise. By moving qi and harmonizing the meridians, acupuncture restores flow and clears stagnation.[23] From a biomedical view, this correlates to the regulation of neural signaling, vascular flow, and hormonal feedback.

In both systems, the message is the same: when communication in the body is restored, healing follows.

The Brain-Body Connection - Longevity, Acupuncture, and the Central Nervous System

Longevity is not just about living longer. It is about living well. In longevity science, one of the most important discoveries is the link between nervous system regulation and lifespan. People who maintain a regulated nervous system and greater neuroplasticity tend to live longer and healthier lives. Neuroplasticity refers to the brain's ability to adapt and reorganize. A well-functioning Central Nervous System (CNS) is essential to this process. It helps regulate heart rate, hormone cycles, memory, emotional resilience, and immune coordination.[24]

As we age, the CNS becomes more vulnerable to inflammation, chronic stress, and neurodegeneration, all of which can disrupt homeostasis. Over time, this dysregulation contributes to the development of conditions such as cardiovascular disease, Alzheimer's, metabolic syndrome, and depression. Many of these conditions are closely tied to accelerated aging.[25]

Acupuncture offers a powerful intervention point here. Acupuncture stimulates specific points along the spine, scalp, and extremities. This stimulation directly modulates CNS activity. It calms the brain's stress centers and enhances the function of the hypothalamus and prefrontal cortex. This helps calm the sympathetic system and reduce inflammation. It increases the release of calming neurotransmitters, including serotonin, GABA, and natural opioids. These support emotional well-being, mental clarity, and deep relaxation.[26]

From the lens of TCM, supporting the brain and nervous system means working through the organ systems most closely tied to them. The kidneys store jing, which generates Marrow to nourish the Brain, known as the *"Sea of Marrow."* The heart houses the Shen, the spirit that governs consciousness and mental activity. The liver ensures the smooth flow of qi, calming emotional tension and supporting the Hun, which influences sleep and vision. When these systems are harmonized, the Shen is clear, the Brain is well nourished, and the nervous system remains adaptable.[27] In both medical systems, the brain is connected to the body, reflecting internal harmony or disharmony.

Modern tools like HRV (heart rate variability) monitors, EEG, and fMRI now show us in real time how acupuncture helps restore this brain-body connection. When the CNS becomes more adaptable, the body follows. This adaptability is the root of longevity. It is found not in resisting aging, but in returning to balance with each cycle of change.[28]

Rewiring for Resilience

The nervous system is at the core of how we experience life. It receives, interprets, and responds to everything we encounter, from pain and temperature to thought and emotion. In this chapter, we explored the central and peripheral branches of this vast network and saw how deeply they influence health, balance, and aging. When this communication system is working well, the body adapts with ease, heals efficiently, and maintains its internal rhythm. When it falters, chronic stress, pain, and disease often take root.

Acupuncture engages this system in vast ways. By interacting with sensory pathways, brain centers, and peripheral nerves, it helps reset maladaptive patterns and restore the flow of information on which homeostasis depends. As we have seen in both ancient medicine and modern science, this reset is not about symptom relief. It is a foundation for longevity, resilience, and vitality.

The story of the nervous system doesn't stop here. In the next chapter, we'll look more into the ANS, the silent regulator that governs everything from your heartbeat to your digestive fire. Understanding how acupuncture restores balance within the ANS is key to understanding how it transforms the body from the inside out, and activates your body's blueprint for longevity.

3

The Autonomic Nervous System - The Hidden Healer

At the core of every breath, heartbeat, and digestive rhythm is the silent guardian known as the Autonomic Nervous System (ANS). As a key branch of the Peripheral Nervous System (PNS), alongside the Somatic Nervous System (SNS), the ANS manages the body's automatic functions without conscious effort. [1] While the somatic system governs voluntary movement, the autonomic system controls the background operations that keep us alive, including breathing, circulation, digestion, and sexual function.[2]

Whispers Beneath Awareness

One of the most beautiful aspects of the ANS is its constant adaptability. According to recent observations, it integrates signals from both the internal and external environment to adjust physiological processes in real time, making it a core player in maintaining homeostasis.[3] This includes regulating smooth muscle in the blood vessels, cardiac muscle in the heart, and glandular secretions that influence immune, hormonal, and digestive activity.[4]

With its widespread reach, the ANS influences nearly every system in the body. It helps regulate heart rate, respiratory rhythm, digestion, perspiration, immune responses, pupil dilation, and reproductive functions.[5] It also sends and receives continuous feedback between the organs and the brain, which is essential for adapting to life's changing demands.[6]

A clear grasp of the ANS is essential to understanding how acupuncture works. The next section examines the two major divisions of this system, sympathetic and parasympathetic, and explains how acupuncture helps restore their balance to support healing, longevity, and emotional resilience.

The Two Branches of the ANS - Yin and Yang in Motion

The ANS is composed of two distinct yet interrelated subdivisions: the sympathetic and parasympathetic nervous systems.[7] These two systems work together in a dynamic balance to regulate the body's internal environment. One activates and mobilizes energy, the other calms and restores it. Western physiology often describes them as stimulating versus inhibiting, or as fight-or-flight versus rest-and-digest.[8]

This dynamic illustrates the principle of yin and yang, a foundational concept in TCM. Just as yang represents action, heat, and outward movement, the sympathetic nervous system triggers alertness, increases heart rate, and prepares the body for stress or survival. In contrast, yin reflects rest, cooling, and inward flow, qualities mirrored by the parasympathetic nervous system, which supports digestion, recovery, and immune function.[9]

When the sympathetic and parasympathetic systems lose balance, homeostasis begins to break down. Factors such as chronic stress, poor sleep, trauma, and emotional strain can shift the system toward sympathetic dominance. Over time, this leads to inflammation, tension, and exhaustion. Both Chinese and Western medicine recognize this imbalance as a key contributor to many modern diseases.[10]

Needles That Weave Balance

Acupuncture is described as helping restore equilibrium. Rather than only stimulating or sedating, it appears to regulate, guiding the body toward its natural rhythm. By restoring the flow of qi and balancing yin and yang, acupuncture may help realign the sympathetic and parasympathetic systems. In both clinical practice and research, it has been observed to support conditions such as anxiety, digestive disorders, hypertension, and insomnia.[11]

When viewed through both lenses, Eastern and Western, the ANS is not just a passive system. It is a bridge between inner and outer worlds, one that acupuncture can access to help the body return to its innate intelligence.

The Rhythm of Vital Years

Longevity isn't merely about extending the number of years we live. It's about increasing the number of vital, resilient, and adaptive years we enjoy. At the center of this resilience is the ANS, which quietly governs the rhythms of life: heart rate, digestion, breath, sleep, immune function, and even emotional regulation. Research in longevity science indicates that the adaptability of the ANS, reflected in its ability to shift fluidly between stress and relaxation, strongly predicts healthy aging and resistance to disease.[12]

One of the most reliable markers of ANS balance is HRV. This is the subtle beat-to-beat variation in your heartbeat. A higher HRV indicates that the parasympathetic nervous system is active and that the body can recover quickly from stress. Lower HRV reflects dominance of the sympathetic nervous system. This branch governs the body's stress response. When it stays overactive, it is linked to aging, chronic disease, inflammation, and a reduced ability to cope with physical and emotional challenges.[13]

How Acupuncture Talks to the Brain

Recent insights suggests that acupuncture may increase HRV, modulate vagal tone, and improve autonomic flexibility.[14] Acupuncture has been shown to activate afferent nerves by stimulating specific points along meridians. These nerves connect to the brainstem, hypothalamus, and vagus nerve, which all contribute to regulating the ANS.[15] This results in measurable improvements in parasympathetic activity, a reduction in sympathetic overdrive, and enhanced capacity for recovery.

By improving autonomic balance, acupuncture helps reawaken the body's innate intelligence. It supports not only healing in the moment, but also creates the conditions required for long-term vitality and longevity.

Acupuncture and ANS Regulation in Practice

While the mechanisms behind acupuncture's effects on the nervous system are compelling, what truly affirms its value is what practitioners and researchers witness in the clinic every day. Whether it's calming anxiety, improving sleep, easing chronic digestive issues, or helping someone recover from burnout, acupuncture consistently demonstrates its ability to regulate the ANS and restore balance.

One of the clearest examples is its effect on chronic stress and anxiety. In patients with generalized anxiety disorder, acupuncture has been shown to reduce symptoms by modulating activity in the limbic system. It also increases parasympathetic tone, which leads to decreased heart rate, lowered cortisol levels, and enhanced emotional resilience.[16]

In clinical settings, patients with chronic pain often report that after a series of treatments, their pain intensity decreases, but so does their reactivity to stress, muscle tension, and fatigue. These outcomes are consistent with studies showing that acupuncture affects the hypothalamic-pituitary-adrenal (HPA) axis. It reduces inflammatory cytokines and improves HRV.[17]

The Gut–Brain–Nerve Connection

Acupuncture has also been used successfully in treating irritable bowel syndrome (IBS) and other functional gastrointestinal disorders, which are often tied to autonomic dysregulation and emotional stress. Clinical trials indicate that acupuncture may help normalize gut motility, reduce visceral hypersensitivity, and increase vagal activity. This illustrates the deep connection between the brain, gut, and nervous system.[18]

Acupuncture's influence on the ANS is supported by both research and clinical observation. Many patients report benefits daily, and studies continue to explore and affirm these effects.When the nervous system is guided back to balance, the entire organism can return to its natural state of vitality.

The Pathway to Regulation

The ANS is the body's silent architect. It is constantly regulating, adjusting, and responding quietly in the background of our conscious awareness. When balanced, it allows us to adapt to stress, recover from illness, and maintain the internal harmony that underlies true health. When dysregulated, it can trigger a cascade of chronic conditions, emotional instability, and disconnection from the self. Acupuncture engages directly with this system, guiding it back to rhythm through subtle recalibration rather than force.

As we move forward, we will explore the vagus nerve, often called the "wandering nerve," and its central role in the parasympathetic nervous system. The vagus is not only one of the body's primary pathway of relaxation and recovery; it is also the gateway through which acupuncture influences breath, digestion, mood, and inflammation. The role of this single nerve may hold the key to explaining how acupuncture restores balance so deeply and completely

4

The Vagus Nerve - The Body's Healing Superhighway

The vagus nerve, known as the tenth cranial nerve, is one of the body's most remarkable pathways of connection. Originating in the brainstem and winding through the neck and chest into the abdomen, it unites the brain with the heart, lungs, and digestive organs, weaving a living thread between thought and physiology. [1]

The vagus nerve is part of the parasympathetic branch of the ANS. This is the division responsible for rest, recovery, and repair. It is a mixed nerve composed of both afferent (sensory) and efferent (motor) fibers. Its function, however, is predominantly sensory. Approximately 80 percent of its fibers carry information from the body to the brain.[2] This means that the vagus nerve does not simply send commands outward. It is constantly listening to the body's internal environment and informing the brain how to respond.[3]

By influencing critical processes like heart rate, breathing, and digestion, the vagus nerve plays a central role in maintaining homeostasis. It allows the brain to receive detailed information from the viscera and respond with regulatory signals that keep internal functions stable and adaptive.[4]

Listening Inward - How the Vagus Nerve Senses and Regulates

Damage to the vagus nerve can disrupt vital processes and has been linked to life-threatening dysfunction, highlighting its essential role in supporting visceral organ function.[5] In contrast, stimulation of the vagus nerve through practices such as breathwork, meditation, or acupuncture can promote healing. Clinical findings have shown that vagus nerve activity is involved in regulating inflammation, mood, and gut function.[6] In fact, vagus nerve stimulation is now being explored as a treatment for conditions such as epilepsy, depression, and chronic inflammatory diseases, which serves as a testament to its influence across multiple systems.

As we will explore in this chapter, the vagus nerve is far more than a structural pathway. It is a communicator between the body and brain. Through this connection, acupuncture supports regulation, recovery, and longevity.

A Bridge Between Worlds - Acupuncture and the Vagus Nerve

Acupuncture's ability to restore homeostasis is not mystical; it's neurological. One of the key pathways through which acupuncture exerts its healing effects is by stimulating the vagus nerve, a primary channel for parasympathetic activation and the body-brain communication loop.

Studies using fMRI and HRV analysis has shown that acupuncture can activate brain regions and nerve pathways directly associated with the vagus nerve. Points such as Yintang, PC6, ST36, and Ear Shen Men have been observed to increase vagal tone, reduce sympathetic arousal, and promote parasympathetic dominance. This shifts the body from a state of reactivity into one of restoration.[7]

How Points Become Portals

Anatomically, this makes sense. Many acupuncture points lie near nerve branches, fascial planes, or vascular regions rich in mechanoreceptors. When stimulated, these points send afferent signals to the brainstem, particularly the nucleus tractus solitarius (NTS), which serves as a central relay for vagal input. From there, the information spreads to regulate heart rate, respiratory rhythm, inflammation, and digestion.[8]

In TCM, these physiological effects are understood as the restoration of the smooth flow of qi and blood. They also appear as the settling of the Shen and the rebalancing of the organ systems.[9] The heart, liver, lung and gastrointestinal tract are especially involved, and all are profoundly innervated by the vagus nerve. When stress, trauma, or deficiency disrupts these organs, the result is often vagal suppression. This can show up as insomnia, anxiety, digestive disturbances, cold hands and feet, and heightened emotional reactivity.[10]

By carefully selecting synergistic point combinations, acupuncture helps regulate internal imbalances and promote autonomic harmony. Clinically effective pairings like Yintang with HT7 or BL15 with BL23 are often chosen for their calming, heart-regulating, and parasympathetic supportive effects, while research-backed points like PC6 and ST36 enhance physiological recovery and nervous system resilience. The nervous system is reminded of how to self-regulate. This helps re-establish the internal environment needed for healing, growth, and longevity.[11]

Acupuncture does not override the body. It listens to it. Through the vagus nerve, it helps the body remember how to heal.

Vagal Tone, HRV, and the Rhythm of Resilience

In longevity science and integrative medicine, vagal tone and HRV have emerged as two of the most reliable indicators of nervous system health and adaptability. Both reflect the balance of the ANS, specifically the body's ability to shift between sympathetic activation and parasympathetic restoration.[12]

Vagal tone refers to the functional strength of the vagus nerve and its ability to slow the heart, regulate inflammation, and restore calm after stress. HRV, a closely related concept, measures the variation between individual heartbeats. Although it may seem counter intuitive, greater variability indicates a more resilient nervous system that can adapt to change and recover from stress more efficiently.[13]

Low HRV is associated with a range of chronic conditions such as anxiety, depression, cardiovascular disease, autoimmune disorders, and even accelerated biological aging.[14] Conversely, higher HRV is associated with longevity, emotional flexibility, and improved immune function. These are markers of a nervous system that is balanced, regulated, and responsive.[15]

Modern Tools, Ancient Truths: Tracking the Shift to Balance

Findings indicates that acupuncture can enhance HRV and support vagal tone through the stimulation of specific points known to influence the parasympathetic nervous system.[16] In clinical practice, patients often describe feeling calmer, more grounded, or 'reset.' These subjective experiences are now supported by objective data from wearable devices and biometric monitoring.

Some practitioners now use HRV-tracking apps, smartwatches, or pulse variability tools to measure changes in nervous system regulation before and after acupuncture sessions . These tools help quantify what Chinese medicine has always known: that true health is not a static state, but a dynamic ability to return to balance.[17]

By improving vagal tone, acupuncture does more than relieve symptoms. It strengthens the body's ability to heal, adapt, and grow. In doing so, it helps restore the rhythm of resilience that supports both vitality and longevity.

The following case study illustrates how disturbances in autonomic regulation can manifest as a wide spectrum of symptoms, and how TCM and acupuncture can be applied to address them.

Clinical Insight - Reawakening the Vagus Nerve

It is not uncommon to see a pattern of symptoms that gradually build over time. Fatigue, bloating, mild anxiety, poor sleep, irregular digestion, and a sense of always being "on" often appear together. A person may feel disconnected from their body, breathe shallowly without noticing, and rarely feel rested, even after a full night's sleep.

In many cases, medical tests return normal results, and these experiences are attributed to stress or described as functional. Through the lens of autonomic regulation, this pattern reflects vagal suppression and sympathetic dominance. The system remains alert and unable to fully return to rest and repair.

From the perspective of Chinese medicine, this presentation mirrors Liver Qi stagnation, Spleen deficiency, and disturbance of the Heart Shen. The tongue may appear pale with a slight red tip and scalloped edges. The pulse often feels thin and wiry.

Treatment focuses on supporting vagal activity, calming sympathetic overdrive, and anchoring the spirit. These approaches help guide the body back toward balance and regulation.

The Pulse of Inner Peace

The vagus nerve is more than a structure. It is the thread that weaves together breath, emotion, digestion, and presence.[18] It holds the quiet intelligence beneath healing, serving as the pathway through which the body communicates safety and as the access point for regulation, resilience, and renewal.[19] When this nerve is activated and flowing, the entire system responds. Pain softens, digestion regulates, the mind calms, and the spirit returns to the body.[20]

Acupuncture works in harmony with our nervous system. It does not override it but instead listens, guides, and gently invites it back into rhythm. As modern science and ancient medicine come together, we are discovering that the vagus nerve may be one of the most powerful gateways to balance and longevity. Perhaps most importantly, it reminds us that healing does not require force. It only requires the right signal.

In the next chapters, we'll explore how to recognize signs of autonomic imbalance through both clinical observation and subtle energetic patterns. Sections II and III draw parallels between classical Chinese medical texts and modern scientific research, revealing a shared language of regulation and rhythm. This foundation leads us into Section IV, where we'll look at the emotional landscape of each organ system and uncover how the nervous system reflects and responds to our inner emotional world.

II

When Survival Becomes the Pattern

Healing the Hidden Wounds of the Nervous System

*" Now, since antiquity, that which communicates with heaven,
the basis of life, is based in yin and yang"*
— Haung Di
"The Liver is the organ system occupying the first line of
emotional defense for the entire body."
—Leon Hammer

5

Yin and Yang in the Nervous System - Ancient Insights, Modern Maps

Acupuncture's role in treating chronic pain and disease brings us back to a core principle of Chinese medicine. Health depends on the balance of yin and yang. Long before the development of modern physiology or neurology, ancient Chinese physicians understood that health was maintained through balance, and illness was the result of its disruption.

One of the earliest and most influential texts on this subject is the *Huang Di Nei Jing*, or *The Yellow Emperor's Classic of Internal Medicine*. Sometimes referred to by its full name, *Huang Di Nei Jing Su Wen* (*Basic Questions of the Inner Classic*), this foundational work outlines the meridian system, the nature of disease, and the use of acupuncture as a means of restoring equilibrium.[1]

According to the *Nei Jing*, health is achieved when yin and yang are in balance and all physiological systems are in harmony with natural rhythms. These rhythms include day and night, activity and rest, expansion and contraction. Disease arises when this balance is disrupted. This disruption can be caused by external forces such as climate or trauma, or by internal factors such as emotion, diet, or overwork.[2]

Huang Di, the legendary Yellow Emperor, emphasizes throughout the text that understanding yin and yang is essential to understanding the foundation of life itself. This perspective resonates deeply with the modern concept of homeostasis.[3] In this view, health is not a fixed state. It is a continual process of regulation, adjustment, and return.

In this framework, acupuncture serves as a guidepost. It helps realign the body when it strays from balance. It also supports the internal mechanisms that restore flow, rhythm, and coherence.

Yin, Yang, and the Physiology of Balance

The ideal state of health, both in Classical Chinese Medicine and in modern physiology, is one of dynamic harmony. The *Huang Di Nei Jing* teaches that the body flourishes when its internal systems are in balance. This balance is not fixed. It is constantly adjusting, like a scale that tips and recalibrates to maintain its center.[4]

Harmony arises from the balance between opposites, such as yin and yang. Just as night transforms into day and rest supports activity, the body must also alternate between tension and release, rest and action, alertness and sleep.[5] Health is not a static endpoint, but a continuous process of regulating these forces in response to internal needs and external changes.

In modern neurophysiology, this ancient model finds a powerful analogue in the ANS, particularly in the balance between the sympathetic and parasympathetic branches. The sympathetic branch is associated with yang. It activates alertness and action. The parasympathetic branch is associated with yin. It supports rest, repair, and digestion. Just as yin and yang govern cycles in Chinese medicine, these two arms of the ANS regulate the body's response to stress, safety, and adaptation.[6]

In The *Ling Shu*, one of the classical texts of acupuncture, describes how fine needles are used to open the conduits and vessels. This restores the body's harmony by guiding qi back into flow.[7] In modern terms, acupuncture modulates nerve signaling, blood flow, and inflammatory response. It helps restore equilibrium in patients whose systems are stuck in sympathetic overdrive or parasympathetic withdrawal.[8]

We can find Remarkable parallels between the ancient teachings of yin and yang and the findings of modern science. As researchers uncover the mechanisms that regulate stress, inflammation, and adaptation, they are echoing what The *Huang Di Nei Jing* described thousands of years ago. Health is not a fixed state. It is a rhythm of opposites, constantly adjusting to maintain harmony. The principles of balance, flow, and regulation are not only philosophical. They are also physiological. In the sections that follow, we explore how the core concepts of Classical Chinese Medicine correspond with modern clinical insights. These include the workings of the ANS, circadian rhythms, and the body's complex feedback networks. Together, these findings affirm that the wisdom of yin and yang continues to live on in today's scientific understanding of homeostasis, resilience, and healing.

This dynamic relationship maps closely onto the ANS. When there is imbalance, it can lead to chronic dysregulation. Overactive sympathetic dominance, or yang excess, and parasympathetic withdrawal, or yin deficiency, are implicated in anxiety, fatigue, and inflammatory disorders. Acupuncture helps recalibrate this system by modulating vagal tone and brain network activity. It facilitates a shift toward balance and internal flow.[9]

Circadian Rhythms - The Daily Dance of Yin and Yang

The cyclical nature of yin and yang also lives within the body's circadian biology. Just as yin governs night and rest, and yang governs day and activity, internal clocks orchestrate daily fluctuations in hormones, temperature, digestion, and immune function. Melatonin rises as night approaches, signaling rest and repair. Cortisol peaks in the morning, preparing the body for alertness and motion. These rhythms are essential for maintaining physiological balance. When disrupted by factors like shift work, jet lag, or chronic stress, the result can be sleep disorders, inflammation, and emotional instability. Acupuncture has been shown to help regulate circadian patterns, improving sleep, hormonal balance, and mood stability.[10]

Modern Feedback Systems and Ancient Parallels

Ancient frameworks of health anticipated many of the principles that modern science is now beginning to articulate with increasing precision. The *Huang Di Nei Jing* described health as a continual process of regulating opposing forces, shaped by rhythm, polarity, and adaptive flow. Today, physiology affirms this perspective. Homeostasis is no longer seen as a fixed endpoint, but as a process maintained by the nervous, endocrine, and immune systems. As experts explore how the body preserves internal balance, they are uncovering mechanisms that echo the foundational insights of Chinese medicine. The following examples from neuroendocrinology, immunology, and psychoneuroimmunology illustrate how modern science continues to reflect the core dynamics of yin and yang theory.

Systems in Dialogue - How the Nervous, Endocrine, and Immune Networks Sustain Balance

Modern research in neuroendocrinology and immunology shows that homeostasis is maintained through complex feedback systems involving the nervous, endocrine, and immune networks. These systems rely on signaling molecules, such as hormones and cytokines, to continuously monitor the body's internal environment and adjust its responses to changing conditions.[11] This process closely reflects the ancient perspective described in the *Nei Jing*, where health is viewed as a balance between opposing forces that must be actively regulated. One example is the discovery of the "inflammatory reflex," which shows how neural circuits help modulate immune responses and restore equilibrium.

Psychoneuroimmunology has shown that the brain and immune system are in constant communication, forming a network that responds to both emotional and physical experiences. This modern insight supports the ancient view that health depends on the continuous integration of the body's systems. Scientist have found that stress and emotions can influence immune function through neuroendocrine pathways.[12] This mirrors the *Nei Jing*'s core teaching that balance and adaptability are essential for maintaining health.

Returning to Rhythm

Health, like nature, is cyclical. Yin gives way to yang, just as winter yields to spring. In our overstimulated world, we often forget how to move with these natural shifts. Acupuncture does not force balance. It reminds the body of its original rhythm. Healing happens when we realign with our own current, and lets the body remember how to rest, rise, and renew.

The next chapter will further explore the correspondence between yin/yang regulation and autonomic balance, examining how acupuncture not only restores energy flow but helps the body re-establish homeostasis, physiologically and energetically.

6

Trauma and the ANS - Rewiring the Survival Response

The body's stress response is designed to protect us. When we encounter danger, the sympathetic nervous system activates immediately. It sharpens our senses, accelerating the heart, to direct blood flow toward the muscles.[1] This is the familiar "fight-or-flight" reaction, a survival mechanism as old as humanity itself.

This system is designed for short-term mobilization, but it becomes harmful when activated continuously without resolution. When the body remains in a prolonged state of stress, the response shifts from protective to damaging. Energy reserves are depleted. Digestion slows. Muscles stay chronically tense. Blood pressure rises. Instead of returning to balance, the system becomes stuck in overdrive.[2]

This extended state of sympathetic dominance leads to what's often called the exhaustion stage. This is when the body's ability to regulate begins to fail. When homeostasis falters, symptoms begin to emerge. Tension settles in the neck, back, and jaw. The stomach becomes distressed. Emotions grow unpredictable. The nervous system speaks in sensation. Over time, the body's pain threshold begins to lower.[3] The longer this state persists, the more deeply it imprints in the nervous system, often laying the foundation for chronic pain and long-term disease.

Trauma amplifies this pattern. Whether sudden or cumulative, it can lock the body into a state of physiological alarm even after the threat has passed. In these situations, the body is not broken. It is adapting to survive, although that adaptation often comes at a cost. Acupuncture offers a path back by regulating qi, restoring yin-yang balance, and re-patterning the autonomic response.[4]

How Trauma Becomes Patterned in the Body

Trauma is not only experienced in the moment. It can become biologically patterned into the nervous system.. Repeated or overwhelming stress creates fear-based neurophysiological imprints that alter the brain's regulatory patterns. When the body cannot return to homeostasis after the stressor resolves, the ANS remains in a heightened state of activation.[5]

In Chinese medicine, this reflects a breakdown in the body's ability to restore yin-yang balance. Chronic tension and internal agitation disrupt the flow of liver qi, which governs the sinews and musculoskeletal system. As this imbalance persists, it can contribute to stiffness, tightness, and musculoskeletal discomfort.[6]

The liver and gallbladder, which govern the ligaments and tendons, become strained under this pressure. The result is not only physical tightness, but emotional rigidity as well. When the system cannot reset, a feedback loop develops. Emotional trauma leads to muscular tension, and the tension, in turn, reinforces the emotional trauma.[7]

Neurophysiologically, this pattern aligns with the body's fight-or-flight response, orchestrated by the sympathetic nervous system. When the body senses a threat, it prepares for survival. The pupils dilate, heart rate and respiration increase. Glucose is mobilized, and circulation shifts toward the muscles and away from digestion and reproduction.[8] At the same time, brain activity shifts from the prefrontal cortex. This region is responsible for higher thinking. Activity moves toward the limbic and brainstem circuits, which control immediate and instinctive reactions.[9]

Over time, these survival adaptations become chronic states. The immune system weakens. Creative thought narrows. The body forgets how to rest. In Chinese medicine, this is understood as liver qi stagnation with secondary deficiency, or yang rising due to yin depletion. In this state, the body lacks the cooling and restorative forces needed to counterbalance the heat of prolonged stress.[10]

Understanding what is happening physiologically during stress helps us better appreciate how acupuncture reintroduces regulation, not just symptom relief. The body is not malfunctioning. It is stuck in a survival mode it was never meant to live in.

The Nervous System's Response to Acute Stress

When the body perceives immediate danger, the ANS responds in an instant. This acute activation, often described as the fight-or-flight response, is the body's way of mobilizing resources to confront or escape a threat.[11] The signal begins in the brain and cascades through the body, prompting both physiological and psychological responses.[12]

Physically, the body shifts into survival mode. Breathing becomes shallow or erratic. The heart races. Blood vessels constrict or dilate depending on the tissue. Muscle tone increases, sometimes leading to tremors or even paralysis. Sweating may intensify, and digestion slows as the body redirects energy toward movement and heightened alertness.[13]

Psychologically, the experience is marked by feelings of dread, hypervigilance, and apprehension.[14] Internal sensations are just as real and measurable as the physical ones.[15] The mind narrows. The emotional body tenses. It is the nervous system's way of signaling that safety has not yet been restored.[16]

TCM has long described similar responses in energetic terms. Acute fear is said to disrupt the kidneys, the organ system responsible for storing essence (jing) and governing our root survival.[17] When the stress is intense or sudden, the heart, which houses the Shen (spirit), is also affected. This can lead to emotional unrest, insomnia, or palpitations.[18] These patterns mirror what we now understand about how trauma moves through the body. It is not just a mental event, but a full-body experience that imprints on the nervous, emotional, and energetic systems simultaneously.[19]

Understanding both the neurobiological and energetic perspectives empowers us to treat the whole person. It reminds us that the stress response is not a flaw in the system, but a protective function. Healing begins when the body feels safe enough to let go.

When the Mind Becomes the Body

Emotional experiences do not live only in the mind. They shape the body. As modern neurobiology confirms, psychological stress has profound physiological consequences. It alters breathing, increases heart rate, raises blood pressure, disrupts digestion, and weakens the immune system.[20] Over time, this mind-body connection can contribute to what is often called a psychosomatic disorder, in which emotional strain manifests as functional or structural disease.[21]

This response is controlled by the involuntary nervous system. It is driven primarily by the sympathetic branch of the ANS, which reacts automatically to emotional stimuli. During prolonged stress, rage, or fear, the body continues to release stress hormones. It redirects circulation and alters its biochemistry, even when no real danger is present. If the emotional charge is not discharged or processed, the body holds on to the unresolved state. Over time, this can show up as physical symptoms. [22]

High blood pressure, immune dysregulation, chronic digestive issues, muscle pain, and even autoimmune conditions can all be traced back to nervous system dysregulation driven by unprocessed psychological stress.[23] In Chinese medicine, this understanding is reflected in the belief that emotions are stored in the organs. Anger is said to affect the liver, fear the kidneys, worry the spleen, and grief the lungs.[24]

The longer these emotions remain stagnant, the more they restrict the flow of qi and blood, setting the stage for chronic pain and internal disharmony. The body, in this framework, is not separate from the mind, it is an expression of it. In order to restore health, both must be brought back into communication.

7

The Liver, the Mind, and the Movement of Qi

In TCM, the liver-gallbladder system governs more than just detoxification and digestion. It is intimately tied to the nervous system, muscular tone, and emotional processing. The liver is responsible for maintaining the smooth flow of qi throughout the body, and by extension, for the regulation of the sympathetic and parasympathetic branches of the ANS.[1]

When emotions are repressed, prolonged, or unexpressed, the liver system becomes over burdened, leading to a state of nervous system tension and hyperactivity.[2] This disrupts not only physical processes like digestion and circulation, but also the sense of psychological ease. The result is tranquility, an energetic equilibrium where the heart and liver are in harmonious communication.[3]

If emotions cannot be released, whether through movement (liver) or expression (heart), the body stores them. This storage creates muscular tension and pressure on the nervous system. Findings indicates that increased sympathetic nervous system (SNS) activity correlates with elevated heart rates and physical symptoms such as lower back pain, neck tension, shoulder stiffness, and fibromyalgia. These symptoms were also associated with reduced parasympathetic activity, showing a clear picture of autonomic imbalance.[5]

As tension accumulates, the liver demands more nourishment to regulate the musculoskeletal system. This increases the circulatory workload, particularly on the heart, which attempts to meet this demand by accelerating blood flow. The result is elevated blood pressure, internal heat, and further hyper excitability of the nervous system.[6]

In both Chinese and Western frameworks, this pattern reflects a progression from stagnation to over activation. Emotional holding can lead to muscular tension, which places increasing strain on the nervous system and contributes to chronic pain, particularly in the neck, shoulders, back, and internal organs.[7] InTCMe, when the liver's movement is impaired, the entire system may slow down, become strained, or generate excess heat. Acupuncture offers a path back by freeing the liver, calming the heart, and reminding the nervous system how to soften its grip.

When Emotion Becomes Illness

Mounting research continues to affirm what Chinese medicine has long taught, emotional states and physiological health are deeply connected. Psychological disorders such as anxiety and depression are now widely understood to stem, at least in part, from ANS dysregulation.[8] Because the ANS governs critical processes like heart rate, digestion, immune function, and temperature regulation, its imbalance can manifest as a range of physical illnesses.

Emotional strain, especially when related to chronic stress, fear, or anxiety, activates the sympathetic nervous system and places the body in a prolonged state of readiness.

If this activation becomes habitual, the resulting symptoms include muscle tension, headaches, hypertension, and increased sensitivity to pain.[9] Many patients also experience symptoms of digestive dysregulation, such as IBS, chronic abdominal pain, and functional dyspepsia. These conditions are closely associated with impaired vagal tone and heightened sympathetic activity.[10]

This connection between mind and body is a central tenet of TCM. Emotions that are not acknowledged, expressed, or resolved can disrupt qi flow and organ function, particularly in the liver, heart, and spleen systems.

Over time, these disruptions evolve into tangible physical symptoms.[11]

As emotional stress increases in modern society, so does the prevalence of chronic disease, a pattern well-documented in both medical literature and clinical observation.[12]

Acupuncture offers a profound therapeutic response to these patterns. Studies show that acupuncture can regulate the ANS, reduce cortisol levels, enhance vagal tone, and ease both the psychological and physical manifestations of stress.[13] Conditions such as migraines, insomnia, depression, constipation, and mood disorders have all been shown to improve through targeted acupuncture treatment. What begins as energetic rebalancing often results in measurable, lasting relief.

The following case studies highlight how stress, trauma, and imbalance in the ANS manifest as diverse physical and emotional symptoms. Each example demonstrates how acupuncture, understood through both TCM and the lens of the nervous system, opens pathways back to regulation and balance.

Clinical Insight: When Stress Becomes the Symptom

A patient sought acupuncture for daily headaches, restless sleep, chronic constipation, and persistent tension in her chest and shoulders. Though they had no formal medical diagnosis, they felt mentally tense, emotionally drained, and physically worn down. Thier symptoms began shortly after ending a high-conflict relationship and taking on a demanding workload with little time to recover.

Medical tests showed nothing abnormal. But their body told another story.

From a nervous system perspective, their symptoms reflected a prolonged stress response, characterized by heightened sympathetic activity and low vagal tone. In TCM, their presentation revealed patterns of liver qi stagnation, heart yin deficiency, and spleen qi depletion. This constellation is often linked to emotional suppression, internal heat, and disruption of digestion and Shen, or spirit.

After several sessions they began noticing a profound shift. Their sleep became more restful, digestion normalized, and the headaches diminished.

But what stood out most was emotional release. "I didn't realize how tightly I was holding everything in, "until I finally let go."

This case exemplifies how emotional stress, when unresolved, migrates into the body. But it also reveals something deeper: the nervous system remembers how to heal, when it is given the right conditions and support. Acupuncture provided the cue their body needed to shift out of survival and return to regulation.

Clinical Insight: A Case of Palpitations and Anxiety

A patient came in for acupuncture due to recurring palpitations, chest tightness, and nighttime restlessness accompanied by anxiety. They described difficulty falling asleep, waking with a racing heart, and feeling "on edge" even during calm moments. Despite undergoing EKGs and full blood panels, no structural abnormalities were found. they were told it was likely "stress-related."

From a lens of the ANS, this reflected classic signs of autonomic imbalance, where sympathetic over activation disrupts heart rhythm, sleep, and emotional regulation. Through the lens of Chinese medicine, her pattern reflected heart yin deficiency and liver qi stagnation, manifesting as internal heat and Shen disturbance. They also noted night sweats and lower back weakness, indicating an underlying depletion contributing to her symptoms.

Treatment focused on calming the nervous system, supporting parasympathetic tone, and restoring the heart-kidney axis. Over a series of sessions, They reported deeper sleep, reduced nighttime palpitations, and a sense of emotional steadiness she hadn't felt in years.

At a follow-up, they said, "It's like I've finally come down from a ledge I didn't even realize I was standing on." That shift, from constant vigilance to inner calm, marked the beginning of their healing.

This case illustrates how acupuncture works on multiple levels. It restores the flow of qi, modulates neural activity, and helps re-establish harmony between the heart and the nervous system. It also demonstrates how classical theory and modern neurophysiology reflect the same principles, once we learn how to interpret them together.

Clinical Insight: A Case of IBS and Sympathetic Overdrive

A patient came in for acupuncture treatment for irritable bowel syndrome (IBS). They experienced abdominal bloating, alternating constipation and diarrhea, and sharp cramping that worsened under stress. They also described difficulty relaxing, shallow breathing, and a persistent sense of tension "in his gut." Though gastrointestinal testing showed no signs of inflammation or structural issues, these symptoms had been disrupting his life for years.

When asked about their emotional landscape, they shared that they were navigating a deeply stressful chapter, marked by life transitions, disrupted sleep, and racing thoughts that kept him up at night.

From a TCM perspective, his presentation reflected a disharmony between the liver and spleen, where emotional stress constrained qi flow and weakened digestive resilience. Through the lens of the nervous system, this was a clear case of sympathetic overdrive suppressing parasympathetic digestive function, a common pattern in high-stress modern lifestyles.

Treatment focused on calming the nervous system, restoring digestive rhythm, and gently shifting the body out of a prolonged stress response. Over the course of several sessions, he reported fewer episodes of cramping, improved regularity, and a noticeable softening in his emotional and physical tension.

They summed it up this way: "For the first time in years, my gut and my mind aren't at war."

These case stories remind us that acupuncture is not just a technique, but it is restoration, remembrance, and reconnection. Whether addressing palpitations, digestive imbalance, or fertility challenges, the pathway of healing begins not with symptom suppression but with the rediscovery of inner rhythm. When we stimulate the Shu points, modulate nerve signals, or release constrained qi, we're helping the body do what it was always meant to do: self-regulate, self-heal, and return to coherence.

Remembering the Path to Balance

The human nervous system is exquisitely sensitive, not only to trauma, but to joy, touch, rhythm, and presence. It records what we suppress and what we express. When emotional stress remains unresolved, it can take root in the body as pain, tension, insomnia, digestive disorders, and fatigue. These symptoms are not signs of failure. They are messages from the body, calling for help, for space, and for regulation.

We have seen how ANS dysregulation plays a central role in many chronic conditions. This same pattern has been recognized for thousands of years in Chinese medicine. Unresolved emotions are understood to disrupt the flow of qi, overburden the liver, weaken the spleen, and agitate the heart. Healing is possible. In fact, the body is always seeking balance.

Acupuncture is one of the most powerful tools we have for restoring balance in the body. It does more than mask symptoms. It communicates directly with the nervous system, organ networks, and energy channels to reset internal rhythms, restore yin-yang harmony, and help the body remember how to self-regulate and heal.

In Section III, we turn our attention to the nerve pathways, spinal column, and meridians. This structural focus sets the foundation for Section IV, where we will explore how emotions influence all five organ systems and their associated physiological patterns.

The relationship between emotion, qi flow, and nervous system regulation is not abstract. It lives in the tissues. For thousands of years, TCM has described a system of conduit vessels that carry energy and information throughout the body. First recorded in the *Huang Di Nei Jing*, these pathways closely follow modern anatomical structures. What early physicians recognized as meridians now align with neural pathways, fascial planes, and vascular channels. The bladder meridian, for example, travels along the spine beside the major nerve roots that influence internal organ function.

As we move forward, we will explore how these classical conduits reflect the structure and function of the ANS. This intersection of ancient mapping and modern physiology shows us that acupuncture restores balance not only energetically, but through precise and measurable communication within the body.

III

The Channels of Regulation

Where Ancient Pathways Meet the Nervous System

"The conduit vessels enable one to determine death and survival, to cope with the hundred diseases, and to balance depletion and repletion."
— *Huang Di*

8

Channels and Nerves - Where Ancient Pathways Meet Neuroanatomy

The previous chapter explored how health arises from balance. This includes the interplay of yin and yang, the rhythmic exchange between sympathetic and parasympathetic forces, and the body's natural ability to adapt to stress and return to a state of regulation. Now, we shift our focus from philosophical foundations to the structural realities beneath the skin. This chapter explores how acupuncture works at the level of nerves, fascia, and internal communication pathways. It draws connections between classical descriptions of the conduit vessels and modern discoveries in neuroanatomy.

As reviewed in earlier chapters, the ANS consists of two branches. These branches govern our response to stress and our ability to recover. The sympathetic system activates during threat and mobilizes the body for survival. The parasympathetic system supports rest, repair, and restoration.[1] In the *Ling Shu*, the ancient conduit vessels appear to describe a similar regulatory framework. Huang Di writes, *"The conduit vessels enable one to determine death and survival, to cope with the hundred diseases, and to balance depletion and repletion"*.[2]

Acupoints and Peripheral Nerve Pathways

Acupuncture points have long been described as energetic sites along meridians, yet modern anatomical studies have begun to reveal a deeper truth beneath the skin. Acupuncture points are not random locations on the body. They are carefully positioned along anatomically and neurologically significant pathways. They appear to align with known neurological structures, particularly peripheral nerves and nerve plexuses. This realization offers a physiological foundation for acupuncture's effects, especially in terms of how needling influences internal organ function, muscle tone, and pain regulation.[3]

The Large Intestine Meridian - An Ancient Route Along Modern Nerves

Descriptions of the large intestine channel in the *Ling Shu* are remarkably consistent with peripheral nerve pathways documented in modern anatomy. In classical texts, this meridian begins at the tip of the index finger, travels along the outer edge of the hand, passes through He Gu (LI4), and ascends through the forearm, shoulder, and neck to the cheeks and nasal passages.[4] Modern anatomical studies reveal that this pathway closely parallels the radial, median, and ulnar nerves, which traverse the arm and influence regions of the face and head. This alignment offers a compelling example of how ancient meridian theory mirrors contemporary neurological understanding.[5]

LI4, as noted above, is one of the most clinically significant points along this route. Anatomically situated near type II afferent fibers and branches of the radial nerve, LI4 is frequently used to treat headaches, sinus congestion, facial pain, and disorders of the mouth and nose. Its effects on the trigeminal nerve system and autonomic regulation have been supported by modern studies, affirming classical descriptions of the large intestine channel's internal branches to the face and sensory organs.[6]

Stimulation of LI4 has also been shown to activate regions of the brain involved in pain modulation and autonomic regulation. Functional MRI studies reveal that needling this point can influence the hypothalamus, limbic system, and brainstem nuclei associated with stress, emotion, and visceral function.[7] This convergence of ancient use and modern data exemplifies how acupuncture engages both energetic and neurological systems to restore balance.

The Inner Arm Corridor - How the Pericardial Meridian Mirrors the Median Nerve

The Pericardial meridian includes several powerful points on the forearm that align directly with the path of the median nerve. Among these, PC-5 (Jianshi) and PC-6 (Neiguan) are especially noteworthy. These two acupoints are located over the deep median nerve as it runs through the anterior forearm. When stimulated with a needle, these points can activate the sensory fibers of the nerve, sending signals toward the central nervous system. This neural activation is believed to influence cardiovascular and autonomic functions, which may explain the traditional use of PC-6 for calming the heart, relieving nausea, and regulating emotional distress. The depth and accuracy of the point location ensure that the stimulation reaches deeper neural layers, not just the skin or muscle.[8]

In classical texts such as the *Ling Shu*, the pathways of the yin vessels associated with the heart are described as descending through the diaphragm and extending into the chest. From there, they travel along the inner surface of the upper arms, following a route that mirrors what we now identify as the Pericardium meridian. These vessels continue through the elbow and run between the sinews of the forearm, eventually entering the palm and tracing a line to the tip of the middle finger.[9] This traditional description corresponds closely to the anatomical path of the median nerve, which courses down the inner arm and forearm, passing through the carpal tunnel and into the hand. The Pericardium points PC-5 and PC-6, both located along this channel, lie directly above the deep median nerve. When stimulated, they engage this neural pathway, bridging ancient meridian theory with modern neuroanatomy.[10] This alignment supports the classical notion that these vessels govern the chest and the heart, while also highlighting how their stimulation influences autonomic and cardiovascular regulation through the median nerve.

The Stomach Meridian, the Peroneal Nerve, and Autonomic Regulation

In the *Ling Shu*, the stomach meridian, also known as the foot yang brightness vessel, is described as beginning near the base of the nose. It travels through the upper jaw and around the mouth, extending to the cheeks and into the jaw, eventually reaching the ears. Branches of this meridian descend through the throat, pass through the diaphragm, and connect with the stomach while encircling the spleen. From there, the primary pathway continues down through the chest and toward the navel. One branch is said to begin at the opening of the stomach and descend through the abdomen, entering the region known as qi chong. It then moves into the hip joint, travels down the side of the thigh, and passes through the kneecap. From the knee, the channel continues along the outer border of the shin, descends across the top of the foot, and reaches the middle toe.[11]

This traditional trajectory closely parallels the path of the deep peroneal nerve, which branches from the sciatic nerve and travels down the anterior aspect of the lower leg. Along its course, this nerve runs beneath acupuncture points such as ST-36 (Zusanli) and ST-37 (Shangjuxu), both of which are classically used to regulate digestion, boost energy, and support immune function. The alignment between the classical meridian and the deep peroneal nerve suggests that stimulation of these points influences visceral regulation through somato-visceral reflexes. It reflects a profound anatomical awareness embedded in the meridian system, long before modern neuroanatomy confirmed its pathways.[12]

Although often labeled a somatic nerve, the deep peroneal nerve also carries sympathetic fibers. These fibers belong to the ANS. They help regulate involuntary processes such as blood flow and sweating in the lower leg and foot.[13] This means the peroneal nerve is not limited to motor and sensory function. It also connects to autonomic regulation, especially through the sympathetic branch.

Microneurography studies have recorded bursts of sympathetic nerve activity from the peroneal nerve in the skin of the foot. These bursts corresponded with sweating and vasodilation, both of which are involuntary processes governed by the ANS.[14] Other research confirms that sympathetic fibers within the peroneal nerve innervate blood vessels and skin, regulating circulation and temperature in the lower limbs.[15]

This connection offers modern insight into the systemic effects of acupuncture. When points like ST-36 and ST-37 are needled, they do more than influence local tissue. They may engage both sensory and autonomic pathways through their relationship with the deep peroneal nerve. This activation can ripple throughout the body, promoting digestive balance, reducing inflammation, and supporting overall homeostasis.

Liver 3 and the Peroneal Nerve

Further research on the peroneal nerve has revealed new insights into the anatomical basis of acupuncture point Liver 3 (LR3). Located between the first and second metatarsal bones on the top of the foot, LR3 has long been used to support circulation and calm the nervous system. A branch of the deep peroneal nerve runs through this area and sends fibers directly to the dorsal pedis artery. These fibers contain sympathetic components that help regulate blood vessel tone and autonomic function. LR3 lies in close proximity to this neurovascular network. This connection helps explain how stimulating LR3 may influence both blood flow and the body's stress response. It highlights the convergence of ancient Chinese medicine and modern anatomy, showing that acupuncture points can affect energy, circulation, and nervous system regulation through direct neural pathways.[16]

The ancient path of the stomach and liver meridians mirrors the anatomical course of this nerve. It suggests that early practitioners understood, through observation and experience, the body's capacity to regulate itself when properly stimulated. Today, science confirms what the classics described. The deep peroneal nerve and the stomach channel are connected through structure, function, and therapeutic potential.

Reflex Pathways and Efferent Activation

Even though much of the focus in acupuncture research is placed on sensory or afferent nerve activation, it is important to consider the entire reflex arc. When sensory fibers are stimulated at the acupoint level, they transmit signals to the spinal cord or brainstem. These signals then engage interneurons that can activate efferent pathways, sending responses back out through motor or autonomic nerves. This closed-loop system explains why acupuncture can affect blood flow, muscle tone, glandular secretion, and visceral organ activity. Points like PC-6 and ST-36 not only initiate sensory signals, but also elicit autonomic responses that regulate the internal environment. This dynamic reflects the body's innate ability to maintain balance through neural feedback loops, a concept that mirrors the classical Chinese idea of restoring harmony and flow.[17]

Efferent Signals and Ancient Conduits - Acupuncture's Role in Autonomic Regulation

The overlap between classical channel theory and modern neurophysiology becomes especially clear in studies examining acupuncture's effect on the ANS. Clinical findings have demonstrated that needling specific points, particularly ST36 and PC6, can activate efferent vagal neurons in the brainstem. This stimulation contributes to the release of catecholamines from the adrenal glands, which helps suppress systemic inflammation and supports internal regulation.[18]

Electroacupuncture at these sites has also been shown to influence gastrointestinal motility and cardiovascular function. By adjusting the frequency and intensity of stimulation, practitioners can engage either vagal or sympathetic efferent pathways. Both play key roles in balancing inflammation, modulating stress responses, and restoring autonomic stability.[19] These findings echo the *Huang Di Nei Jing's* assertion that the flow of qi through the conduits *supports* the entire organism in adapting to internal and external change.

From a physiological standpoint, acupuncture works not only by regulating energy, but by guiding the body back toward homeostasis through multi-system signaling. The conduit vessels, once thought to be energetic constructs, are now understood as integrated channels of fascia, nerve, and fluid. Each is responsive to touch, pressure, and intention.

The Vagus Nerve and the Large Intestine Meridian - Ancient Maps of Parasympathetic Flow

As previously noted, the vagus nerve plays a vital role in parasympathetic regulation. It serves as the primary communication pathway of the parasympathetic nervous system, originating in the brainstem and traveling through the neck and chest into the abdominal cavity. Along this route, it innervates the lungs, heart, liver, digestive system, and other internal organs.

Several acupuncture points correspond closely with key anatomical regions of the vagus nerve. One of the clearest examples can be seen by examining the pathway of the large intestine meridian. In the *Ling Shu*, this meridian is described as extending from the fingertips, traveling up the arm, into the neck, and continuing into the face. This conduit passage shares notable similarities with the course of the facial nerves. In a study by Zhou and Benharash (2014), the authors note that acupuncture points along the vagus nerve align closely with the pathway of the large intestine channel.[20]

A clear example of this connection is acupuncture point LI18, located on the lateral side of the neck. LI18 corresponds with a major cervical branch of the vagus nerve. Stimulation of this point has been shown to enhance vagal tone, reduce physiological stress responses, and activate the parasympathetic nervous system.[21] This alignment suggests that early Chinese medicine practitioners may have been perceiving more than energetic flow. Through sensory awareness and clinical observation, they were likely mapping internal networks of regulation, sensation, and communication that closely mirror modern anatomical understanding.

Toward a Unified Understanding of Acupuncture

The alignment of acupuncture points with peripheral nerve structures offers a powerful bridge between Eastern and Western frameworks of medicine. It provides a mechanistic explanation for many traditional claims, while preserving the elegance of the meridian system. Rather than viewing meridians as mystical or metaphorical, we may begin to understand them as maps of neuroanatomical pathways. These maps guide practitioners to precise locations where therapeutic stimulation can influence the nervous system. As ongoing trials continues to validate these connections, acupuncture may be increasingly seen not just as an ancient art but as a precise form of neuromodulation.

In the next chapter, we will explore how these regulatory pathways deepen through the use of specific back Shu points. These points are anatomical landmarks and gateways to deeper regulation of the nervous system and the spirit.

9

Spinal Pathways and the Energetics of Organ Regulation

In Chinese medicine, healing begins with flow. When the movement of qi through the five elements is disrupted by shock, trauma, grief, or chronic emotional strain, the sheng cycle can lose its natural coherence and rhythm.[1]

In *The Clinical Practice of Chinese Medicine,* Lonny S. Jarrett writes about a state he calls aggressive energy (AE), where stagnant or pathological qi begins to injure organ function. When this state persists, it can manifest as mental illness, cancer, heart disease, or other degenerative conditions.[2]

Aggressive energy reflects a deep-level disturbance in the body's energetic hierarchy. It is not surface tension, but a disruption of constitutional harmony, often rooted in emotional trauma or systemic depletion. According to Jarrett, one of the most effective ways to address this is by using the Back Shu points of the zang organs. These are specific acupuncture points located along the bladder meridian on the back.[3]

What makes the bladder meridian so uniquely powerful is its anatomical and energetic resonance. Running bilaterally along the spine, the bladder channel is the longest meridian in the body and lies directly over the afferent and efferent nerve roots for the entire spinal column.[4] These correspond to the sympathetic ganglia of the ANS.[5] When a practitioner needles along this channel, especially at the Shu points, they are not only stimulating the flow of qi. They are also engaging with the neurological pathways that govern autonomic regulation.

Western physiology echoes this precision. There are 33 pairs of spinal nerves that exit the spinal cord and regulate the function of muscles, glands, and internal organs.[6] Each nerve root mirrors the function of a zang-fu organ in Chinese medicine, making the Shu points a gateway to both energetic and neurological healing. In this way, acupuncture acts like a tuning fork, restoring coherence between the body's electrical and energetic systems. It does not force balance; instead, it invites it through subtle resonance and regulation.

Activating the Nervous System Through Shu and Jiaji Points

Each of the zang-fu organs in Chinese medicine is associated with a corresponding Shu point along the bladder meridian, which runs in parallel lines along either side of the spine.[7] These Shu points provide access to the energetic blueprint of the organ and also interface directly with neurological structures that regulate organ function. In addition to the Shu points, another powerful set of points known as the Huatuojiaji points can be used to further engage the ANS.

These points, located just lateral to the spinal column, are named after the legendary physician Hua Tuo and are anatomically positioned near the nerve roots that exit the spine.[8] The name Huatuojiaji literally translates to "next to the spinal column," and they are known for their ability to treat neurological, visceral, and muscular dysfunction.

Stimulation of the Huatuojiaji points allows practitioners to target the spinal plexuses. These are clusters of nerves within the sympathetic nervous system that extend into key regions of the body, including the heart, abdomen, and pelvic organs.[9] These plexuses act as hubs where neural messages from the spinal cord are relayed to internal organs. This makes the Huatuojiaji points an ideal therapeutic access point for restoring autonomic balance.[10]

When Shu points are used, they connect directly to the organs through their associated meridians. Huatuojiaji points, on the other hand, influence the nervous system pathways that serve those same organs. By combining these two sets of points, acupuncture can regulate the flow of qi while also modulating neurological function.[11] This dual action is especially valuable in treating chronic conditions where emotional, physical, and nervous system imbalances intersect.

By activating the Shu and Huatuojiaji points, acupuncture taps into a powerful convergence of ancient wisdom and neurological precision. These spinal points do more than move qi. They engage the same nerve pathways that regulate internal organs and autonomic responses. This bridge between energy flow and nerve signaling gives us a deeper understanding of how acupuncture influences the entire system. The next section will explore how these back points align with the efferent and afferent nerves, offering crucial insight into how acupuncture stimulates the ANS through the spine.

10

Spinal Gateways - The Ling Shu and the ANS

The spine is a structural axis and a living conduit for the flow of energy, sensation, and communication between the brain and the body. Along its length, both ancient physicians and modern anatomists have found gateways of influence. These are regions where touch, pressure, and needling produce significant internal effects. In TCM, this understanding is embodied in the Shu points of the bladder meridian. In Western neuroanatomy, it is reflected in spinal nerves, sympathetic ganglia, and visceral reflex arcs. These two systems, once separated by time and language, now reveal profound similarities. When viewed together, they form a unified map of how acupuncture may influence the body's deepest regulatory functions.

The Spine, Shu Points, and the Sympathetic System - An Ancient-Modern Dialogue

Acupuncture points along the trunk do more than rest atop the body. Many of them correspond directly with the spinal nerve plexuses. This is especially true in the neck, thorax, abdomen, lower back, and sacrum. These points often mirror dermatomal patterns and segmental innervation. This creates a significant overlap between TCM and neuroanatomy.

Spinal nerves that emerge from the vertebral column branch out to influence skin, muscle, and internal organs. This alignment helps explain the phenomenon of referred pain. It also supports the long-standing observation in acupuncture that points on the back can influence kidney function, while abdominal points affect the intestines.[1]

Classical Chinese medicine recognized this connection over two thousand years ago. In Chapter 51 of the *Ling Shu*, transport points, known as Shu points, are described along the back near specific vertebrae:

"The transport [openings] of the lungs are located near the third vertebrae.

The transport [openings] of the heart are located near the fifth vertebrae.

The transport [openings] of the diaphragm are located near the seventh vertebrae.

The transport [openings] of the liver are near the ninth vertebrae.

The transport [openings] of the spleen are located near the eleventh vertebra.

The transport [openings] of the kidneys are located near the fourteenth vertebra.

They all are located to the side of the spine in the distance of approximately 3 inches".[2]

These Shu points correspond closely with modern descriptions of spinal segmental innervation. The sympathetic trunk runs alongside the spine and controls organ function. Spinal nerves also supply the skin and fascia of the back and abdomen. This reflects the path of the bladder meridian, which carries the Shu points in Chinese medicine.[3]

Segmental Wisdom - Shu Points, Spinal Nerves, and the Heart's Regulation

Each internal organ has a Shu point located roughly 1.5 cun lateral to the spinous processes. These points serve as energetic gateways. They are essential in both diagnostic palpation and therapeutic treatment.[4] For example, the Shu point of the heart lies near the fifth thoracic vertebra, or T5. This level corresponds with the sympathetic ganglia from T1 to T5. These nerves regulate the myocardium and coronary arteries.[5] The heart is regulated by both sympathetic and parasympathetic branches of the nervous system. One speeds up the heart rate. The other slows it down. This duality reflects the principle of yin and yang. It shows the body's dynamic balance between activity and rest.

When the Body Speaks - Sensory Signals, Shu Points, and Homeostasis

Scientific studies now confirm what Chinese medicine has long taught. Acupuncture can regulate heart rate, blood pressure, and vagal tone. These effects demonstrate how restoring flow in the body supports the return of health.[6] Transport points can be seen as energetic doors. They give access to organ function, emotional states, and even aspects of the spirit. This understanding aligns with what modern neuroanatomy reveals about spinal nerve influence over visceral organs.[7]

Acupuncture points often become tender or reactive when homeostasis declines. These points are rich in sensory nerves. They act like signals, letting us know when something is off. During early autonomic imbalance, tenderness is often found between T1 and T9. T5 is frequently the first tender point.[8] This corresponds exactly to where the sympathetic nerves innervate the heart.

Chronic pain can become "wired" within the spinal cord, creating persistent patterns of discomfort. Acupuncture addresses this by stimulating the Huatuo Jiaji and Shu points, areas rich in nerve fibers arising from the posterior primary rami of the spinal nerves.[9] These regions become critical areas to address when working with chronic disease. This tactile reality is beautifully supported by another quote from The *Ling Shu*. Huang Di states:

"To test whether one has found the right location, one presses it with the finger. When the patient feels reaction there, and if an existing pain is resolved, that is the transport opening."

This classical method of confirmation mirrors what modern anatomy has revealed. The body often speaks through sensitivity. When homeostasis fails, the nerves at these spinal levels light up. Acupuncturists have long known this. Now we can explain it through both energy and science.

The Sympathetic Pathways - Highways of Stress and Regulation

The sympathetic nervous system manages the fight-or-flight response. It begins in the spinal cord, between T1 through L2. As mentioned before, if these points are tender this is a sign that homeostasis is declining in the body. From here, preganglionic fibers leave the cord, travel through the ventral roots, and briefly follow the spinal nerves. They then split off and enter a structure called the sympathetic trunk. This trunk is a chain of ganglia that runs from the base of the skull to the pelvis.[11]

Once inside the trunk, these fibers have options. They may synapse right away. They may travel up or down the trunk to synapse elsewhere. Or, they may skip the trunk and pass through it to reach ganglia closer to the organs they serve.[12] After the synapse, postganglionic fibers continue on their path. Some rejoin spinal nerves and travel to blood vessels, sweat glands, or hair-raising muscles. Others become splanchnic nerves. These bypass the spinal nerves and go directly to internal organs.[13] The splanchnic nerves are crucial for sympathetic control. Each one originates from a specific spinal level and targets specific organs: The splanchnic nerves arise from distinct levels of the spinal cord and carry sympathetic fibers to the abdominal and pelvic organs. The greater splanchnic nerves, originating from T5 to T9, travel to the stomach, liver, pancreas, and spleen. The lesser splanchnic nerves, arising from T10 to T11, innervate the kidneys and portions of the upper intestines. The least splanchnic nerves, from T12, reach the kidneys and adrenal glands. From the lumbar region, the lumbar splanchnic nerves (L1 to L2) connect with the lower intestines and pelvic organs. Finally, the sacral splanchnic nerves, arising from S2 to S4, project to the pelvic organs.

During stress, these nerves allow the body to act fast. The heart rate increases. Breathing deepens. Blood moves to the muscles. Digestion slows. The adrenal medulla releases adrenaline. The body is mobilized for action.[14]

The Sympathetic Trunk and the Bladder Meridian - A Shared Pathway

The source of these signals is known as the thoracolumbar outflow. Preganglionic neurons send their messages through the sympathetic trunk. The system works in two steps: the first neuron reaches the ganglion, and the second carries the message to the target tissue.

The adrenal glands are an exception. Here, preganglionic neurons connect directly to chromaffin cells in the adrenal medulla. These cells release epinephrine and norepinephrine directly into the bloodstream. The effect is systemic and immediate.[15]

This entire system runs through a physical structure called the sympathetic trunk. Preganglionic fibers enter through the white rami communicates. Postganglionic fibers exit through the gray rami. These connections mirror the arrangement of acupuncture pathways. The bladder meridian travels along the spine in almost the same path. Shu points, placed along this meridian, align with sympathetic ganglia and spinal nerves.[16] When a needle is inserted, it may influence not only energy, but neural balance as well. Acupuncture does not work in opposition to this system. It works with it. Channel theory and sympathetic pathways are two languages describing the same truth. One uses qi. The other uses nerves. Together, they reveal the full story.

In the next section, we turn our attention to one of the most profound frontiers of healing. This is where emotions shape the biology and where unseen pain reveals itself through the body. Psychosomatic disorders are not imagined. They are deeply embodied. Acupuncture offers a way to gently unwind their imprint from both the nervous system and the soul.

IV

The Emotional Body

Psychosomatics, Trauma, and the Spirit-Body Connection

*"Whenever a person is frightened, fearful, angry, or overworked,
whether one is active or quiet, all this causes changes"*
— *Huang Di*

11

When Emotions Take Shape - The Psychosomatic Roots of Disease

To better understand the emotional and spiritual layers of the ANS, this section brings together classical Chinese medical theory and modern neuroscience. Ancient Chinese Medical texts have long recognized the relationship between the organs and specific emotional states. Grief is linked with the lungs. Fear is associated with the kidneys. Contemporary science is beginning to validate these connections through the lens of neurobiology and trauma-informed care.

One of the most significant intersections between mind and body is found in the realm of psychosomatic disorders. These are conditions in which emotional distress manifests through physical symptoms. At the center of these conditions lies the ANS.

The Liver Remembers - Emotional Regulation and the ANS

Dr. Hammer states, "understanding the psychosomatic mechanisms lies in the ANS." The ANS doesn't just regulate physical functions, it also translates emotional input into physiological output, often without conscious awareness.[1] When dysregulated, it can give rise to both physical illnesses and emotional imbalances. Studies show clear links between ANS dysfunction and disorders such as depression and anxiety, highlighting the bidirectional nature of emotional and autonomic regulation.[2]

As previously discussed in Chapter 7, the liver and gallbladder are seen as the primary organ systems overseeing the nervous system. When emotional tension rises, particularly from repressed frustration, resentment, or anger, it generates internal heat in the liver. This internal heat then agitates the nervous system. This tension often accumulates in the sinews and chest, leading to symptoms such as chest tightness, insomnia, muscular stiffness, and even cardiovascular or digestive disruptions.[3]

The liver, however, is also regarded as one of the most resilient organs due to its connection with blood storage and renewal. It serves as the body's first line of defense against emotional trauma, metabolizing psychic tension just as much as it metabolizes toxins.[4]

The *Huang Di Nei Jing* offers vivid descriptions of how unresolved emotion becomes disease. It teaches that repeated anger causes qi to rise in a disordered way, leading to blood stagnation and weakening of the sinews. Over time, this disrupts the delicate flow between the liver and the heart, causing qi and blood to "battle" within the chest. These imbalances may manifest as chest pain, palpitations, migraines, or even paralysis if left unresolved.[5]

This ancient view is not merely metaphorical. It reveals an early recognition that emotional strain shapes both circulation and structure, pressing itself into the tissues when left unchecked. In both models, the treatment begins by restoring regulation of qi, the nervous system, and of the heart-mind connection.

Emotions as Energy - How Anger, Grief, and Fear Shape the Body

The *Ling Shu* carries this teaching further, offering timeless guidance on the impact of unresolved emotion. It explains that intense anger causes the qi to rise, disturbing the liver and potentially leading to long-term illness. Grief, fear, and worry are also thought to damage qi, throwing off internal harmony and weakening the body's life force. Repeated emotional strain doesn't just affect mood, it also shapes posture, breath, and organ function. According to the *Ling Shu*, excessive rage not only clouds the mind but also creates rigidity in the spine and lower back. This is both an emotional and physiological observation of how holding emotions can manifest as physical stiffness.[6]

Modern observations mirrors these insights. Studies show that suppressed anger often manifests as chest tension, breath restriction, and discomfort, particularly in the upper body.[7] These symptoms correlate with over-activation of the sympathetic nervous system. This is the same system responsible for fight-or-flight responses and the physiological effects of chronic stress. Patients with this pattern often report neck pain, shoulder stiffness, and lower back discomfort, all of which reflect autonomic dysregulation.[8]

Acupuncture offers relief by treating symptoms and modulating the nervous system. It has been shown to reduce sympathetic activation, enhance parasympathetic tone, and ease pain caused by emotional and physical tension.[9] From both classical and modern perspectives, this is how acupuncture helps restore the free movement of qi, blood, and emotion.

The Body Remembers What the Mind Forgets

Psychosomatic disorders remind us that the body is not just a passive vessel. It reflects the emotional experiences we carry. When emotions are unprocessed or suppressed, they do not disappear. Instead, they take shape in the body through patterns of tension, altered posture, or persistent pain.[10] In TCM, anger is said to injure the liver, grief to disturb the lungs, and fear to weaken the kidneys.[11] Neurobiology offers a complementary view, showing how these emotional patterns are regulated by the ANS, which continuously governs our internal state and responses.[12]

Acupuncture stands at the intersection of ancient wisdom and modern science, helping to restore the body's internal rhythm. It does not divide the emotional from the physical. It treats them as parts of a unified system. Increasingly, data supports what practitioners have long observed: acupuncture can regulate heart rate, reduce anxiety, calm inflammation, and remind the body what safety feels like.

Where the Organs Speak Emotion

To fully understand how the ANS mirrors our emotional landscape, we must turn toward the inner terrain of the body. Each organ in TCM is not only a physiological system, but also a spiritual steward, a vessel for emotional expression and regulation. Just as the liver processes anger and the kidneys hold fear, the heart, lungs, and spleen carry their own emotional imprints, shaped by joy, grief, worry, and will. In the sections ahead, we will explore how these organ-emotion pairings form a map of the emotional body. They reveal how dysregulation in spirit, qi, or feeling can shape the tone of the nervous system itself. Guided by both classical texts and emerging research, we will travel through the wisdom of the Zhi of the kidneys, the Shen of the heart, the Po of the lungs, the Yi of the spleen, and the Hun of the liver. Together, we will discover how emotional vitality or distress becomes somatic experience, and how acupuncture helps restore flow, coherence, and balance.

12

Quieting the Storm - Acupuncture, Autonomic Balance, and Emotional Well-Being

Psychological stress has far-reaching effects on the ANS. It often tips the body into sympathetic overdrive[1]. From a TCM perspective, emotional disturbances disrupt the flow of qi. These imbalances particularly affect the heart, liver, and kidney systems, which are understood to govern the spirit, the movement of emotions, and the will to act.[2]

This classical understanding is reflected in the *Ling Shu*, where it is written:

"Grief, fear, fury, and rage harm the qi. When the qi harms a long-term depot, it causes disease in that depot." [3]

With specific regard to the heart, the text further states,

"Anxiety, grief, fear, and dread will harm the Heart."[4]

In modern scientific terms, such disruptions are reflected in patterns of vagal dysregulation, reduced HRV, and diminished resilience. Findings confirm that chronic stress alters ANS activity and contributes to both emotional and physical dysfunction.[5]

The parallels echo the principles described in the *Huang Di Nei Jing*, which emphasize that emotional excess can injure the internal organs and disturb systemic harmony. Ancient insights into the relationship between emotions, qi, and the organ systems continue to resonate with contemporary understandings of psychophysiological stress.

Stress, however, does not arise from emotions alone. It can also emerge when we fall out of alignment with the natural cycles that support physiological balance. Just as emotional excess can disturb the internal organs and spirit, a disconnection from rhythms like the rising and setting of the sun can unsettle the body's yang qi. This disruption not only weakens its protective function, it also contributes to chronic stress by disturbing the heart and nervous system. We will take a deeper look at this by exploring how night shift workers, whose lives operate out of rhythm with the sun, experience extreme stress and physiological imbalance.

Where the Heart Finds Rest - Acupuncture and the Night Worker's Nervous System

In the *Su Wen*, it is written:

"If the sun were to lose its location, then this would reduce the longevity of a man, and his physical appearance would not look fine. The fact is, the movements of the celestial bodies in heaven require the sun to be lustrous and brilliant. Hence, the yang qi follows the sun and rises. It is that which protects the outside."[6]

This passage reflects the cosmological foundations of TCM, where human health is closely tied to celestial rhythms. When a person becomes disconnected from the natural cycle of day and night, the body's yang qi, which governs vitality and outward protection, may become disrupted. This concept is especially relevant to night shift workers whose biological rhythms are often misaligned with the rising of the sun. This ancient view of physiological balance being influenced by natural cycles finds modern relevance in clinical observations, particularly in studies examining how circadian disruption impacts autonomic regulation and emotional health.

In a randomized controlled trial, Wu et al. (2009) investigated the physiological effects of laser acupuncture on night shift workers.[7] This population is particularly vulnerable to chronic stress. Their disrupted sleep-wake cycles contribute to autonomic imbalance and emotional dysregulation. The study focused on Pericardium 6, or PC6. This point is traditionally used in Chinese medicine to calm the spirit, regulate the heart, and relieve symptoms such as nausea and palpitations. PC6 is also known for its effect on the ANS. It helps restore balance between sympathetic activity and parasympathetic rest.

The trial included forty-five healthy male participants, all of whom worked rotating night shifts. Participants were randomly assigned to either the laser acupuncture group or a control group. The intervention involved low-level laser stimulation applied bilaterally to PC6. Each session lasted twenty minutes. Treatments were administered three times per week for two consecutive weeks. To assess changes in autonomic function, measurements of HRV were recorded. This is a widely accepted, non-invasive biomarker that reflects the dynamic balance between sympathetic drive and parasympathetic recovery.

The results revealed that those who received laser acupuncture at PC6 experienced a statistically significant increase in high-frequency HRV components. This increase reflected enhanced vagal tone and a clear shift toward parasympathetic dominance. At the same time, there was a notable reduction in low-frequency HRV components and the LF to HF ratio. These changes indicated a decrease in sympathetic nervous system activity. In short, PC6 stimulation promoted a more relaxed physiological state. It calmed the cardiovascular system and supported emotional regulation.

The relationship between the heart and pericardium described in Chinese medicine is increasingly supported by modern findings. In classical theory, the Pericardium functions as the protector of the heart. It shields the heart from emotional excess and internal disruption. This helps preserve the integrity of the Shen, the spirit housed within the heart. When stress threatens this inner harmony, the Pericardium steps in to regulate and restore balance.

This idea is supported in the *Spiritual Axis* (*Ling Shu*), Chapter 71, which states:

"*If the Heart is attacked by a pathogenic factor, the Mind suffers, which can lead to death. If a pathogenic factor does attack the Heart, it will be deviated to attack the Pericardium instead.*"[8]

By activating Pericardium 6 (PC6), the practitioner engages this protective channel. The nervous system softens. The spirit calms. The heart is unburdened. Balance is restored.

Emerging findings affirm the classical use of PC6 and highlights acupuncture's influence on the nervous system. Through the precise stimulation of classical points, acupuncture bridges ancient wisdom and modern science. Its purpose is not just symptom relief. It is the restoration of harmony within the body and mind.

Psychosomatic Harmony - Acupuncture and the Stress–Body Connection

When emotional stress becomes chronic and unresolved, it does not only affect the mind. It imprints on the body. In TCM, this is understood through the interconnectedness of the Shen, qi, and blood flow. Emotions like anger, grief, and worry can stagnate the liver qi, disturb the heart, or weaken the spleen. This disruption gives rise to emotional symptoms as well as physical imbalances that reflect psychosomatic distress.[9] The *Nei Jing* teaches that excessive emotional states can damage the organs and disrupt internal harmony.[10] Recent scientific investigations now support this ancient view. Studies in psychoneuroimmunology and trauma science have shown that chronic emotional stress alters neurochemical pathways and leads to measurable ANS dysfunction.[11]

Restoring the Current - Electroacupuncture and Emotional Repair

Stress leaves its mark on both body and mind. For centuries, healers have turned to acupuncture not only to calm the spirit but also to ease the somatic weight of worry, tension, and fatigue. In recent decades, electroacupuncture has emerged as a particularly powerful method, combining the ancient practice of needling with the subtle force of electrical stimulation. This approach has been studied in depth, offering evidence that the gentle charge applied through classical points can reawaken balance in the nervous system. A comprehensive assessments of its efficacy came from Chen Allen (1992), who reviewed eighty-five clinical studies on acupuncture's impact in the treatment of mental and stress-related disorders.[12]

The analysis spanned a wide range of patient populations, diagnostic categories, and treatment protocols, providing one of the earliest large-scale assessments of acupuncture's role in neuropsychiatric care. Electroacupuncture, which involves applying mild electrical stimulation to acupuncture needles, was found to be highly effective across the board. The data revealed a 78.8 percent success rate in treating mental health conditions such as anxiety, depression, and insomnia. In parallel, a 77.1 percent efficacy rate was reported for the treatment of physical symptoms commonly linked to chronic stress. These included muscle tension, gastrointestinal disturbances, palpitations, and fatigue.

Among the most frequently utilized acupuncture points were ST36, known as Zusanli, and GB20, referred to as Fengchi. ST36 is a classical point located on the lower leg and is traditionally used to tonify qi, regulate digestion, and support immune strength. GB20 is located at the base of the skull and is often used to treat headaches, dizziness, and emotional tension.[13] From a biomedical perspective, both points have been associated with increased intracephalic blood flow. Enhanced cerebral circulation, in turn, supports greater oxygenation and metabolic activity in the brain.[14]

Chen's review highlighted a significant connection between this improved blood flow and the modulation of central neurochemistry. Stimulation of these points was linked to increased release of serotonin in the central nervous system. Serotonin is a key neurotransmitter involved in the regulation of mood, sleep, pain perception, and autonomic balance. This neurochemical shift provides a possible explanation for acupuncture's calming effects on both emotional and physiological symptoms. It also reinforces the TCM understanding that emotional and physical well-being are inseparable.

By improving central circulation and influencing neurotransmitter release, electroacupuncture appears to regulate the nervous system from multiple angles. These findings not only support acupuncture's clinical use for stress-related disorders, it also offers a physiological basis for its effects. The review by Chen Allen remains a cornerstone in literature, bridging the worlds of traditional healing and modern neurobiology.

Soothing the Shen, Freeing the Liver - A TCM Approach to Cultural Distress

Stress weaves itself through both body and mind. It shows up as restless thoughts, tight muscles, disturbed sleep, and fatigue that lingers. Healing, too, must reach into both realms. Electroacupuncture, with its subtle currents and timeless points, has been studied as one way to calm this dual burden. Early large-scale reviews sought to understand how this therapy might ease suffering and restore balance where stress takes root. Clinicians, Choi et al. (2021) explored the effectiveness of acupuncture in treating Hwa-Byung, a Korean culture-bound syndrome often translated as "fire illness" or "suppressed anger syndrome."[15] This condition is characterized by a distinct combination of emotional and physical symptoms. Individuals with Hwa-Byung commonly report sensations of heat rising in the chest, throat tightness or blockage, palpitations, insomnia, pressure in the head and chest, and persistent feelings of injustice, frustration, and resentment. It is recognized within Korean society as a psychosomatic response to prolonged emotional suppression, particularly among women in rigid social or familial structures.

The researchers recruited fifteen participants, all of whom met the diagnostic criteria for Hwa-Byung. Each participant received ten individualized acupuncture sessions over a four-week period. Treatment protocols were based on both classical Korean and TCM principles, emphasizing the regulation of liver qi, calming of the Shen, and harmonization of the heart and spleen. Commonly used points included LI4, LR3, PC6, and HT7. These points are known to release internal constraint, soothe emotional agitation, and regulate the ANS.

To measure the outcomes of treatment, they utilized both subjective assessments and objective physiological markers. Psychological distress was evaluated using standardized mental health questionnaires, while autonomic function was assessed through HRV readings and electrodermal activity. The results were significant. Participants reported marked improvements in emotional well-being, with reductions in irritability, anxiety, and somatic symptoms. Physiological data supported these subjective reports. There was a measurable decrease in sympathetic nervous system activity and a shift toward parasympathetic regulation.

These findings highlight acupuncture's unique role in the treatment of psychosomatic conditions. Hwa-Byung is not simply a mental health issue, nor is it purely physical. It represents a state where unresolved emotional tension becomes embedded in the body. Acupuncture, through its precise engagement with the ANS and meridian pathways, offers a means to untangle this embodied distress. By releasing constraint, improving circulation, and calming the heart, acupuncture not only alleviates symptoms but helps restore the body's innate capacity for emotional integration.

The information from this trial reinforces a growing understanding in both Eastern and Western models of care. Emotional pain is not abstract. It lives in the tissues, the breath, the pulse. When it is not expressed, it is stored. When it is not processed, it alters physiology. Acupuncture, when skillfully applied, becomes more than physical treatment. It becomes a method of emotional unburdening, a bridge between the visible symptoms and the invisible roots of suffering.

Lifting the Weight - Acupuncture's Role in Depression and Autonomic Rebalancing

In both TCM and modern neurology, depression is seen as a state of stagnation. This may involve qi, blood, or emotional energy becoming blocked or deficient. Classical texts associate depression with disruptions in the heart, which governs the Shen or spirit, the liver, which ensures the smooth flow of emotions, and the spleen, which supports thought and emotional processing.[16] Biomedicine, on the other hand, often links depression to dysregulation in the ANS, chronic inflammation, and altered vagal tone. New evidence suggests that acupuncture may provide a therapeutic pathway through both physiological and emotional systems. By engaging the vagus nerve, modulating neuroinflammation, and influencing neurotransmitter release, acupuncture offers a unique bridge between ancient theory and modern neurobiology.[17]

The Ear as a Gateway - Rebalancing Depression with Gentle

Stimulation

A new wave of evidence is revealing how ancient ideas are being validated by modern technology. Transcutaneous auricular vagus nerve stimulation, or taVNS, is one such example. By delivering gentle electrical impulses to specific points on the outer ear, taVNS activates internal pathways long recognized in acupuncture and now increasingly supported by neuroscience.

Researchers at Harvard Medical School and the China Academy of Chinese Medical Sciences explored taVNS as a treatment for major depressive disorder.[18] Patients receiving taVNS showed significant reductions in symptoms such as anxiety, sleep disturbance, psychomotor slowing, and hopelessness. These improvements were measured using the Hamilton Depression Rating Scale and were sustained even after treatment ended.

What makes taVNS unique is its multi-system impact. Rather than targeting mood through a single mechanism, taVNS appears to shift the entire internal landscape. It influences brain regions involved in emotion regulation, memory, and self-awareness. These include the amygdala, anterior cingulate cortex, insula, and hippocampus. Brain imaging shows measurable changes in these areas after just a few weeks of treatment. Patients who experienced the strongest improvements in mood also showed the greatest changes in activity within these brain networks.

Scientist believe part of taVNS's effectiveness lies in its ability to calm inflammation. Chronic stress and depression are often linked to immune system overactivation. This can lead to increased production of inflammatory cytokines that affect mood, sleep, energy, and cognition. taVNS appears to interrupt this cycle by helping regulate immune signals and restore balance.

Other mechanisms are also being explored. Early evidence suggests taVNS may support neurogenesis, or the growth of new brain cells, particularly in the hippocampus. It may also improve communication along the gut-brain axis, helping regulate digestion, hormones, and microbiome function. This broad therapeutic reach is what makes taVNS so promising for people experiencing complex symptoms that involve both mind and body.

As we continue to explore the pathways between the ear, brain, and emotional well-being, taVNS invites a new kind of medicine. It is one that listens more closely to the body's subtle rhythms. One that reminds us healing does not always arrive with force, but with gentle signals, consistent attention, and the willingness to reconnect. In that quiet return, profound change begins.

Rebalancing the Inner Pulse - Vagal Tone and Emotional Vitality

Depression touches both mind and body. It clouds thought, unsettles the spirit, and disrupts the rhythms of the nervous system. Healing approaches that address only one side often fall short. Acupuncture offers a pathway that attends to both, reaching into the heart of emotion while also restoring balance to the body's inner currents. In a clinical trial conducted by Noda et al. (2015), clinicians investigated the effects of press needle acupuncture on individuals experiencing depressive symptoms.[19] Press needle acupuncture is a non-invasive technique in which extremely small needles are adhered to the surface of the skin using medical adhesive. These needles remain in place for extended periods and offer continuous, gentle stimulation to specific acupuncture points. The technique is well-tolerated, making it particularly suitable for individuals who are sensitive to traditional needling or who benefit from sustained regulatory input to the nervous system.

The trial included adult participants with mild to moderate depressive symptoms. Each individual received continuous press needle stimulation for seventy-two hours. The selected acupuncture points targeted both emotional regulation and autonomic balance. Although the full protocol was individualized, common points included those traditionally used to calm the Shen, support heart function, and relieve emotional stagnation.

To evaluate the impact of the intervention, the researchers conducted both psychological and physiological assessments before and after the treatment period. Psychological well-being was measured using the Beck Depression Inventory, a validated questionnaire that assesses mood, cognition, and physical symptoms associated with depression. Physiological function was assessed through Holter electrocardiography, a method of continuously recording heart rhythms over a twenty-four-hour period. This allowed the observers to analyze changes in HRV, or HRV, which is widely recognized as a reliable indicator of ANS activity and sympatho-vagal balance.

The findings were notable. Participants who received press needle acupuncture showed a statistically significant increase in high-frequency HRV, reflecting enhanced vagal tone and greater parasympathetic activity. At the same time, there was a measurable reduction in blood pressure, as well as significant improvement in Beck Depression Inventory scores. These results indicate that participants experienced both physiological and emotional benefits. The nervous system shifted away from stress-driven sympathetic activation and toward a calmer, more regulated parasympathetic state. Mood also improved, with participants reporting reduced sadness, irritability, and fatigue.

This research offers compelling evidence for the role of acupuncture in treating depression through a dual mechanism. It not only acts on the emotional centers of the brain but also recalibrates the rhythms of the body through autonomic regulation. Vagal activation, improved cardiovascular coherence, and the gentle, continuous nature of press needle therapy may work together to restore internal harmony. This aligns with TCM principles, which emphasize that emotional and physical healing arise when qi is able to flow freely, and the spirit can rest within a calm and nourished heart.

Acupuncture, Autonomic Balance, and Emotional Well-Being

Emotional well-being is intimately connected to the balance of the ANS. Chronic stress, unresolved grief, and emotional trauma often manifest not only in the mind, but also in the body. These emotional states can disrupt vagal tone, alter HRV, and disturb the body's capacity for internal regulation. TCM has long recognized this profound mind-body connection. It views the heart, liver, and kidney systems as essential to both emotional and energetic health.

This chapter explored how acupuncture supports both emotional and physiological balance by regulating the ANS. Across a range of psychological conditions such as chronic stress, depression, and psychosomatic symptoms, research consistently demonstrates that acupuncture plays a meaningful role in promoting nervous system stability and restoring homeostasis.

Scientific studies have shown that the insertion of an acupuncture needle initiates a complex sequence of neurophysiological responses. These responses are mediated through the sympathetic and parasympathetic branches of the ANS. Together, these systems influence almost every aspect of internal regulation, including heart rate, digestion, respiration, immune function, skin conductance, and body temperature.

When the ANS becomes imbalanced, the effects are often both emotional and physical. Anxiety, low mood, digestive issues, respiratory symptoms, and cardiovascular disturbances may all arise as the body struggles to maintain equilibrium. The research reviewed in this chapter shows that acupuncture, through specific point selection and stimulation, can gently guide the nervous system back toward balance. This shift supports symptom relief while also enhancing the body's long-term capacity for resilience and repair.

These findings echo what TCM has taught for thousands of years. Emotional and physical well-being are not separate. They move together. Healing begins not only in the mind, but also in the body's rhythms. When those rhythms are restored, the spirit has space to settle, and the body remembers how to heal.

Among all the organ systems, none bears the emotional weight of the human experience more than the heart. In the next chapter, we explore the Shen, the spirit housed within the heart, and how its balance determines the radiance of our emotional and spiritual well-being.

13

The Spirit and the Shen – Emotional Regulation in Classical Chinese Medicine

TCM does not separate the mind from the body or emotions from physical health. Instead, they are viewed as interconnected threads within a unified system. This holistic view is embodied in the concept of the Shen, the spirit that resides in the heart and reflects one's mental, emotional, and spiritual vitality.[1] As stated in the *Su Wen*, "The Heart is the basis of life. It is responsible for the changes of the spirit."[2]

The Heart Knows the Way

Where Western psychology often locates the mind in the brain, Chinese medicine roots consciousness and emotional vitality in the heart. The heart in TCM is not simply the organ that pumps blood. It is a sacred vessel. It is considered the sovereign of the body because it reflects the influence of all five yin organs and embodies the emotional and spiritual qualities of each.[3] In the *Su Wen*, Chapter 8, "The heart is the official functioning as ruler. Spirit brilliance originates in it." [4] The heart is entrusted with holding the Shen. The Shen is the spark of awareness, perception, and joy.

The Shen governs more than emotion. It is a reflection of one's vitality, revealed in bright eyes, a calm presence, and harmony between thought, feeling, and action. When disturbed, however, it may manifest as anxiety, restlessness, insomnia, heart palpitations, dissociation, or forgetfulness.[5] According to the *Huang Di Nei Jing*, "the Heart stores the spirit," a concept understood as the Shen. When heart qi is abundant and regulated, the Shen is anchored. But when the heart is unsettled by excessive emotions, internal heat, or underlying weakness, the Shen becomes unrooted, giving rise to these imbalances.[6]

This classical understanding has modern parallels. Emotional trauma can disrupt autonomic balance and trigger a cascade of physiological responses. Symptoms like racing thoughts, poor sleep, and a heightened startle reflex often reflect sympathetic overactivation, which aligns with the traditional concept of Shen disturbance.[7]

Tracking the Spirit Through the Nervous System

In neurobiological terms, the Shen reflects the central regulation of autonomic tone. This refers to the balance between the sympathetic nervous system, which prepares the body for defense and action, and the parasympathetic system, which supports recovery and rest. When emotional stress is ongoing or unresolved, this balance becomes strained. The body may remain in a heightened state of alert, even in the absence of danger, mirroring the ancient Chinese view of a Shen that is no longer rooted.[8]

The ancient understanding of the Shen provides a powerful lens for interpreting emotional and physiological distress. In recent years, scientific studies have begun to reflect this wisdom by exploring how emotional trauma, nervous system dysregulation, and insomnia may be linked to measurable imbalances in autonomic tone. While the terminology differs, both traditions describe the same reality. TCM speaks of Shen and modern science speaks of autonomic regulation. Both point to the same truth, that disturbances of the spirit reveal themselves through the body's rhythms. The Shen, when disturbed, can now be tracked through changes in vagal activity, heart rhythm, and sleep quality. What follows are examples of how acupuncture, rooted in the classical aim of calming the spirit, is being used in clinical settings to restore these rhythms and support healing.

The Return of Rhythm and Shen

In both classical and modern views, healing the spirit begins with restoring rhythm to the body. Modern science offers a parallel explanation through the lens of ANS regulation. When emotional trauma disrupts vagal tone and elevates sympathetic activity, the body becomes stuck in a state of chronic arousal. This state of dysregulation mirrors the classical idea of Shen disturbance.

A 2024 case series published in *Medical Acupuncture* explored acupuncture treatment for generalized anxiety disorder.[9] The study followed patients who received acupuncture twice a week for four weeks. Results showed significant reductions in anxiety symptoms along with improvements in heart-rate coherence, a key marker of vagal regulation. The authors concluded that acupuncture may reduce sympathetic overactivation by stimulating the vagus nerve. This provides a measurable biological pathway through which acupuncture helps restore emotional balance and nervous system resilience.

Though the language is different, the insight is the same. Restoring internal harmony calms the spirit, quiets the mind, and roots the Shen.

Restoring Sleep Through Shen and the Blood

Insomnia is more than just the inability to fall asleep. In TCM, it is often understood as a sign that the spirit, or Shen, cannot settle. When the Shen is disturbed, the mind stays restless, thoughts race, and the body cannot descend into the stillness of sleep. This imbalance may arise from a deficiency in heart blood, which normally anchors the Shen, or from internal heat that agitates the spirit.

A 2020 study by Tong Zheng Hong expands on this classical view by identifying a set of Shen-related acupuncture points frequently used in the treatment of insomnia.[10] In addition to HT7 (Shenmen), the protocol included points such as Baihui (DU-20), Shenting (DU-24), Benshen (GB-13), Sishencong (EX-HN1), Neiguan (PC6), Sanyinjiao (SP6). These points were chosen not just for their anatomical location but for their energetic meaning. The study emphasized the importance of understanding Chinese character-based point names, which reveal deeper symbolic and functional connections such as the relationship between kidney jing, spleen qi, and heart blood in calming the Shen.

Researchers describe insomnia as a disharmony of the Three Treasures, which include jing, qi, and Shen. When jing and qi are depleted, blood becomes insufficient. Without blood to nourish the heart, the Shen loses its home. Wind may also arise internally due to spleen deficiency and poor digestion, further disturbing sleep.

Acupuncture, when applied with a deep understanding of pattern differentiation and Shen-related points, helps restore this balance. It strengthens blood, calms wind, and re-establishes the settling rhythm that allows the spirit to return to rest. By focusing on the root, whether jing, qi, or blood, practitioners can guide the Shen back into its home and help the nervous system re-enter parasympathetic restoration.

This research demonstrates that treating insomnia depends on more than selecting a single point. While Shenmen (HT7) remains central, seven additional Shen-related acupoints can be chosen according to the severity and underlying pattern. The Chinese names of these points reveal functions that guide their use, reminding practitioners that the meaning of each acupoint carries clinical weight. Effective treatment rests on accurate pattern identification and on restoring harmony between jing, qi, blood, and Shen. These are the foundations that allow the spirit to settle and sleep to return.

Modern Tools for an Ancient Spirit

From the Chinese medicine perspective, calming the Shen involves more than just physical regulation. It includes nourishing the heart, soothing emotional constraint, and grounding the will. When heart blood is deficient, the Shen has no home.[11] When liver qi is stagnant, emotions can rise without clarity.[12] When kidney essence is depleted, the will weakens and the spirit feels unanchored.[13] These classical patterns offer a holistic map for understanding emotional and energetic balance in the body.

Current research now provides biological language for these same patterns. A 2021 meta-analysis by Yang et al. reviewed 20 randomized controlled trials involving over 1,800 participants.[14] The researchers found that acupuncture significantly reduced anxiety symptoms across a range of anxiety disorders. The results revealed a medium effect size favoring acupuncture over control interventions, with additional improvements in sleep quality. While the study focused on generalized anxiety disorder, the findings are relevant to trauma-related conditions that involve chronic dysregulation of the hypothalamic-pituitary-adrenal (HPA) axis and impaired autonomic balance. These disruptions can be measured using biomarkers such as HRV, which reflect vagal tone and stress resilience. In essence, these physiological imbalances mirror what Chinese medicine has long described as disturbances of the Shen, the spiritual and emotional aspect of the heart. Acupuncture's ability to modulate the stress response, restore autonomic balance, and promote neurohormonal regulation positions it as a powerful tool for trauma recovery and emotional healing. In this way, ancient and modern systems align. Calming the Shen is not only metaphorical but also measurable.

Understanding the Shen through both classical theory and emerging research reveals it not as a singular entity, but as the integrated expression of psychological, physiological, and relational coherence. In TCM, the Shen reflects one's capacity for presence, emotional stability, and connection to self and others. When the Shen is disturbed, individuals may experience anxiety, restlessness, insomnia, or emotional disconnection. These symptoms closely parallel what occurs during ANS dysregulation, particularly when the body is locked in prolonged sympathetic activation. Studies on generalized anxiety disorder, trauma, and insomnia have demonstrated that acupuncture can reduce sympathetic arousal, increase vagal tone, and improve biomarkers such as heart-rate variability and sleep quality. These outcomes reflect measurable pathways by which Shen regulation occurs.

Whether described as Shen disturbance, heart fire, HPA axis dysregulation, or vagal suppression, the underlying pattern is one of imbalance between activation and restoration. Acupuncture offers a clinical intervention that bridges these worlds. By restoring autonomic tone and supporting the body's capacity for self-regulation, it provides a therapeutic method for both physiological recovery and emotional healing. In this way, the ancient aim of calming the Shen is affirmed by modern evidence. It is not only a metaphor for spiritual harmony, but a measurable process within the nervous system.

The Shen, the Nervous System, and the Path to Longevity

When the Shen is calm and the nervous system is regulated, the body is no longer living in survival mode. In TCM, this state of internal harmony is considered essential for cultivating jing, the essence that supports growth, vitality, and lifespan. Chronic Shen disturbance, whether from trauma, emotional suppression, or overwork, consumes heart blood, stagnates liver qi, and weakens kidney essence. These are foundational substances that govern resilience and influence the aging process.[15]

Modern science reflects a similar truth. Chronic activation of the sympathetic nervous system, what we understand as long-term stress, has been shown to accelerate biological aging. Research by Epel and colleagues (2004) found that individuals exposed to high levels of emotional stress had shorter telomeres and reduced telomerase activity. These changes impair cellular repair and regeneration, increase oxidative stress, and compromise immune function. What Chinese medicine views as the depletion of essence and disturbance of spirit can also be measured through biological markers of stress and aging. Whether seen through the lens of the Three Treasures or cellular physiology, the message is the same. Calm the mind, regulate the nervous system, and nourish the Shen to preserve vitality over time.[16]

HRV, a modern biomarker of vagal tone, has been shown to correlate with both emotional regulation and longevity.[17] The higher the vagal tone, the more adaptable the nervous system becomes, and the more resilient the body is in the face of aging. Calming the Shen and supporting parasympathetic regulation can help patients feel more emotionally grounded. Practices such as acupuncture, breathwork, touch, and ritual create conditions for the nervous system to shift out of survival mode. Over time, these interventions may also slow the aging process at both the cellular and energetic levels. Longevity, then, is not merely about adding years to life, but restoring the quality of presence within each moment. It is the fruit of balance, coherence, and the return of spirit to body.

While the science reveals how chronic stress accelerates aging and how vagal tone supports vitality, Chinese medicine reminds us that the most profound transformations begin in stillness. It is not enough to understand longevity through data alone. True healing is experienced in the moments when we return to ourselves, through breath, ritual, and the quiet medicine of presence.

Restoring Parasympathetic Balance Through Ritual

Through acupuncture, ritual, intentional presence, and safe therapeutic touch, the Shen is gently guided back to its home in the heart. As the body softens, the breath deepens, and the parasympathetic nervous system begins to engage, the conditions for healing and regulation are re-established. This transition from sympathetic dominance to parasympathetic support reflects what Chinese medicine describes as calming the Shen and nourishing heart blood, inviting stillness, clarity, and reconnection.[18] In this space of nervous system safety and energetic balance, the individual begins to reconnect with a deeper sense of self. That self has always existed beneath the layers of trauma, stress, and fragmentation. This is the heart of integrative medicine. Presence becomes practice. Remembering becomes a path toward wholeness.

Healing is more than treating physical symptoms. It is about creating a space where the body and mind can find ease. In moments of true rest, the spirit begins to return to stillness. Within this quiet, the heart, both as a living organ and as a symbol of our inner life, can feel safe enough to open.[19] This safety is not only emotional but neurological, as the regulation of the ANS through presence, breath, and touch allows the body to shift from a state of survival into a state of restoration.[20] In Chinese medicine, this is known as calming the Shen and anchoring it in the heart, which allows for clarity, joy, and coherence to reemerge.[21] In this sacred pause, healing unfolds on multiple levels. The nervous system recalibrates, the spirit reorients, and the individual begins to remember their innate wholeness. This is the true medicine of presence. It is a moment not just of physiological repair, but of spiritual return.

14

Trauma and the Po – Grief, the Lungs, and Somatic Release

Grief does not always arrive with tears. Sometimes it moves quietly, settling into the breath and the body. It can linger beneath the surface, held in the chest where even the kindest words cannot reach. As the *Su Wen* teaches, "When one is sad, the qi is dispersed".[1]

In Chinese medicine, this experience is embodied in the Po, the corporeal soul that resides in the lungs. The *Su Wen* states, *"The Lungs are basis of qi; it is the location of the Po-soul"*.[2] The Po governs our instinctual nature. It regulates the breath, controls reflexive movement, and guides our ability to feel and release grief.[3]

The Po is the most embodied of the Five Spirits. The *Ling Shu* describes the Po as the spirit that moves with the essence, closely tied to the rhythms of inhalation and exhalation.[4] It is formed at birth and remains rooted in the body, entering and exiting in harmony with the breath.[5] Through its relationship with the lungs, the Po helps anchors presence, and connects us to the felt experience of life. While the Shen reaches upward toward spirit and abstraction, the Po grounds us in form. It draws awareness into the present moment through sensation, respiration, and embodiment.[6]

The ancient text *Ling Shu* states, *"The origin of life is called essence... That which enters and leaves together with the essence, that is called the Po-soul"*.[7]

While breath is not directly mentioned, the Po's close connection to the lungs links it to the rhythm of respiration. We can understand this as the Po moving with the breath, a symbolic reflection of how spirit and body remain connected through each inhale and exhale. This teaching describes more than physical respiration. It points to a deeper truth. The body's wisdom is born of breath.

The Lungs and the Language of Loss

In Chinese medicine, the lungs are seen as more than organs of respiration. They govern not only breath, but also rhythm, immunity, emotional clarity, and the boundaries that define our sense of self.[8] The lungs are responsible for receiving the pure qi of Heaven. As Qi Bo states in the *Su Wen*, "*The qi of Heaven communicates with the Lungs*".[9] This Heavenly qi is then distributed throughout the body, supporting dignity, self-protection, and connection to the world.[10]

When lung qi is strong, we feel upright, present, and in sync with life. We breathe with ease and move through the world with resilience and clear emotional boundaries. When the lungs are weakened, especially by sadness or unresolved grief, this rhythm is disrupted. The Po is especially sensitive to these emotional states. Maciocia writes, "The corporeal soul (Po) is responsible for physical sensations, feelings, and general somatic expressions".[11] Prolonged sorrow constrains lung qi, leading to shallow breathing, fatigue, frequent sighing, dry skin, or increased susceptibility to respiratory and immune disorders.[12]

This classical view is echoed in the *Su Wen*, where Qi Bo states, "*When one is sad, then the heart connection is tense. The lobes of the Lungs spread open and rise, and the upper burner is impassible*".[13] Grief, in this view, rises and blocks the normal descent of lung qi, resulting in breath obstruction and chest tightness.

Recent research supports these ancient insights. Trauma specialists describe a condition known as somatic dissociation, where the breath becomes shallow, the chest contracts, and the body maintains a defensive posture. In this state, the nervous system limits emotional expression in order to protect itself. Grief that is unexpressed, especially when linked to childhood loss or ancestral trauma, often becomes stored in the body. Research by Li and colleagues (2025) found that individuals with high levels of trauma-related dissociation were significantly more likely to experience chronic somatic symptoms such as chest pain, fatigue, and muscle tension. Among nearly one thousand female mental health service users, those with PTSD and dissociation were more than twice as likely to report these physical complaints. These findings confirm that emotional trauma often becomes biologically embedded.[14]

These expressions of grief are not just metaphorical. Grief is both psychological and physiological. Acute grief may show up as disturbed sleep, appetite changes, fatigue, and chest or throat tightness. While these are common during mourning, they can worsen when grief remains unresolved. In such cases, the hypothalamic-pituitary-adrenal axis may become dysregulated, inflammation may rise, and cardiovascular risk can increase. Neuroimaging reveals that grief activates brain regions associated with pain and emotional regulation. When left untreated, complicated grief can impair immune function and raise the risk of early mortality.[15]

Both classical and modern systems remind us that breath is not merely mechanical. It is the bridge between spirit and body. When lung qi is supported and the breath is allowed to soften and descend, emotional release becomes possible, and the healing process begins.

The Body Remembers Grief

Grief is not only an emotion of the heart. It settles into the body, altering breath, sleep, and the steady rhythms that sustain health. When loss remains unresolved, its weight can be carried not just in memory but in physiology. Research has begun to trace how unprocessed grief shapes both mind and body, revealing patterns that echo what ancient traditions have long observed. In the study, *Traumatic Grief as a Risk Factor for Mental and Physical Morbidity*, Prigerson et al (1997). identified traumatic or complicated grief as a distinct clinical condition that significantly impacts both mental and physical health.[16] It was found that individuals experiencing high levels of unresolved grief were more likely to suffer from depression, anxiety, sleep disturbances, and substance use. More importantly, traumatic grief was linked to increased physical illness and a higher risk of early mortality. Bereaved individuals often showed signs of chronic disease, reduced functioning, and a diminished quality of life. The authors proposed that ongoing activation of the body's stress-response systems, including the ANS and inflammatory pathways, may explain the long-term physiological burden of grief.

Although the study did not focus solely on the ANS, it clearly described a pattern of persistent physiological arousal. Symptoms such as restlessness, elevated heart rate, disrupted sleep, and difficulty concentrating reflect the kind of nervous system imbalance that is commonly seen in trauma. These signs point to a state of sympathetic dominance, where the body remains in a prolonged fight-or-flight mode and struggles to return to a state of calm and repair.

Additional insight comes from research conducted by Sahar, Shalev, and Porges, which examined vagal regulation in individuals with posttraumatic stress disorder. Participants with PTSD failed to show the normal increase in respiratory sinus arrhythmia (RSA) during mental stress. RSA is a key indicator of vagal tone and parasympathetic function. Those without PTSD showed healthy vagal flexibility, allowing them to recover from stress more effectively. However, the PTSD group remained stuck in sympathetic activation. Their heart rate was not modulated by parasympathetic input, revealing a diminished capacity to regulate and return to baseline.[17]

These findings suggest that unresolved grief may result in a breakdown of autonomic flexibility. This contributes to the development of cardiovascular issues, immune dysfunction, and metabolic problems often observed in grieving individuals. When the parasympathetic nervous system cannot adequately counterbalance prolonged sympathetic arousal, the body loses its ability to restore balance. Over time, this chronic state of dysregulation may lead to illness, accelerated aging, and early death. Grief, when left unprocessed, becomes more than an emotional wound. It imprints itself biologically and alters the body's capacity to heal.

This connection is further supported by findings that focused on recently bereaved women. Using functional MRI, researchers measured both resting vagal tone and brain activity during grief-related stimuli. Participants with lower baseline vagal tone exhibited significantly higher activation in the posterior cingulate cortex (PCC), a region associated with self-referential emotional processing. They also showed stronger connectivity between the PCC and the subgenual anterior cingulate cortex (sACC), areas linked to emotional pain and depressive rumination. These patterns suggest that when vagal tone is low, the brain becomes more reactive and emotionally overwhelmed by grief. The nervous system struggles to self-regulate, and the body's ability to recover is impaired.[18]

This pattern aligns closely with Chinese medicine's classical description of constrained lung qi and disruption of the Po. According to this view, unresolved emotional pain becomes embedded in the body when the natural movement of qi is impaired. In both frameworks, grief contracts the chest, restricts breath, and creates a state of inner holding. Shallow breathing, poor vagal tone, and sympathetic dominance are the physiological language of what the ancients described as blocked qi and a spirit unable to return to rest.

TCM holds that the lungs are central to the process of emotional release and physiological regulation. The lungs govern breath, support the circulation of qi, and help regulate the nervous and immune systems through the distribution of zong qi (gathering qi) and wei qi (defensive qi). When lung qi is strong, vitality circulates freely, emotional boundaries are maintained, and the inner world remains resilient. When lung qi is weak or constrained, the body becomes vulnerable to external invasion, and emotional stagnation begins to affect physical health. This framework echoes modern findings in psychoneuroimmunology, which show that reduced vagal tone, shallow breathing, and chronic stress weaken immune defense and disturb internal rhythm. When the Po is suppressed, the breath becomes tight, the skin and boundaries weaken, and the unresolved grief of the past lives in the present moment.[19]

Both systems agree that the path toward healing begins with restoring breath, supporting internal regulation, and creating safe passage for grief to move and transform. Whether described as vagal tone or lung qi, the goal is the same, help the body remember its rhythm and return to a state of calm awareness.

Acupuncture and Breath - Releasing the Po

As Qi Bo states in the *Huang Di Nei Jing*, "The lung qi: if depleted, then the nose will be blocked. The [breath qi] do not flow freely, with shortness of [breath] qi".[20]

Sadness and grief directly affect the breath. These emotions disrupt the natural rhythm of the corporeal soul, causing it to pulsate irregularly. As the lung qi becomes constrained, respiration is suspended. This often results in shallow or rapid breathing, which further depletes the qi in the chest. Symptoms such as tightness, breathlessness, or emotional collapse can follow. Treating the lungs is essential in cases of emotional imbalance related to depression, bereavement, or unprocessed grief.[21]

Recent findings continue to echo ancient wisdom. Grief activates the body's stress response, engaging the sympathetic nervous system and flooding the body with cortisol and other stress hormones. Blood flow shifts toward vital organs and large muscle groups, while functions like digestion and immunity slow down. Physical symptoms may include cold hands and feet, headaches, digestive discomfort, and diffuse body aches. Breathing often becomes shallow and irregular, sometimes so subtle that it goes unnoticed, leading to sensations of light headedness, tingling, or dissociation. These reactions are not metaphorical but biological expressions of autonomic imbalance. When grief remains unresolved, its imprint can linger in the body, manifesting as chronic physical and emotional strain.[22]

By viewing grief through both ancient and modern perspectives, a clear truth emerges. Healing begins with the breath. Restoring respiratory rhythm, calming the nervous system, and supporting the descending function of the lungs are essential steps toward emotional regulation and physiological balance. Breath work, somatic practices, and acupuncture can all support this restoration.

Among these options, acupuncture has gained recognition as a safe and effective approach. A 2021 systematic review by Zhang and colleagues examined 45 clinical studies and found that acupuncture significantly reduced symptoms of depression.[23] It also improved sleep, mood, and overall quality of life. In many cases, acupuncture was as effective as antidepressant medications, with fewer side effects. The authors also noted high treatment satisfaction and patient compliance, making acupuncture an accessible and well-tolerated therapy. Their findings confirm what Chinese medicine has taught for centuries. When the lung qi is supported, the breath softens, the spirit descends, and healing becomes possible.

A growing body of evidence continues to show that acupuncture can support respiratory rhythm during periods of physical and emotional stress. Several studies, which will be explored more fully in the chapter on respiration, have found that acupuncture improves breathing function and helps regulate autonomic balance in patients under prolonged strain. These findings reflect what Chinese medicine has long understood. When the breath is supported and allowed to move freely, the body begins to return to a state of harmony.

Longevity Through the Breath of Release

In both TCM and modern trauma science, we find a shared truth. Long life relies not only on cellular health or diet, but also on emotional flow and nervous system regulation. The lungs, as described in Chinese medicine, are guardians of vitality. They do more than breathe. They release. The lungs help the body shed what is no longer needed, from pathogens to pain. This act of letting go, of exhaling fully, is more than emotional liberation. It is a form of cellular preservation.[24]

When the Po is held in safety and the lungs are free to move qi and release grief, the body regains its deep rhythm. This gentle internal rhythm mirrors what Chinese medicine calls the body's internal clock of health. Current biomedical science affirms that autonomic markers such as HRV, vagal tone, and regulated breathing not only reflect resilience but also predict longevity. When grief remains unresolved, it does not only affect emotions. It gradually disrupts the body's deeper systems. Studies shows that prolonged sorrow can suppress immune function, strain the heart, and interfere with restful sleep. Over time, these imbalances make it harder for the body to recover from stress. The result is a greater risk of chronic illness, physical decline, and shortened lifespan. Studies also demonstrate that persistent grief can dysregulate the ANS, elevate systemic inflammation, and alter brain activity in regions related to emotional pain and attachment. These disruptions cumulatively reduce resilience and accelerate aging. The long-term toll of unresolved grief is not only emotional but deeply biological, confirming that the regulation of breath and emotion is foundational to health. Supporting the lungs and restoring the movement of the Po may be essential not just for emotional integration, but for longevity itself.[25]

In Chinese medicine, the natural descent and dispersal of lung qi is considered vital for well-being. When this function is restored, it reflects more than physical balance. It shows that the body has returned to its internal rhythm. Breath moves with ease, emotions begin to settle, and a quiet stability takes root within. This is also reflected in measurable changes in nervous system regulation. Scientific studies confirm that grief activates the sympathetic nervous system. The heart rate increases. Blood pressure rises. Breathing becomes shallow. While these shifts may be adaptive in the short term, prolonged activation can lead to reduced vagal tone, suppressed immunity, and increased vulnerability to illness and early mortality.[26]

When grief becomes chronic, it settles into the body in quiet and persistent ways. Appetite fades. Sleep becomes light or restless. The chest holds pressure. Digestion slows. Energy wanes. The body forgets how to exhale. It lives in a state of waiting. Unable to release. Practices that gently invite the parasympathetic nervous system to return, such as breathwork, ritual journaling, mindful movement, and intentional nourishment, can help restore a sense of inner rhythm and safety.[27]

Slow and conscious breathing is one of the most accessible ways to support this restoration. A meta-analysis of voluntary breathing practices found that techniques such as diaphragmatic and paced breathing significantly improve HRV. These changes not only reduce acute stress but also promote long-term nervous system resilience.[28]

Acupuncture adds another layer of support. Systematic reviews have shown that it can reduce depressive symptoms, improve emotional stability, enhance sleep, and regulate autonomic function.[29] Clinical trials have also demonstrated its capacity to calm sympathetic activity and support cardiovascular and respiratory health during physical or emotional distress.[30]

Grief touches every system in the body. It changes the breath, tightens the chest, alters the sleep cycle, and clouds the spirit. Healing does not come from silencing these responses. It comes from reawakening the rhythm beneath them. When breath is no longer held and tears are welcomed, the Po begins to stir again. The body, once frozen in sorrow, becomes a sanctuary of transformation. From that sanctuary, the path toward longevity begins.

The Breath of Resilience

When grief constricts the breath and the Po cannot descend, the nervous system loses its rhythm. The body enters a state of hypervigilance, locking the breath and holding tension deep within the chest. Yet breath itself holds the key to restoration. Slow breathing techniques have been shown to enhance emotional well-being and support autonomic balance. A recent randomized controlled trial published in *Cell Reports Medicine (2022)* found that daily five-minute cyclic sighing reduced respiratory rate and significantly boosted mood and positive affect more than mindfulness meditation. Over four weeks, participants practicing exhale-focused breathwork also reported larger decreases in anxiety and negative emotion, reflecting a clear shift toward parasympathetic dominance.[32]

Other studies echo this truth. Even a single session of deep, slow breathing has been shown to calm anxiety and steady the heart, with the greatest ease arising in older adults.[33] Slow diaphragmatic breathing appears to awaken the vagus nerve, softening the grip of sympathetic arousal and inviting the body into a state of repair.[34] Most recently, emerging evidence has revealed that structured deep breathing can harmonize heart rhythms and lower blood pressure in older adults, a reminder of how something as simple as breath can reshape the nervous system in the present moment.[35]

When integrated into daily life, these practices become more than stress relief. They become rituals of remembrance. Each exhale helps release what the body carries. Each inhale invites vitality to return. When the Po is given space to move and breath is no longer held, the body reclaims its rhythm. In this return, healing begins. Intentional breathwork interrupts the stress response and steers the body out of survival mode into a state of rest, repair, and emotional integration. This creates a foundation for resilience and longevity. Grief, when left unresolved, can lock the system in chronic defense, weaken immunity, and slowly erode inner harmony. But when it is honored through acupuncture, breathwork, ritual, and rest, vitality is renewed.

Longevity is not the absence of loss. It is the presence of resilience. It is not found in resistance or avoidance, but in the sacred art of release. By tending to the Po, we attend to the breath of the soul. In doing so, we restore the body's natural capacity to thrive across the decades.

The Sacred Act of Exhalation

In the framework of Chinese medicine, healing the lungs involves more than restoring physiological function. It is also a spiritual and ritual process. The lungs govern the energy of release, and true healing requires engaging with that release both internally and externally. Practitioners may invite patients into symbolic or seasonal rituals that reflect nature's own wisdom. These can include breath practices, such as extended exhalations that mimic the body's natural sigh and soften internal tension. Journaling or writing letters to the departed, or to parts of oneself that feel lost or unacknowledged, can offer grief a voice and a path forward.

Even the act of witnessing the seasonal shift into autumn, when trees surrender their leaves and the air grows still, reminds us of something essential. Letting go is not an end. It is a sacred transformation. Trauma may teach the body to hold its breath. The chest contracts. Expression falters. But healing begins when we remember that we are meant to exhale. The lungs, in their quiet rhythm, reveal the wisdom of release. Once the Po is at ease, the breath naturally returns. The chest opens and what once lingered in silence begins to move. In that soft unraveling, the body becomes more than tissue and tension. It becomes an altar. Pain becomes breath. Breath becomes prayer. And in that prayer, we return to ourselves.

This return is not only emotional. It is physiological. It is the restoration of rhythm. And as we now turn to the subject of longevity, we will see that rhythm is not only a path to healing. It is the foundation of a long and balanced life.

All of these findings confirm what Chinese medicine has long taught. Grief lives not just in the mind. It also lives in the breath, the skin, and the pulse of life itself. To heal, we must come home to the body.

The Sacred Art of Release

There comes a moment in healing when the body no longer needs to hold it all. Grief begins to soften. The breath deepens. What once felt stuck starts to move again. Supporting the Po helps the breath come back with ease. The chest opens. The body exhales.

Below is a simple yet powerful practice to help bring the Po into balance and restore the body's memory of safety.

Practice This: Re-patterning the Body's Memory

Find a quiet space where you can sit or lie down comfortably.

1. Anchor the nervous system

Place one hand on your chest, at the center of the heart. Put the other on your lower belly to activate the energy between the two kidneys. Close your eyes. Notice where tension lives without judgment. Just observe.

2. Breathe into Safety:

Take a slow inhale through the nose, letting the breath reach all the way down to your belly.

Exhale gently through the mouth with a soft sigh.

Repeat for 1-3 breaths. With each exhale, imagine letting go of a memory the body no longer needs to hold.

3. Affirmation of Return:

Silently repeat:
It is safe to feel.
It is safe to soften.
My body remembers how to rest.

4. Ground the Spirit:

With your next inhale, imagine a gentle light gathering at the center of your chest (the heart), calming the Shen.

On the exhale, let that light descend to the soles of your feet, grounding the Po and anchoring you to the Earth.

5. Journal Prompt:

- *Where in my body do I store the past?*
- *What can I do to make my body feel safe right now?*
- *What new memory would I like to create inside myself today?*

Come back to this practice any time the nervous system feels flooded or the past echoes too loudly. Healing happens in small returns to the present.

15

Digesting Life - The Spleen, the Yi, and the Nervous System

We are not only digesting food. We are also digesting life. Every emotion, memory, and event we encounter is metabolized through our entire being. This process moves not only through the mind but through the rhythm of our breath, the intelligence of our gut, and the quiet resilience of our nervous system.

In TCM, the spleen governs more than just digestion. It is the center of transformation, turning food into energy, thoughts into clarity, and experience into wisdom. As the *Huang Di Nei Jing* states, *"The Spleen stores the sentiments"*.[1] This ancient insight reveals the spleen's deeper emotional role, holding the imprints of our thoughts, feelings, and lived experiences.

When the spleen is strong, we feel centered, grounded, and nourished. When it is weak, we may feel foggy, fatigued, and emotionally unanchored. Overthinking, worry, and mental spinning begin to take root. These insights are rooted in classical Chinese medicine, which describes the spleen as the organ responsible for transformation and transportation of nutrients, as well as the housing of the Yi. This is the residence of the intellect. This is the part of the mind that oversees thinking, generating ideas, focus, and studying.[2]

The spleen is the organ of the Earth element. And Earth is where we return when we need to come home to ourselves. In the *Nei Jing*, it is said that *"The Spleen and the Stomach are the officials responsible for grain storage"*.[3] They are the nourisher and the alchemist, turning what we take in from the outside world into the inner fuel that sustains body and mind.

The Spleen in Chinese Medicine

The spleen is at the heart of postnatal qi, the energy we generate after birth from the food we eat and the air we breathe. While Western medicine views the spleen primarily as a lymphatic organ, in TCM it is considered the ruler of digestion, nutrient absorption, and mental clarity. The spleen extracts the essence of nourishment from what we consume and helps distribute that nourishment throughout the body.[4]

Emotionally, the spleen is impacted by worry, obsessive thinking, and mental overwork. When we ruminate, loop on problems, or try to control the uncontrollable, we weaken the spleen's ability to transform. This doesn't just result in digestive upset; it shows up as fatigue, muscle heaviness, poor concentration, and emotional overwhelm.[5]

The spleen is considered the master of transformation. It is responsible not only for processing food and fluids but also for refining and directing vital energy throughout the body. It uplifts clear qi to support mental focus and organ stability, contributes to the generation and containment of blood, and houses the Yi, the aspect of consciousness responsible for thought, intention, and focus.[6]

The *Nei Jing* expands on this role, stating, *"The Spleen (and the Stomach, the Large Intestine, the Triple Burner, and the Urinary Bladder) is the basis of grain storage. It is the location of the Camp Qi. It is where substances are turned, and where entry and exit occur"*.[7] This passage affirms the spleen's central role in the transformation not only of food into qi, but also of emotional and sensory experience into meaning. The Yi, as the spleen's associated spirit, helps orchestrate this inner refinement by determining what thoughts are absorbed, what is let go, and how the mind remains grounded in clarity.[8]

The Mind that Digests - Understanding the Yi

In the system of the Five Spirits, the Yi is associated with mental focus and cognitive intention. The Yi is responsible for our capacity to focus, study, contemplate, and integrate knowledge. It governs applied thought, how we direct our attention, hold intentions, process ideas, and transform experience into understanding. When balanced, it brings grounded cognition, clarity, and purpose to our mental efforts. It is the part of us that reflects, learns, and remembers with care and steadiness.[9]

The Yi also offers organization and integration. It helps us transform mental activity into practical steps, giving shape to our thoughts and anchoring the creative impulses of the spirit in concrete reality. Its function closely mirrors the spleen's physiological role in digestion: just as the spleen extracts the pure essence from food, the Yi extracts meaning and wisdom from experience.[10]

When the spleen is deficient, the Yi may become overburdened or scattered. This can manifest obsessive thinking, overstudying without retention, difficulty concentrating, and mental fatigue. People may feel overwhelmed by too much information or stuck in cycles of analysis without resolution. When the spleen is strong, however, the Yi functions as a gentle but steady compass. It can hold focus, drawing insight from experience, and moving forward with thoughtful intention. In this way, the Yi plays a crucial role in emotional digestion, helping the mind and spirit make sense of life's input, and offering the stability needed for growth and transformation.[11]

The Overthinking Body - Worry, Digestion, and the Disrupted Center

Worry and chronic stress are frequent emotional patterns observed in clinic. In recent years, rapid shifts across our social, economic, and environmental landscapes have contributed to a widespread sense of uncertainty. Many people live in a state of quiet urgency, rushing between obligations with minds clouded by persistent, low-level anxieties. Moments of stillness are rare. Breath becomes shallow, and the body forgets how to fully relax. Although worry may appear subtle, the effects build over time and leave a significant imprint on the body.

Classical Chinese medicine recognized this link centuries ago. The *Ling Shu*, in Chapter 8, explains that worry obstructs the smooth flow of qi, resulting in stagnation and internal blockage.[12] These ancient observations are echoed in modern physiology. The ANS, which regulates breath, heart rate, and muscle tone, often becomes dysregulated in states of chronic worry. Symptoms like chest tightness, shortness of breath, and tension in the shoulders reflect the body's difficulty returning to a calm, parasympathetic state. From both traditional and scientific perspectives, ongoing worry places the system in a prolonged state of strain that slowly diminishes vitality and resilience.

Worry primarily affects the lungs and spleen. It interrupts the natural movement of qi and weakens digestion. This can lead to symptoms like fatigue, bloating, loss of appetite, and a sense of heaviness in the body.[13] As we explored in Chapters 3 and 4, the ANS orchestrates digestion. When a person is caught in repetitive thoughts and chronic concern, the body moves out of rest and digest and into subtle defense.

Worry is considered the emotional counterpart of the spleen's mental energy. When that energy is excessive or taxed, the spleen cannot properly transform and transport not only food but also experience. The result is stagnation, both physical and emotional. Over time, this state of imbalance can interfere with vitality, clarity, and the body's ability to restore itself.[14]

Worry, Digestion, and the ANS

This is where Eastern and Western paradigms align. TCM has long recognized the digestive system as a central hub of vitality and wisdom. As stated at the beginning of this chapter, the spleen and stomach are considered the "root of postnatal qi" in TCM. They form the energetic foundation from which we draw vitality, clarity, and resilience throughout life.[15] Repeating this concept here highlights the vital role that healthy digestion and emotional regulation play not only in supporting daily function but also in promoting long-term health and graceful aging. Similarly, Western science has begun to explore the enteric nervous system, often referred to as the "second brain," which contains over 100 million neurons embedded in the gut wall. This system operates semi-independently and plays a major role in regulating digestive function, mood, and overall health.[16]

While Chapter 3 outlined the structure of the ANS, this section shifts focus to how emotional states affect digestion. In particular, it explores how worry disrupts gut function through the pathways of the ANS. Worry is more than a passing mental habit. It is a physiological signal that keeps the body alert, guarded, and mobilized. When worry becomes chronic, it gradually shifts the body out of parasympathetic regulation. This leads to a prolonged stress response, even when there is no immediate threat.

This shift has direct consequences for digestion. The parasympathetic branch of the ANS supports rest, repair, and nutrient absorption. It helps regulate gut motility, digestive enzyme secretion, and the rhythmic contractions that move food through the digestive tract. When worry takes hold, the sympathetic branch becomes more dominant. Blood is redirected away from the intestines and toward the muscles. Enzyme output decreases. The smooth, wave-like movements of digestion become irregular or halted. Even when food is present, the body may struggle to break it down and absorb its nourishment.

Modern medicine continues to confirm this link. Chronic worry is associated with reduced vagal tone, decreased HRV, and symptoms such as bloating, abdominal pain, and irregular bowel movements. These autonomic patterns are frequently observed in conditions like irritable bowel syndrome (IBS) and other functional gut disorders. At the same time, a growing number of studies show that acupuncture can help restore balance within the ANS. It can reduce sympathetic overactivity, support parasympathetic tone, and ease the physical symptoms that arise when emotional strain interferes with digestive function.

The following studies explore this connection in greater depth. Together, they illustrate how worry impacts the nervous system, how these effects ripple into the gut, and how acupuncture may provide a therapeutic bridge back to balance.

How Worry Alters the ANS

Worry is often thought of as a mental loop, yet its imprint reaches far beyond the mind. It alters breath, digestion, and the subtle rhythms of the nervous system. When worry becomes chronic, the body itself begins to carry the pattern, revealing how emotion and physiology are inseparable.

Modern research has started to map this connection, showing how persistent mental strain reshapes the body's inner regulation. Research has shown how chronic worry influences the ANS and disrupts the body's natural ability to regulate itself. Persistent, repetitive thought patterns create a state of internal tension that keeps the body alert, even in the absence of external threat.[17]

Findings reveal that individuals experiencing ongoing worry tend to have lower parasympathetic activity and reduced HRV compared to those who are calm or emotionally balanced. As explored in previous chapters, HRV is one of the most reliable indicators of autonomic balance and vagal tone, both of which support rest, digestion, emotional regulation, and resilience.

This pattern suggests that worry does not affect only the mind. It may play a role in reshaping the nervous system, keeping the body in a subtle state of defense. These physiological effects mirror the view in TCM that worry interrupts the smooth flow of qi, weakens the spleen, and interferes with the body's capacity to transform experience with ease.

Over time, this imbalance may appear as digestive discomfort, shallow breathing, fatigue, or emotional exhaustion. Whether described as qi stagnation or reduced vagal activity, the outcome is the same. Chronic worry drains the body's reserves and prevents it from returning to its natural rhythm of regulation and renewal.

The Impact of Worry on Gut Homeostasis

Worry does not live in the mind alone. It has ripple effects that extend throughout the body, particularly into the digestive system. While the nervous system serves as the bridge between thought and physiology, the gut itself reflects the subtle disturbances of emotional imbalance. Recent scientific findings are beginning to confirm what TCM has long observed. When worry becomes persistent, the digestive system becomes compromised.

Recent research has explored how psychological stress influences gut homeostasis, especially through the lens of cognitive and emotional patterns.[18] Stress acts like a repetitive mental loop that reshapes the internal landscape of the gut. It interferes with the delicate communication between the brain and digestive system, disrupting the balance of the microbiome. People experiencing chronic stress often show changes in gut motility, a decline in microbial diversity, and signs of low-grade intestinal inflammation. These effects are not random. They mirror shifts in ANS function.

Under normal conditions, the parasympathetic branch of the ANS supports digestion, microbial balance, and intestinal repair. However, when stress takes hold, the nervous system shifts. The sympathetic branch becomes more active. Blood flow is redirected, digestive secretions decrease, and the gut lining becomes more vulnerable to permeability and inflammation. Research has identified psychological stress (including emotions such as worry) as a factor that may cause vagal suppression, reduced mucosal immunity, and microbial imbalance. While 'worry' is not singled out in the review, these mechanisms apply to a range of stress-related states.

We can see this in observations in both biomedicine and Chinese medicine. Patients struggling with chronic stress and emotions, like worry, may start to experience irregular digestion. Common symptoms include bloating, abdominal discomfort, fatigue, and food sensitivities. Over time, the gut may lose its resilience.

Research has also examined that gut health cannot be restored through diet alone. Lasting digestive balance requires nervous system regulation. This is where interventions such as acupuncture become deeply relevant. As we will see throughout this book, calming sympathetic over activity and supporting parasympathetic function, acupuncture helps restore the gut's internal rhythm. It encourages better motility, improved enzyme secretion, and a more stable microbial environment. In doing so, it provides not only symptom relief, but a path to deeper regulation and resilience.

What is starting to be observed is the immense effects that chronic stress has on the body. The enteric nervous system does not simply react to what we eat. It responds to how we think and how we feel. Restoring balance, therefore, requires attention to both gut and mind. Through the integration of nervous system science and TCM, a more complete picture of digestive health begins to emerge.

Acupuncture and the Physiology of Worry

Worry weaves itself quietly into the fabric of daily life. Though subtle at first, it begins to tighten the threads of qi, constricting the flow of vitality. In biomedical terms, worry reflects the persistent activation of thought patterns that trigger autonomic imbalance. It engages the body's alert systems long after external threats have passed, creating chronic internal strain. Understanding how to relieve this tension at its root is essential for restoring nervous system regulation.

A 2021 systematic review and meta-analysis published in *Annals of General Psychiatry* examined the effectiveness of acupuncture in the treatment of anxiety disorders.[19] The analysis included 20 randomized controlled trials and over 1,700 participants. While the studies used the clinical framework of anxiety, many of the symptoms reported, racing thoughts, chest tightness, digestive disturbance, insomnia, and fatigue, are strongly linked to what Chinese medicine identifies as chronic worry.

The results were consistent. Acupuncture was found to significantly reduce anxiety symptoms across multiple measures, including both psychological and physiological indicators. Participants receiving acupuncture experienced greater reductions in anxiety scores than those in control groups, including those receiving standard pharmacological treatment or cognitive behavioral therapy alone. Importantly, the improvements were not only statistical. They were also described as clinically meaningful. Patients reported feeling calmer, more grounded, and less mentally overactive. Their symptoms of worry began to quiet.

From a physiological perspective, acupuncture's effectiveness is believed to stem in part from its ability to regulate autonomic function. The review highlighted mechanisms such as improved HRV, reduced sympathetic activation, and increased parasympathetic tone. These changes align with what is needed to interrupt the physical feedback loop of worry. By calming overactive neural circuits and supporting vagal recovery, acupuncture helps the body shift from vigilance into rest.

In TCM, the goal of treatment is not simply to stop the mind from worrying. It is to restore the center. When the spleen is nourished and the qi flows freely, thoughts become lighter, and digestion becomes stronger. The findings from this meta-analysis affirm that acupuncture offers a powerful tool for treating worry not just as an emotion, but as a full-body condition rooted in nervous system imbalance. By bringing balance to the body, the mind begins to settle.

Quieting Worry Through the Vagus Nerve

Worry is not always loud or dramatic. It often moves quietly beneath the surface, shaping how the body holds tension and how the mind loops through thought. In Chinese medicine, it is understood to constrict internal flow. In modern clinical terms, it frequently appears as generalized anxiety disorder. This pattern is marked by mental overactivity and low parasympathetic function. Treatments that improve vagal tone, such as acupuncture, help guide the body back toward balance and calm.

A 2024 case series, by Soledade Soleil Meira do Valle and Harry Hong, explored this connection through the lens of acupuncture.[20] They followed individuals diagnosed with generalized anxiety disorder who exhibited symptoms strongly linked to chronic worry, racing thoughts, shallow breathing, digestive discomfort, and tension in the chest. Acupuncture was applied using protocols designed to activate the vagus nerve and improve autonomic regulation.

The outcomes were significant. Participants showed increased HRV and improved heart rhythm coherence. These are measurable indicators of a shift from sympathetic dominance to parasympathetic recovery. Clinically, patients reported feeling more grounded, less mentally agitated, and better able to rest. These results support the growing body of evidence that acupuncture can directly influence vagal tone and restore physiological calm.

This case series offers a powerful confirmation of what Chinese medicine has long observed. Worry disrupts internal flow. It scatters the mind and stagnates the center. But with the right support, the body can return to coherence. Through gentle regulation of the nervous system, acupuncture helps restore the quiet rhythm beneath the noise.

When Worry Disrupts the Gut

In both TCM and modern neurogastroenterology, worry disturbs digestion. Persistent worry is thought to tax the spleen and lead to qi stagnation, which may lead to symptoms such as bloating, fatigue, poor appetite, and epigastric discomfort. In Western terms, worry dampens parasympathetic tone, interfering with healthy gut movement. Though the language differs, both systems describe the same phenomenon. Emotional strain interrupts the natural flow of digestion.

Experts have brought this connection into focus. Acupuncture has been shown to influence the ANS in cases of gastrointestinal dysmotility. Chronic worry can disrupt gut rhythm, slowing gastric emptying, altering intestinal contractions, and impairing secretory function. These patterns reveal how emotional imbalance can shape physical function and how regulating the nervous system through acupuncture may help restore the body's natural harmony. [21]

The parasympathetic nervous system is responsible for coordinating the subtle, wave-like movements that propel food through the digestive tract. When vagal activity is strong, digestion tends to be smooth and efficient. But worry activates sympathetic responses that override this natural rhythm. Blood flow is reduced to the gut. Enzymatic secretions decline. The digestive process becomes irregular or halted. This pattern closely mirrors what TCM refers to as spleen qi deficiency and damp stagnation

Acupuncture can restore autonomic balance through multiple mechanisms. Acupuncture stimulates vagal afferent pathways, modulates gastrointestinal reflexes, and improves the rhythmic contractions of the gut. Clinical results included measurable improvements in gut motility, symptom relief, and reduced autonomic arousal. These findings point to acupuncture as a meaningful therapy for worry-related digestive dysfunction. It does not simply mask symptoms. It works at the level of nervous system regulation to restore the body's internal harmony.

Worry is not just emotional. It is deeply physiological. It affects breath, thought, and digestion in ways that can be tracked, measured, and treated. Acupuncture offers a bridge between emotional recovery and physical relief, helping the body remember how to digest again, not only food, but experience.

Chronic Worry, Digestive Dysregulation, and the Loss of Safety

Polyvagal Theory offers a deeper understanding of how the ANS influences digestion. In addition to the sympathetic and parasympathetic branches, this model introduces the ventral vagal system, a pathway that supports feelings of safety, social connection, and emotional regulation. When the nervous system senses safety, digestion improves. Blood flows freely to the gut. Motility increases. Nutrient absorption is optimized. But when we feel isolated, threatened, or emotionally dysregulated, digestive function begins to decline. Stress signals divert energy away from nourishment and toward defense. The ability to digest food is closely tied to our ability to digest experience. In this context, nervous system regulation becomes essential to both emotional health and physical resilience.[22]

Building on this understanding, clinical findings indicate that traumatic stress affects gastrointestinal function and chronic pain.[23] Long-term exposure to threat reduces vagal tone, measured by lowered respiratory sinus arrhythmia. This indicates a disruption in ventral vagal activity, the branch of the nervous system responsible for physiological safety, rest, and internal regulation. When this system is weakened, digestive function declines. Peristalsis becomes erratic. Inflammatory responses increase. Even in the absence of physical disease, symptoms emerge that reflect a nervous system struggling to find its balance.

Although these patterns are often studied in trauma, the same mechanisms apply to chronic worry. Worry acts as a quiet but continuous signal of threat. It activates the body's protective systems and prevents full engagement with rest and nourishment. Over time, this state of guardedness can impair digestion, leading to symptoms such as bloating, constipation, and abdominal pain. These disruptions often reflect autonomic imbalance rather than structural damage.

TCM describes a similar pattern through the lens of the spleen. When the spleen becomes weakened by overthinking or emotional strain, digestion falters. qi stagnates. The body becomes heavy, the mind cloudy, and food difficult to process. In both systems, chronic emotional activation disrupts the ability to metabolize not just nutrients but life itself.[24]

Recovery begins with restoring a sense of internal safety. As you will see throughout this book, several interventions can support ventral vagal tone. Practices such as acupuncture, breathwork, and safe human connection play a key role in helping the body re-establish autonomic balance. As the body shifts out of defense, digestion often begins to restore itself. The process of receiving, transforming, and letting go becomes possible again, both physically and emotionally.

Pensiveness and the Weight of Unfinished Thought

When the nervous system becomes tense and overwhelmed, the body's ability to digest, both physically and mentally, begins to falter. As stated earlier, the spleen governs transformation. It turns nourishment into usable energy and thought into clarity. But under emotional strain, this capacity is weakened. A tight, overactive nervous system often creates tension in the epigastric region, just below the ribs. This inner constriction mirrors the difficulty we may have in absorbing food, ideas, or emotional experience. Thoughts feel fragmented or incomplete, like information we cannot quite process. On a physical level, this may show up as bloating, abdominal discomfort, fatigue after eating, or cravings for sugar and stimulation. On a mental and emotional level, it often manifests as repetitive thinking, poor concentration, and a sense of being mentally stuck. Worry, confusion, and unresolved emotion circulate without resolution. The body feels heavy, the mind noisy, and digestion of both life and nourishment becomes incomplete.

In this state, a more subtle emotion may begin to take root. Pensiveness is closely related to worry, but it carries a distinct tone. It is marked by brooding, obsessive reflection, and ongoing preoccupation with past events or people. Individuals may disconnect from the present moment, caught in loops of memory, regret, or longing. Over time, this inward fixation can lead to compulsive thinking patterns that are difficult to interrupt. In Chinese medicine, pensiveness is known to injure the spleen. Pensiveness can cause epigastric pain, poor digestion, and fatigue.[25] Ruminating while eating is especially damaging, as it prevents the spleen from fully transforming food into qi.[26] When we eat while mentally preoccupied, the body cannot fully absorb nourishment. Digestion slows, and the benefits of food are diminished.

The *Su Wen*, Chapter 39, offers further insight. It states, *"When one is pensive, the qi lumps together"*.[27] Thought becomes heavy, and qi no longer flows with ease. The body, like the mind, holds on to what it cannot process. Pensiveness is not just a mental tendency. It is a physiological pattern that affects clarity, vitality, and the rhythm of digestion. Healing begins by calming the nervous system, quieting the mind, and restoring the spleen's ability to transform. When thought becomes steady and rhythm is re-established, the body regains its capacity to digest not only food, but the deeper layers of life itself.

Pensiveness, Motility, and the Disruption of Digestive Harmony

In Chinese medicine, pensiveness is not merely emotional. It is a state that affects the entire body. When a person becomes consumed with unresolved thoughts, the mind begins to loop. Reflection turns into rumination. Memory becomes fixation. This mental repetition places a burden on the spleen and weakens the body's ability to process nourishment and experience. From a physiological standpoint, this state of mental preoccupation can also disrupt the rhythm of the gut.

Science now recognizes that psychological stress can directly affect intestinal motility and gut hormone function.[28] Prolonged emotional strain alters the movement of the small intestine and disrupted the balance of key regulatory substances in the body. Specifically, subjects exposed to persistent stress showed a significant reduction in small intestinal peristalsis, the natural wave-like contractions that propel food through the digestive tract. Alongside this change in motility, levels of cholecystokinin (CCK) and vasoactive intestinal polypeptide (VIP), two important hormones involved in digestion, were also altered in both plasma and intestinal tissue.

These physiological changes closely mirror the classical classical Chinese medicine understanding of the spleen's role. Pensiveness slows the natural flow of qi. It interferes with the body's ability to transform food and absorb its essence. In clinical terms, this may present as sluggish digestion, abdominal tension, bloating, and fatigue after meals. But beneath the symptoms lies a deeper pattern. The spleen becomes overburdened not only by food that is hard to digest, but by thoughts and memories that remain unprocessed. The mind holds on. The gut slows down.

Viewed through this lens, the emotional weight of pensiveness can be understood in physiological terms. Mental overstimulation, worry, and brooding disrupt the hormonal rhythms that support gut function. They weaken peristalsis and create stagnation both energetically and physically. The spleen, which thrives on clarity and consistency, becomes confused. Its ability to nourish the body and mind begins to wane.

To restore digestive harmony, treating pensiveness not only as an emotional state, but as a disruption in rhythm and flow, can help bring balance. Practices that calm the nervous system, quiet the mind, and release the grip of circular thinking are essential. Through this understanding, acupuncture, breath-based practices, and intentional eating become not just supportive, but necessary for restoring the spleen's capacity to transform. When thoughts soften and inner movement returns, the gut responds. Digestion becomes smoother, and with it, the ability to absorb both nutrients and life itself.

Pensiveness, Rumination, and the Gut-Brain Disturbance

While stress is often understood in physical or emotional terms, its lingering cognitive patterns, such as pensiveness and rumination, can significantly disturb digestive function. These mental states, marked by repeated internal loops of thought, unresolved concerns, and over-analysis of past events, place a continuous load on the ANS and the gut-brain axis. In both TCM and modern neurogastroenterology, such patterns are recognized not as harmless overthinking, but as physiological disruptors that alter gut function at the cellular and systemic level.

Research continues to reveal how psychological stress contributes to bowel dysfunction. Prolonged mental and emotional strain alters gut motility, disrupts mucosal immunity, and reshapes the microbiome. These disruptions are not limited to moments of acute stress. They often result from sustained internalized thought patterns, such as chronic worry or pensiveness. When the body remains caught in this state, it continues to respond as if under threat long after the original trigger has passed.[29]

Many individuals with digestive imbalance report high levels of mental preoccupation. Thoughts loop endlessly. The mind processes and reprocesses without rest. In modern physiology, this may appear as dysregulation of the hypothalamic-pituitary-adrenal axis or reduced vagal tone. In TCM, it reflects a pattern of pensiveness that burdens the spleen and slows digestion. Although described in different terms, both perspectives point to the same truth: the digestive system becomes overworked and under-supported when the mind cannot release.

Pensiveness and rumination, in TCM, are not just patterns of thought. They become embodied states. The mind loops and the gut tightens. The spleen struggles to transform both food and experience. Over time, chronic internal tension weakens digestion, disrupts the microbiome, and leads to symptoms such as bloating, irregular bowel movements, and sensitivity to food. Healing begins when we interrupt the cycle, when the mind becomes quieter and the nervous system remembers how to rest.

This growing convergence between ancient and modern medicine reminds us that digestive healing involves more than diet alone. Thought itself must be tended to. Whether through acupuncture, mindfulness, breath practices, or daily rhythms that restore calm, balance returns when we quiet the overactive mind and allow both body and spirit to find their natural flow again.

Calming the Overthinking Mind - Acupuncture, Obsessive Thought, and Pensiveness

In both Chinese Medicine and modern neuropsychiatry, obsessive thinking is understood not simply as a mental quirk, but as a physiological pattern that disrupts the body's rhythm. When the mind loops uncontrollably, caught in persistent thoughts, compulsions, or repetitive anxieties, there is often an underlying imbalance in the nervous system and a deeper emotional disconnection from the body. In TCM, this mental agitation is recognized as a form of *pensiveness* that injures the spleen and scatters the Yi, the spirit of intellect. The result is mental fatigue, emotional stagnation, and disrupted digestion. Over time, the system becomes depleted, ungrounded, and unable to transform either nourishment or thought.

Recent research has begun to explore the combined effects of acupuncture, moxibustion, and conventional medicine in treating obsessive-compulsive disorder and related emotional conditions. This growing body of work focuses on how these therapies influence obsessive thought patterns, anxiety, and nervous system regulation.[30]

The design of these studies reflects an increasing awareness of the limitations of medication alone, particularly for conditions rooted in both mind and body. While pharmacological treatments may ease symptoms temporarily, they often fail to reach the deeper energetic and physiological imbalances that sustain obsessive looping. Acupuncture and moxibustion are known to calm the Shen, regulate the flow of qi, and nourish both the spleen and heart systems. Together, these approaches help release tension stored in the body, ground overactive mental energy, and restore emotional steadiness.

What makes this emerging research especially relevant is its integrative perspective. Rather than viewing Eastern and Western medicine as separate, it seeks to understand how they can complement one another. Acupuncture and moxibustion may enhance the effectiveness of conventional treatments while reducing side effects. By modulating autonomic tone, easing sympathetic overactivity, and supporting parasympathetic recovery, they help rebuild the internal sense of safety that obsessive thought patterns often erode.

This integrative approach marks a shift in how emotional health is understood. Obsessive-compulsive tendencies and chronic pensiveness are not simply mental conditions. They are embodied, neurobiological, and energetic patterns that require holistic care. For those caught in cycles of overthinking or emotional fixation, unable to rest or digest experience fully, acupuncture offers not just relief but regulation. It communicates with the nervous system in the language of rhythm, stillness, and coherence.

As we consider the role of the spleen, the Yi, and the overactive mind, this research invites a new understanding of healing. It reminds us that recovery does not come from stopping thought, but from restoring flow. When qi moves freely and the nervous system feels safe, the mind softens its grasp. In that softening, transformation begins.

Transcending the Loop - Acupoint Stimulation and the Overactive Mind

Obsessive thought patterns are often misunderstood as purely psychological disturbances. Yet TCM has long recognized that obsessive thinking and pensiveness disturb not only the mind, but also the body. These mental loops knot the qi of the spleen, impair digestion, and scatter the spirit of intention, known as the Yi. When thoughts spiral endlessly, clarity dissolves, and the body begins to echo this inner fragmentation. The nervous system becomes tense. The digestive tract slows. Emotional energy becomes stuck in place.

A 2016 randomized controlled trial by Bin Feng and fellow clinicians, published in the *Journal of Psychiatric Research* examined the effects of transcutaneous electrical acupoint stimulation (TEAS) as an adjunct treatment for obsessive-compulsive disorder (OCD).[31] TEAS is a non-invasive form of acupuncture that uses electrical impulses applied to traditional acupoints through surface electrodes. This technique merges ancient meridian theory with modern neurostimulation, offering an innovative way to calm the nervous system without needles.

Participants diagnosed with OCD were randomly assigned to either a standard pharmacological treatment group or a group receiving both standard care and adjunct TEAS therapy. Over the course of treatment, those who received TEAS showed significantly greater improvements in obsessive-compulsive symptoms, anxiety scores, and overall clinical functioning.

One of the most insightful findings was that TEAS appeared to modulate

ANS activity. Participants demonstrated enhanced vagal tone, greater parasympathetic regulation, and improved HRV. These are key physiological indicators of nervous system balance, and they mirror the classical TCM goals of calming the Shen and regulating qi flow.

From a TCM perspective, this makes intuitive sense. Acupoint stimulation at sites such as Neiguan (PC6), Shenmen (HT7), and Sanyinjiao (SP6) targets the heart, spleen, and kidney systems, organs deeply connected to emotional processing and thought regulation. When these points are activated, the body is guided out of mental entanglement and toward coherence. The nervous system softens. The breath slows. The obsessive loop begins to unwind.

These findings offer more than data. It offers hope for those caught in cycles of overthinking, worry, and mental restlessness. It validates that obsessive thinking is not just a mental issue. It is an embodied state, and one that responds beautifully to therapies that restore rhythm to the nervous system and flow to the mind.

Longevity and Digestive Resilience

Longevity is not simply a matter of adding years to life. It is about cultivating vitality, clarity, and connection throughout those years. A key pillar of this quality of life is the ability to nourish and regulate the digestive system.

The health of the gut is foundational to both physical and emotional well-being. When the spleen and stomach are functioning optimally, qi and blood are produced in abundance. This supports the nourishment and renewal of all organ systems. A strong digestive system ensures that the body is well-supplied with energy and has the resources needed for tissue repair, immune regulation, and mental clarity.

When digestive function is impaired, however, a cascade of imbalances can follow. Contemporary studies show that compromised gut health is linked to systemic inflammation, chronic fatigue, metabolic dysfunction, and accelerated aging. Disruptions in the gut microbiota have been associated with neurodegenerative diseases and reduced immune function, highlighting the importance of maintaining digestive resilience across the lifespan.³²

When the Mind Won't Rest - Aging, the ANS, and the Spleen

Worry often hides in plain sight. It can seem quiet, internal, even reasonable. Yet beneath the surface, worry creates ripples across the body's systems. Modern science is now beginning to confirm what TCM has observed for centuries. Persistent mental strain, especially when rooted in rumination and pensiveness, disrupts internal rhythms and accelerates the aging process from within.

A recent study (2023) explored this connection by following more than 400 individuals between the ages of 19 and 50.³³ Blood samples were used to measure biological age through epigenetic clocks, while psychological assessments captured each participant's level of chronic stress and emotional resilience. Even when adjusting for factors like income, smoking, and body weight, the data revealed a clear pattern. Those with elevated levels of psychological stress showed signs of accelerated biological aging, including changes in insulin sensitivity and cellular markers of wear.

This insight echoes the principles of Chinese medicine. The spleen, known as the organ of thought and digestion, is said to become weakened by excessive mental activity. When thoughts loop without resolution, they tie up qi, slowing the body's ability to process both nourishment and experience. Over time, this can manifest as fatigue after meals, sugar cravings, abdominal discomfort, and a foggy or restless mind.

Yet not everyone in the study was equally affected. Individuals who demonstrated strong emotional regulation and self-control appeared more resistant to the aging effects of stress. From a TCM perspective, they had internal systems that were more resilient. Their qi likely flowed with greater ease, their spleen energy more stable, their nervous system better able to return to balance after disruption.

This supports a growing understanding that emotional health is not separate from physical health. The nervous system, the digestive system, and the mind are deeply intertwined. Practices that nourish regulation, like acupuncture, breathwork, and moments of embodied stillness, can create measurable shifts across these domains. They reduce physiological stress responses, improve digestion, and help quiet the mental noise that depletes energy over time.

In the pursuit of longevity, this connection cannot be ignored. To age well is to live in rhythm. It is to tend to the invisible forces that guide digestion, immunity, clarity, and restoration. When we address worry at its roots, when we bring calm to the mind and coherence to the nervous system, we do more than feel better in the moment. We activate the body's natural intelligence for preservation. We nourish the spleen. We slow the inner clock. And we return to the wisdom of both ancient and modern medicine, where true longevity begins with regulation.

From Ruminating to Radiating - A Path to Longevity

How we hold our thoughts shapes how we hold our years. Hope, trust, and a quiet expectation of goodness lighten the load the body must carry. Fear and rumination, by contrast, press heavily on both mind and physiology. Modern medicine is beginning to confirm what wisdom traditions have long suggested. The way we meet life inwardly has the power to influence how long and how well we live. Research published in *Proceedings of the National Academy of Sciences* (2019) examined two large epidemiologic cohorts, one of women and one of men, over several decades.[34] The researchers discovered a profound pattern. Individuals who scored higher in optimism, defined as a general expectation that good things will happen, were significantly more likely to live to age 85 or older. This correlation held even after adjusting for health behaviors, chronic illnesses, and socioeconomic status. Optimism appeared to be an independent predictor of exceptional longevity.

The implications of this study speak to more than just personality traits. Optimism tends to be accompanied by lower levels of chronic worry and reduced rumination. It is a mindset characterized by psychological flexibility, trust in the future, and the ability to reframe challenges without becoming trapped in repetitive or self-defeating thought loops.

From the perspective of TCM, this is more than a cognitive state. Worry and pensiveness are seen as emotional patterns that directly weaken the spleen, the organ responsible for digestion, clarity, and transformation. When the spleen is overburdened by repetitive thought or excessive rumination, qi becomes stagnant. Digestion falters. The mind feels heavy and the body fatigued. Over time, this contributes to systemic depletion and internal imbalance.

Chronic worry activates the sympathetic nervous system and suppresses vagal tone, disrupting sleep, immunity, and digestion. By contrast, optimism has been linked to healthier nervous system regulation, lower inflammation, and better metabolic outcomes.

In this light, optimism is not simply a personality quirk. It is a physiological ally. Cultivating a hopeful orientation toward life, training the mind to dwell less on fear and more on possibility, may help preserve the body's internal rhythm. It protects the spleen, stabilizes the ANS, and supports the deep biological harmony needed for healthy aging. Longevity, then, is not only a matter of diet or genetics. It is also shaped by how lightly or heavily we carry our thoughts.

Nourishing the Center - The Gut Microbiome as a Key to Healthy Aging

At the core of life is the act of digestion, the way we transform what is taken in and turn it into energy, clarity, and strength. Ancient teachings place the spleen and stomach at the center of this process, while modern science now turns to the gut microbiome. Both perspectives point to the same truth. The health of this inner terrain shapes not only how we feel today, but also how we age across a lifetime.

Recent insights in microbiome science offers a substantial look at how gut health shapes the process of aging.[35] The findings reveal that aging is not simply the accumulation of years but the gradual decline of resilience across multiple systems including immune, metabolic, cognitive, and emotional. One of the key factors influencing this decline is the composition of the gut microbiota. This vast ecosystem of microbes affects nearly every aspect of physiology, from energy production and inflammation regulation to hormone balance and mental clarity. In older adults, a loss of microbial diversity is consistently linked to frailty, chronic inflammation, and metabolic dysfunction. Yet the opposite is also true. A balanced and diverse microbiome can buffer the effects of aging, strengthen the immune system, and enhance quality of life.

In TCM, the spleen and stomach are regarded as the body's center of transformation. They digest not only food but also thoughts, emotions, and experience. This inner alchemy mirrors what modern science reveals about the microbiome's influence on both mental and physical vitality. When the digestive center is strong, the body feels nourished and the mind remains clear. When it weakens, energy wanes, emotions stagnate, and the spirit feels heavy. Modern findings on the microbiome reflect this ancient truth that balance within the gut is expressed as strength, clarity, and emotional steadiness throughout life.

Central to this connection are short-chain fatty acids, beneficial compounds produced by gut microbes during the fermentation of dietary fiber. These metabolites reduce inflammation, maintain gut barrier integrity, and modulate immune responses. Each of these functions supports longevity. When their production declines, the body's ability to regulate inflammation and sustain vitality diminishes. From a TCM perspective, this could be understood as a depletion of spleen qi and yin, resulting in poor nourishment and internal heat.

Dietary diversity and whole, plant-based foods are essential for cultivating a resilient microbiome. Just as TCM emphasizes eating with the seasons to harmonize the spleen and stomach, modern research supports a diet rooted in natural variety. Processed foods high in fat and sugar disrupt this balance. They reduce microbial diversity and foster chronic low-grade inflammation. Over time, these patterns weaken the foundation of vitality and accelerate aging.

Research also highlights the deep relationship between the gut and brain. The microbiome communicates through neurotransmitters and immune-modulating compounds that influence mood, cognition, and emotional stability. In TCM, this aligns with the belief that the spleen governs thought and that digestive health directly shapes mental clarity and emotional harmony.

Looking ahead, scientists envision future approaches to longevity that include targeted modulation of the microbiome through prebiotics, probiotics, fermented foods, and individualized nutrition. Yet the essence of this insight remains timeless. How we nourish our center determines how we age. Whether viewed through the lens of microbiota or the movement of qi, true longevity arises from harmony within.

Alchemy of Clarity - Transforming Thought, Food, and Longevity

The spleen is regarded as the center of transformation. It turns food into postnatal qi, the vital energy that sustains life after birth. But its role extends far beyond digestion. The spleen is also responsible for processing thought and intention. It is the internal alchemist that helps us absorb not just nutrients, but experience. When the mind becomes caught in worry or pensiveness, this alchemy breaks down. Thoughts begin to loop. Ideas become stuck and heavy. The digestive system reflects this internal state. Bloating, fatigue after eating, sugar cravings, and a tight, uncomfortable sensation in the gut are common signals that the spleen is overburdened.

From a physiological perspective, worry and pensiveness activate stress pathways within the ANS. This pulls the body away from parasympathetic regulation, where rest, digestion, and repair occur. As vagal tone diminishes, digestive motility slows, enzymatic secretion decreases, and nutrient absorption becomes compromised. Over time, these disruptions accumulate. They can weaken immunity, increase systemic inflammation, and impair metabolic function. The link between chronic emotional strain, impaired digestion, and diminished vitality is now supported by a growing body of research across disciplines.

Acupuncture offers a therapeutic pathway to restore this balance. By targeting specific points that influence vagal tone, gut motility, and mental calm, acupuncture helps regulate the nervous system and revitalize spleen function. It settles the overactive mind, releases the knots of pensiveness, and reawakens the body's ability to transform food and thought into energy. When the spleen is supported, digestion becomes smoother, clarity returns, and emotional weight begins to lift.

This restoration is not just about feeling better in the moment. It is a foundation for longevity. In both ancient and modern systems of medicine, vitality is not measured only by the absence of disease, but by the capacity to adapt, recover, and renew. The health of the digestive system, particularly the gut-brain axis, plays a central role in this capacity. By supporting the spleen through acupuncture, nourishment, and emotional regulation, we protect the very systems that preserve vitality across the decades. We do more than calm worry. We strengthen the body's blueprint for resilience and longevity.

Rooted in Rhythm - The Spleen, Spirit, and the Secret of Longevity

In TCM, the spleen and stomach are known as the central axis of postnatal life. They are the great alchemists of the body, transforming food, breath, and rest into the usable qi that sustains us each day. While our prenatal essence, called *jing*, offers the foundation of our vitality, it is postnatal qi that we must actively cultivate to support health, clarity, and aging with grace. This qi is not only produced through digestion, but also through the way we move through life itself. Through how we rest, how we think, and how we care for the rhythm of our days.

The modern world often pulls us away from this center. We eat too quickly. We think too much. We work without pause. Cold, raw foods chill the spleen's digestive fire. Chronic worry and rumination knot the qi, leading to stagnation that is both physical and emotional. The classics are clear. *Su Wen* Chapter 39 states, "When one is pensive, the qi lumps together."[36] We feel this as bloating after meals, sugar cravings, difficulty focusing, and the sensation of being mentally stuck. The nervous system, under strain, mirrors this disruption. When the body cannot rest, the mind struggles to rest as well. When thought loops endlessly, digestion falters. Food remains undigested. So do emotions, memories, and meaning.

The medicine lies in rhythm and return. Warm, cooked meals taken with presence. Breathing with awareness. Creating small spaces of calm between actions. When we honor the spleen's needs, the transformation process resumes. Thoughts begin to settle. The nervous system shifts from vigilance to rest. Energy becomes available once again. Not just to survive, but to heal.

Longevity, in this understanding, is not merely the passage of time. It is the cultivation of harmony. It is the quiet strength of a well-regulated nervous system. It is the nourishment of thoughts that support rather than scatter. It is the steadiness of a center that remembers how to pause, breathe, and transform. To age with vitality is not about resisting change. It is about partnering with it. In every warm meal offered with care, in every breath taken with intention, we return to this harmony. And in that return, we preserve life.

Practices for Nourishing the Spleen and Yi

You don't need to do more to nourish your spleen. You need to do less, with greater presence and steadiness. The spleen thrives in simplicity, rhythm, and gentle consistency. The Yi, the spirit of thought and intention, is nourished not through constant stimulation but through moments of quiet reflection. It settles best when the mind is calm, the body is grounded, and life is approached with mindful clarity.

Here are grounded rituals to restore their balance:

1. Eat Warm, Simple, Regular Meals

The spleen prefers warmth: soups, porridges, steamed vegetables, lightly spiced grains.

Avoid cold, raw, or overly complex meals, which weaken digestion over time.

Eat at the same times daily when possible to build internal rhythm.

2. Honor the Transitions

The Earth element governs the "in-between" times: late summer, the pause between seasons, the moment between inhale and exhale.

Create rituals for transitions: a cup of tea after work, a walk after meals, a breath before speaking.

3. Tend to Your Mental Diet

Limit multitasking and information overload.

Replace worry loops with grounding thoughts or affirmations like:

"I am safe to take one step at a time."

"I nourish my mind with calm."

4. Move Gently and Daily

The spleen loves movement that's rhythmic and intentional: walking, gentle yoga, qigong.

Movement helps "transform and transport" both food and emotion.

5. Breathe Into the Belly

Diaphragmatic breathing stimulates the vagus nerve and calms the nervous system.

Try this daily ritual:

Inhale through your nose filling the belly.

Exhale through your mouth releasing any worry or overthinking.

Try this once before meals or during moments of overthinking.

6. Reflect to Digest Emotion

The spleen digests thought the way the stomach digests food. Journaling can help clarify and release what weighs on the mind.

Try this prompt:

"What am I still trying to digest - emotionally, mentally, or spiritually?

To digest life is to live deeply. To nourish the spleen is to return to center.

16

The Wellspring Within - The Kidneys, Zhi, and the Blueprint for Longevity

In TCM, the kidneys are far more than anatomical filters of fluid and waste. They are considered the *"Root of Life."* They store jing, our inherited essence, and serve as the wellspring of both yin and yang in the body. This jing is foundational. It governs growth, development, fertility, regeneration, and aging. In this way, the kidneys are not only tied to survival but to vitality itself.[1]

When kidney jing is full, the body is resilient, the spirit is steady, and the will is strong. We possess the energy to grow, to heal, and to endure. Kidney yin stores the inherited essence, often described as the "Water of Life."

This essence nourishes the tissues and supports the development of the nervous system. It gives rise to marrow, which in TCM includes bone marrow, the brain, and the spinal cord. As this marrow fills the brain, it anchors memory, supports cognition, and fosters emotional resilience.[2] The connection between jing and the nervous system reveals a deeper truth. Our ability to think clearly, feel steady, and stay present in the body relies on the health of this original essence.

Pre-heaven essence is described as the jing formed at conception through the union of parental energies. This essence determines constitutional strength, vitality, and longevity. It is stored in the kidneys and linked to the Ming Men, or Gate of Life, located between the two kidneys. This area is home to a deep physiological fire that fuels all metabolic processes. It gives rise to kidney yang, which initiates growth and inspires purpose. The Ming Men not only sustains life, but also powers the spirit of will itself.[3]

This ancient view resonates with what we now understand about the adrenal glands, which sit just above the kidneys. These glands regulate hormones, manage stress, and support energy balance. Hammer relates kidney jing to adrenal and endocrine function, describing it as stored energy that supports sympathetic and parasympathetic balance. When this essence is full, the nervous system remains adaptive. Brain function is supported, hormonal rhythms stay steady, and the spirit is able to rest.[4]

The *Huang Di Nei Jing Ling Shu* supports this integration of physical and spiritual health. It states, *"Having entered, it communicates with the Kidneys. It opens an orifice in the two Yin. It stores the essence in the Kidneys".*[5] Essence does not only create marrow and brain tissue. It opens pathways of perception, clarity, and consciousness.

But the kidneys do more than store essence. They also house the Zhi, the spirit of will. The *Suwen* affirms, *"The Kidneys store the will".*[6] Zhi animates endurance and the ability to stay the course. It empowers us to carry out our life's direction and stay true to it, even in the face of fear or fatigue. Zhi governs long-term memory, perseverance, and the internal strength to complete what we begin.[7]

Kidney yang gives rise to this intelligent will. It gives us the ability to act with clarity and purpose, to express one's intentions in the world. When kidney yang is strong, Zhi becomes a deep and steady flame. The person has the ability to face the unknown and walk with courage, regardless of uncertainty.[8]

Fear, however, is the emotion that most directly harms the kidneys. The *Suwen* warns, *"Among the depots it is the Kidneys... Among the states of mind it is fear... If fear causes harm, it harms the Kidneys".*[9] Chronic fear, especially when unacknowledged, depletes essence and disrupts the Zhi. It scatters the spirit, weakens resolve, and leaves the nervous system unmoored. This breakdown of will can be linked to emotional patterns such as phobias, low self-worth, and an inability to face the future. When the Zhi is weakened, fear replaces confidence. Memory falters. The capacity to focus or trust one's inner guidance begins to fade.[10]

The *Suwen* deepens our understanding of fear and its impact on the spirit. *"To be scared in one's ponderings and considerations, this will harm the spirit. When the spirit is harmed, then fears will flow excessively without end".*[11] Fear does more than interrupt our sense of safety. It clouds perception. It weakens decision-making. It scatters the mind and injures the spirit at its core. When fear takes root in the body, it begins to deplete the kidney essence and fragment the Zhi. This results in a profound loss of clarity and direction. The person may feel as if their inner compass has been broken or their will has become unreachable.

In TCM, unresolved fear can give rise to chronic anxiety, obsessive thought patterns, and phobias that feel overwhelming or irrational. When the Zhi becomes depleted through trauma, exhaustion, or long-term imbalance, even small challenges may provoke a sense of dread. The capacity to recover, take initiative, or move forward with confidence begins to weaken. Such disruptions of will often appear as deep hesitation, avoidance, and a diminishing ability to trust in oneself or in the direction of life.[12]

The Zhi as a vital inner force that fuels our ability to pursue life with purpose. When this will is strong, it acts as a steady fire that guides action and direction. When it weakens, the spirit retreats. Without this internal fire, fear begins to dominate. A person may experience growing anxiety, dread, or hesitation in the face of the unknown. As the Zhi diminishes, their ability to see clearly and move forward becomes clouded. The connection to one's life path, once vibrant and intuitive, begins to fade.[13]

The Spirit of Zhi is not simply about pushing through. It is the quiet strength that lives deep inside. It is what allows us to stay in alignment with our truth, even when life becomes difficult. When the kidneys are nourished, and the essence is replenished, the Zhi can return to its steady rhythm. The nervous system finds balance. The breath deepens. The inner compass becomes clear again. It is the harmony of kidney yin and yang that creates the foundation for both stillness and strength. Jing is the root. Zhi is the spark. Together, they support a life of clarity, courage, and conscious direction. In moments of trauma, fatigue, or uncertainty, when the will seems scattered or lost, it is often a call to return to the kidneys. To nourish them is to reconnect to the source. By restoring jing and supporting the Zhi, we remember what it means to walk forward in trust, not fear.

Zhi and the Nervous System - The Interface of Will and Regulation

Contemporary science offers powerful confirmation of what Chinese medicine has long described through the concepts of *jing* and *Zhi*. In neuropsychological terms, the spirit of will, known in classical texts as *Zhi*, shares many functions with the prefrontal cortex, the limbic system, and the hypothalamic-pituitary-adrenal (HPA) axis. Research has shown that regions of the prefrontal cortex help regulate memory, emotion, motivation, and the ability to adapt to stress. These regions shape how we engage with life, respond to challenges, and find meaning in our experiences.[14]

Further evidence indicates that the prefrontal cortex also supports conscious decision-making and long-term planning.[15] The limbic system connects memory with emotional significance, while the HPA axis manages hormonal responses, including the release of cortisol during times of stress or danger. When these systems become dysregulated, such as during prolonged stress or trauma, motivation weakens, focus diminishes, and self-regulation breaks down. In Chinese medicine, this pattern is seen as a weakening of the *Zhi*. The person may feel exhausted, forgetful, emotionally distant, or unsure of their path forward.

This is not merely a metaphor. It is physiological. In classical thought, the kidneys generate marrow, which nourishes the brain and spinal cord. From a developmental perspective, the early formation of the brain and nervous system depends on inherited constitutional strength. In TCM, this is known as pre-heaven essence, the *jing* received at conception that shapes not only physical structure but also the body's capacity for stress regulation and emotional balance.[16] Modern science now recognizes this same idea through genetics and prenatal programming. *Jing* influences the strength and adaptability of the nervous system, including the tone of the vagus nerve.

The *Suwen*, Chapter 8, offers a timeless insight that echoes this understanding: "The Kidneys are the official functioning as operator with force. Technical skills and expertise originate from them."[17] The kidneys are not passive organs. They are initiators of action. They hold the ability to respond with purpose and precision. This aligns with what we now know about the prefrontal cortex and the HPA axis. These systems help us regulate our actions, manage pressure, and carry out skilled responses. When that inner force is compromised, the will falters, and a person may begin to doubt their ability to act at all.

As reviewed in previous chapters, the ANS plays a central role in regulating how we respond to life. At the heart of this system is the vagus nerve, which governs many of the body's restorative functions. It supports sleep, digestion, immune health, and emotional balance. The tone of the vagus nerve reflects our inner resilience. It reveals whether the body feels safe enough to rest, heal, and connect.

When kidney essence is strong, the nervous system adapts with ease. Breath slows, the heart rate stabilizes, and mental clarity returns. But when essence becomes depleted, vagal tone weakens. The body shifts into survival mode, cycling between states of agitation, collapse, or freeze. This physiological pattern mirrors what Chinese medicine identifies as Zhi deficiency, characterized by diminished will, clarity, and centered direction.

Research has highlighted the plasticity and vulnerability of the prefrontal cortex across the lifespan. This region, which is central to working memory, self-regulation, and goal-directed behavior, is profoundly shaped by stress and life experience.[18] Prolonged or early-life stress can alter the structure and function of the prefrontal cortex, disrupting its ability to manage cognition, emotion, and autonomic responses. These disruptions are not always permanent. When stress is reduced, especially in younger individuals, the brain often shows remarkable capacity for recovery.

However, with age, the prefrontal cortex becomes less resilient. The effects of chronic stress deepen, and healing takes longer.

Emerging research continues to confirm what TCM has long described through the lens of *jing* and *Zhi*. The prefrontal cortex and the hypothalamic-pituitary-adrenal (HPA) axis govern motivation, memory, and hormonal regulation. Under prolonged strain, both systems become impaired. The ability to focus, plan, and respond flexibly weakens, reflecting the ancient view of a draining of kidney essence and the withdrawal of the *Zhi*. The will becomes fragile. A person may feel unanchored, unable to move forward, and disconnected from inner purpose. Yet, just as the kidneys store the *jing* and animate the *Zhi*, the brain holds the potential for resilience. With nourishment, rest, and care, restoration is possible, even after depletion.

This loss of inner guidance was described thousands of years ago. In the *Suwen* it is written, "These are the so-called 'five diseases'... When it collects in the Kidneys, fear results."[19] Fear, in this context, is not only an emotion but also a state of energetic and physiological disarray. It signals that the foundation has been weakened and the will has retreated.

By viewing the kidneys through both classical and modern perspectives, a deeper truth emerges. *Jing* is not just a poetic image. It is a reflection of real constitutional vitality. *Zhi* is not just a spiritual idea. It is the coordinated function of the nervous system, the will to act, and the strength behind every meaningful decision. When the kidneys are nourished, spirit and physiology begin to align. The mind clears, the breath finds rhythm, and the will returns.

Modern Science and the Spirit of Will

A growing body of evidence shows what TCM has long understood through the language of jing and Zhi. The kidneys are not isolated filtration organs. They are deeply embedded in the body's regulatory networks, including the central and ANSs. When this communication is healthy, vitality is supported across every system. When it is disrupted, the effects ripple outward, touching everything from cognition to inflammation to emotional resilience.

The relationship between the kidneys and the nervous system can be understood as a form of "cross-talk."[20] The central nervous system regulates kidney function through intricate neuroendocrine signaling, and in turn, changes in kidney health can influence cognitive capacity and brain structure. Chronic kidney disease, for example, is associated with cognitive decline, vascular damage, and increased risk of stroke and dementia. This reflects the classical view in Chinese medicine that *jing* nourishes the brain and that depleted essence leads to memory loss, confusion, and emotional instability.[21]

The ANS is also closely tied to kidney function. Through sympathetic and parasympathetic pathways, the ANS regulates blood flow, filtration, and fluid balance. Within this system, the vagus nerve plays a protective role. It carries messages of calm, modulates inflammation, and supports immune resilience. Stimulation of the vagus nerve has been shown to reduce kidney inflammation, prevent fibrosis, and stabilize autonomic regulation. These findings mirror the TCM understanding that when *jing* is full, the nervous system remains balanced.

What is interesting about the neuro-kidney relationship is that it begins in utero. The early formation of the brain, spinal cord, and vagus nerve is shaped by inherited genetic material and influenced by maternal health, stress levels, and environmental exposure. In TCM, this corresponds to the role of pre-heaven essence. *Jing* received in utero lays the foundation for a lifetime of constitutional strength. It influences not only physical structure but also emotional regulation and the ability to handle stress. The development of the ANS in early gestation reflects the wisdom of TCM, which has always recognized the importance of inherited kidney energy in shaping long-term resilience.

These findings offer an affirmation of the classical idea that *Jing* creates marrow and that marrow nourishes the brain. When kidney essence is strong, the nervous system can function with adaptability and intelligence. When the *Zhi* is intact, the will remains steady even in times of difficulty. But when chronic stress, trauma, or illness weakens this system, both modern science and ancient wisdom point to the same outcome. The brain becomes vulnerable, memory fades, fear increases, and the spirit loses its direction. As the *Suwen* states, *"When one is in fear, then the essence withdraws."*[22] This withdrawal is not just metaphysical. It is physiological. Emerging evidence has shown that prolonged stress, inflammation, and kidney dysfunction disrupt brain function and autonomic regulation.[23] Essence does not vanish all at once. It slowly recedes, taking with it the clarity of thought, the steadiness of breath, and the ability to move through life with conviction.

When the Waters Run Shallow - Jing Depletion and the Fragile Nervous System

The story of resilience begins before our first breath. Within the earliest stages of human development, patterns of circulation, nourishment, and protection shape the organs that will sustain life. Emerging science continues to affirm what TCM has long understood, revealing that early biological patterns leave quiet but lasting impressions on vitality and shape how the kidneys, nervous system, and essence of *jing* sustain health throughout life. Recent studies suggest that variations in early circulatory patterns can affect kidney size and function in childhood.[24] When resources are directed more toward essential neural growth than evenly throughout the body, the developing kidneys may receive less nourishment. This adaptive process, known as neuroendocrine prioritization, reflects the body's innate intelligence to protect core systems during stress. While this mechanism supports immediate survival, it can also influence how energy is distributed and conserved throughout life, offering insight into the classical idea that early experiences shape long-term resilience.

As stated earlier in this chapter, this constitutional reserve is known as *jing*. It shapes the development of the kidneys, bones, brain, and nervous system. This includes the central and autonomic systems and the vagus nerve, which are understood to play central roles in how we process stress and restore equilibrium. When *jing* is strong, the nervous system adapts fluidly. Stress is met with balance. The will remains steady. When early nourishment or protection is limited, the effects may emerge later as emotional sensitivity, fatigue, or difficulty recovering from challenge.

These patterns are not fixed. They reflect how the body remembers and how deeply it can heal when given rest, care, and safety.

The *Suwen* offers a profound reflection on this pattern, *"The Kidneys are responsible for hibernation. They are the basis of seclusion and storage. They are the location of essence. Their effulgence is in the hair on the head. Their fullness manifests itself in the bones. They are the minor yin in the yin."*[25] These lines describe more than physiology. They speak of a sacred reservoir of rest, storage, and renewal. The reference to hibernation resonates with the restorative functions of the parasympathetic nervous system and the vagus nerve, which guide the body into states of deep stillness and repair. The effulgence in the hair and fullness in the bones offer visible signs of internal vitality, reflecting what modern science recognizes as the downstream effects of healthy kidney function and abundant essence.

When kidney growth or function becomes limited, the architecture of the nervous system may also be affected. Fewer nephrons, the tiny filters within the kidneys, are associated with greater vulnerability to hypertension and kidney dysfunction later in life. Yet these influences extend far beyond physical filtration. They touch the adaptability of the ANS, the tone of the vagus nerve, and even the development of higher brain regions involved in focus and regulation. Such early physiological patterns may shape how easily the nervous system manages stress, restores balance, and engages fully with life.[26]

The *Suwen* also teaches that, *"The locations where the five essences collect. When it collects in the Kidneys, fear results."*[27] In this view, fear is not only psychological but also physiological, signaling that the foundation of safety has been unsettled. When *jing* loses its anchor, the nervous system may become reactive, and the spirit uncertain. This reflects modern findings that early or repeated stress can heighten the sensitivity of the stress response system, creating patterns of vigilance or withdrawal. In TCM, these patterns are understood as signs of *Zhi* imbalance, when the will dims and inner direction feels obscured.

In the *Suwen* it was written that, *"When the yin and yang are balanced and sealed, the essence and spirit are in order. When the yin and yang are dissociated, then the flow of essence qi is interrupted."*[28] This wisdom reminds us that harmony is the foundation of vitality. *Jing* cannot circulate without balance between yin and yang, activity and stillness, sympathetic and parasympathetic tone. When this balance is restored through rest, breath, and nourishment, the essence renews itself. The nervous system finds rhythm again, and the spirit begins to settle.

Ultimately, the kidneys are not just physical organs. They are the deep roots of who we are. When *jing* is full, the bones are strong, the mind is clear, and the will is steady. When it becomes depleted, renewal may take time, yet recovery always remains possible. By linking early development, nervous system adaptability, and the spirit of will, both ancient medicine and modern science affirm a shared truth: the kidneys are the origin of resilience. *Jing* is structural, hormonal, neurological, and emotional. *Zhi* is the embodied will to move forward, encoded in the brain and anchored in the body. When we nourish the kidneys through rest, breath, nourishment, and emotional safety, we do more than replenish energy. We help the body remember its design and invite the spirit home again.

The Imprint of Fear – Early Foundations of the Spirit of Will

From the very beginning of life, the body learns how to respond to the world around it. Patterns of safety and strain become written into our physiology, shaping both the nervous system and the essence that sustains it. Contemporary science continues to affirm what Chinese medicine has long understood: early conditions of adaptation leave subtle but lasting impressions on vitality.[29]

Jing is the essence we inherit at the start of life. It forms the blueprint for our physical and emotional foundation. *Zhi*, arises from this essence and guides our capacity for purpose, courage, and endurance. When life's early conditions are harmonious, *jing* settles deeply into the kidneys, nourishing stability and calm. When stress or adversity takes hold, this reserve can become unsettled. The nervous system grows more vigilant, and the will may feel unsteady.[30]

In both classical and modern thought, the body's earliest adaptations are seen as acts of intelligence that preserve life under pressure. Yet these same patterns can shape how we later manage stress, emotion, and recovery.[31] This is the essence of developmental resilience. It reflects the understanding that the body remembers its history but also holds the power to rewrite it through restoration, nourishment, and balance.[32]

The *Suwen* teaches, *"When it collects in the Kidneys, fear results."*[33] In this context, fear is not merely an emotion but a signal from the body that the foundation of safety has been disrupted. It is the echo of essence that could not fully root. Another passage reminds us, *"When the yin and yang are balanced and sealed, the essence and spirit are in order. When the yin and yang are dissociated, then the flow of essence qi is interrupted."*[34] These teachings parallel modern findings that early exposure to stress hormones and inflammation can fragment the coherence of the developing nervous system. In the language of Chinese medicine, the pathways between *jing* and *Zhi*, between essence and will, lose alignment.

A growing body of evidence continues to affirm that early environmental stress can influence both emotional imprinting and organ development. A 2021 scoping review explored connections between psychosocial stress and kidney health across the lifespan.[35] The findings suggest that early exposure to chronic stress may interfere with nephron formation, leading to subtle structural vulnerability. Though further study is needed, the evidence consistently shows that stress leaves an imprint that shapes the way the body manages pressure, recovers from fear, and maintains equilibrium.

Taken together, research reveals a clear pattern. Early stress influences not only emotional development but also the structure of vital systems, particularly the kidneys. Today's science continues to confirm what Chinese medicine has long known. The kidneys form the root of life and hold the essence that gives structure to both body and spirit. When development is disrupted, the effects may not be immediately visible, yet they are carried within the body's deep memory. Patterns such as heightened sensitivity, delayed recovery from stress, or difficulty grounding may reflect essence that did not fully anchor and a will that never found solid ground.

In TCM, the kidneys form the foundation of life. They hold *jing*, the deep essence we inherit, and give rise to *Zhi*. When *jing* becomes scattered through chronic strain, the foundation weakens and the will may feel unsteady. What modern science observes as reduced resilience, ancient medicine understands as the echo of spirit seeking to root more deeply. When we nourish the kidneys, we do more than support organ function. We mend the bond between essence and action. We help the system remember its design and invite the *Zhi*, to return home.

By restoring kidney energy, calming the nervous system, and supporting vagal balance, we nurture the return of clarity and courage. The breath finds rhythm. The spirit of will remembers its path forward.

The Language of Fear and the Wisdom of Calm

Fright is not only a momentary shock to the system. It has the power to fracture the connection between the mind and body, between spirit and will. In *Suwen* Chapter 39, it is written, *"When one is frightened, then the Heart has nothing to lean on, the spirit has nowhere to return, and one's deliberations have nowhere to settle. Hence, the will is in disorder".*[36] This passage describes not just an emotional state, but a physiological unraveling. Modern science now confirms this ancient insight. Research has outlined how fear activates specific pathways in the brain and body designed for immediate protection, but harmful when chronically engaged.[37]

Exposure to a fear-inducing stimulus triggers the amygdala, which initiates a cascade through the hypothalamic-pituitary-adrenal (HPA) axis. As we have seen throughout this chapter, this axis releases stress hormones such as cortisol and activates the sympathetic nervous system. In the short term, this response heightens vigilance, increases heart rate and blood pressure, and sharpens sensory input. It is an adaptive survival mechanism. But when fear persists or becomes internalized through trauma or unresolved stress, this acute reaction becomes a long-standing state of hyperarousal.

Chronic fear disrupts the balance of neurotransmitters like serotonin, dopamine, and norepinephrine. It downregulates the function of the prefrontal cortex, the part of the brain responsible for executive decision-making, emotional regulation, and long-term planning. These shifts may lead to impaired learning, decreased impulse control, and greater reactivity to minor stressors. In children and adults alike, prolonged activation of this fear circuitry can contribute to the development of anxiety disorders, panic attacks, and a sense of internal chaos.

This biological reality mirrors the Suwen's wisdom. *" When one is frightened, then The Heart has nothing to lean on"* when cognitive regulation is hijacked by survival responses. *"The spirit has nowhere to return"* when the Shen becomes unanchored in the storm of unprocessed fear. *"The will is in disorder"* when the Zhi, residing in the kidneys, can no longer organize intention or action due to a dysregulated nervous system.[38]

In TCM, fright is said to directly damage the kidneys. It is believed to scatter the essence and weaken the Zhi, the spirit of will. This correlates with the modern observation that chronic fear alters ANS tone, reduces vagal regulation, and fragments the ability to access states of calm. The kidneys, seen as the foundation of jing and deep inner strength, are especially vulnerable when the sympathetic system dominates. Sleep becomes shallow, digestion slows, and the ability to recover fades. The system becomes wired for defense rather than restoration.

Early-life or repeated exposures to fear can sensitize the HPA axis, leaving the system more prone to overreact in the future. This heightened reactivity may contribute to persistent patterns of hypervigilance and emotional dysregulation. In TCM, this dynamic is viewed as a disturbance in the Shen–Zhi axis. Outwardly the body may appear calm, yet internally there is no true rest, as the spirit remains unanchored.[39]

Ancient and modern medicine converge here. Fright is not simply an emotional event, it is a pattern that can reshape physiology, fracture coherence, and separate essence from expression. Healing requires more than calming the surface. It means reconnecting the heart and kidneys. Restoring Shen and Zhi. Nourishing the jing and soothing the nervous system so that the will can rise again with clarity and strength.

Fear is a full-body event that reshapes the inner landscape of the nervous system. In moments of acute danger, fear serves a vital role. It sharpens the senses, heightens awareness, and prepares the body to respond. Protective responses occur: heart rate increases, muscles tense, attention becomes narrowly focused. They allow the body to act swiftly and survive immediate threats. But when fear lingers, when the stress response does not resolve, it begins to erode the very systems it was designed to protect.

Chronic Fear, Neural Rewiring, and the Loss of Regulation

Fear is a necessary response, guiding us to protect ourselves in moments of danger. Yet when it becomes constant, its weight seeps into every layer of being. It shapes the brain, unsettles the breath, and leaves the heart unsteady. Over time, this state of vigilance touches the spirit itself, changing how we think, feel, and move through the world. Both modern neuroscience and TCM describe the deep imprint fear leaves when it is not resolved. As discussed earlier in this chapter, activation of the hypothalamic-pituitary-adrenal (HPA) axis initiates the body's stress response. When the amygdala, the brain's internal alarm system, perceives danger, it signals this pathway along with the sympathetic nervous system. The resulting surge of stress hormones not only prepares the body for immediate action but also feeds back into the brain, influencing circuits related to memory, emotion, and executive function.[40]

As the amygdala becomes more reactive, the brain enters a prolonged state of vigilance. Over time, the hippocampus begins to shrink. The prefrontal cortex, which governs planning, foresight, and decision-making, loses strength. The body becomes stuck in a reactive loop, less capable of reflection, self-regulation, and repair.

TCM has long recognized this pattern, though it speaks in a different language. The kidneys are seen as the root of life. They store jing, or essence, which gives rise to the marrow. Marrow generates the brain and spinal cord, known in classical texts as the Sea of Marrow. Jing nourishes cognition, emotional strength, and spiritual clarity. The Zhi, is rooted here. It is our capacity to persevere, to act with intention, and to return to stillness when needed.

In TCM, fear injures the kidneys. It scatters the will and drains the essence. In the *Suwen* Chapter 5, it is said that, *"If fear causes harm, it harms the Kidneys."*[41] This core teaching links emotional trauma directly to physiological depletion. Over time, this depletion reaches deep into the marrow and nervous system, affecting the ability to adapt, recover, and feel secure in the body. In the *Suwen* Chapter 39, it is also said, *"When one is in fear, then the qi moves down... When one is frightened, then the qi is in disorder"*.[42] This downward and chaotic movement mirrors what happens when the body is overwhelmed. Energy collapses inward. The vagus nerve loses tone. The heart rhythm becomes unstable. Sleep becomes fragmented. Digestion slows. Over time, the whole system falls out of sync. The person may feel ungrounded, emotionally scattered, or unable to take meaningful action. In TCM, this is when the Shen loses its anchor in the heart. The Zhi becomes unmoored. The will falters. The body cycles through hypervigilance, depletion, and withdrawal.

Healing this pattern is not about eliminating fear. It is about restoring the root. Rebuilding jing, rebalancing the nervous system, and nourishing the kidneys are essential steps in helping the body remember its original coherence. This may involve restorative practices such as deep rest, mineral-rich foods, warming herbs, breath work, gentle acupressure, or simply creating space for safety and stillness.

As qi is guided inward and upward once more, the mind softens. The will steadies. The spirit begins to return. This is the heart of regulation. Not just calming the surface, it tends to the foundation.

Rewiring the System - How Acupuncture Regulates Fear

Fear and unresolved stress are not just emotions that pass through the mind. They have a somatic effect and leave lasting imprints in the body. They change the way we breathe, sleep, digest, and think. Over time, they can disrupt the body's natural rhythms, keeping us locked in a state of tension and overdrive. Chronic stress places continued strain on the HPA axis, the communication loop between the brain and adrenal glands that was discussed earlier, disrupting its ability to maintain balance in the face of ongoing demand.[43]

This stress response system plays a crucial role in survival. When the brain perceives a threat, it sends signals to release hormones like cortisol, which help the body prepare to react. But when stress is constant, the HPA axis can become overactive. The body stays in a heightened state, even when the danger has passed. Sleep becomes restless, thoughts race, the heart beats faster than it should, and the ability to relax fades.

Research by Wang, Zhang, and Qie (2014) explored how acupuncture affects this overactive stress response.[44] Their research found that acupuncture can help calm the HPA axis. It has the ability to reduce the activity of stress hormones and strengthen the body's natural ability to return to balance. In other words, acupuncture doesn't just relieve symptoms, it helps the body remember how to come back to center.

But this balance is not just about hormones. It also involves the ANS, which controls automatic functions like breathing, digestion, and heart rate. When stress is high, the part of the nervous system responsible for action, the sympathetic branch, takes over. This is the system that prepares us to fight or flee. It keeps us alert and ready but also makes it hard to rest, digest, or feel safe. Over time, this creates a loop of exhaustion and tension.

Acupuncture helps shift the body out of the state of fright or flight. By soothing the stress response, it creates space for the parasympathetic branch to come back online. As stress hormones quiet down, the breath deepens, the heartbeat slows, and the inner sense of safety begins to return. This shift supports not just physical healing, but also emotional balance, mental clarity, and a deeper connection to self.

As we have observed in this chapter, in TCM, fear injures the kidneys. Kidneys are the root of our vitality. They store jing, or essence, which fuels all growth, healing, and regulation. Jing nourishes the brain, spinal cord, and nervous system. It supports our ability to stay steady in times of change. The Zhi gives us the strength to move forward and the resilience to return to stillness after disruption.

The findings from this research offer a modern confirmation of this ancient wisdom. By calming the HPA axis and supporting the rest-and-restore functions of the nervous system, acupuncture becomes more than just physical treatment. It becomes a form of medicine rooted in rhythm and restoration. It helps bring the system back into coherence. What we describe today with words like cortisol, vagal tone, or stress circuitry, ancient practitioners observed through the quality of the pulse, the clarity of the spirit, the depth of sleep, and the flow of Qi.

When fear goes unaddressed, the will weakens. The person may feel tired yet unable to rest. The heart races. The mind becomes foggy. The spirit drifts. But when we begin to care for the system intentionally, through practices like acupuncture, nourishing food, rest, and self-reflection, the body begins to remember. The will grows stronger. The heart finds its anchor. The qi begins to flow again, steady and clear.

In this way, acupuncture offers a bridge. It connects the language of modern science with the soul of ancient healing. It reminds us that healing is not just about fixing what is broken. It is about remembering the rhythms that once kept us whole. It is about helping the body, mind, and spirit find their way back home.

Acupuncture, the Kidneys, and Hormonal Longevity

Acupuncture has long been used to promote balance, prevent disease, and support vitality across the lifespan. One of the key ways it may contribute to longevity is through its regulation of the hypothalamic-pituitary-adrenal (HPA) axis. Chronic activation of this axis is known to accelerate biological aging. It weakens immunity, depletes metabolic reserves, impairs sleep, and contributes to neurodegeneration.

The HPA axis is essential for helping the body adapt to challenges, but prolonged activation can cause more harm than good.[45] When stress hormones like CRH and cortisol remain elevated over time, they begin to erode the very systems they were designed to protect. The immune system becomes suppressed and the body's ability to recover weakens.

As we age, the ability to turn off the stress response becomes less efficient. Even after the stressor has passed, the body may continue operating as if it's still under threat. This lingering state of internal alarm shapes not only our physical health but also our emotional landscape. It becomes harder to rest. It's harder to connect. It is harder to feel at ease inside ourselves. Aguilera's work highlights that restoring this regulatory rhythm, learning how to come back to center, is essential for long-term health.

In a 2013 clinical trial, researchers found that acupuncture applied to the point Stomach 36, helped modulate this neuroendocrine stress response.[46] Subjects under chronic physiological stress exhibited elevated levels of CRH, ACTH, and corticosterone, hallmarks of HPA axis overactivation (Eshkevari, Permaul, and Mulroney 2013). Electroacupuncture significantly reduced these hormone levels and calmed the stress circuitry, while no such effect was observed in those receiving sham acupuncture. The treatment also normalized levels of neuropeptide Y, a chemical messenger that rises with sympathetic overactivation. This points to a shift away from the stress-driven sympathetic state and toward parasympathetic restoration. In TCM, this physiological resilience reflects the preservation of jing, the kidney essence, which underlies vitality, emotional stability, and longevity. These findings offer a modern biological explanation for how acupuncture may preserve health at a foundational level, restoring rhythm, regulation, and the body's natural capacity to adapt and thrive.

The Spirit of the Brain - Acupuncture and Cognitive Vitality

Another pathway through which acupuncture may support longevity is by enhancing the brain's capacity for renewal. One of the most important molecules involved in this process is brain-derived neurotrophic factor, or BDNF. This protein supports the growth, survival, and adaptability of neurons and plays a central role in learning, memory, and emotional balance.[47] As levels of BDNF decline, which often occurs with chronic stress and aging, the brain becomes more vulnerable to cognitive decline, emotional dysregulation, and neurodegenerative processes.[48]

Recent research has shown that acupuncture can stimulate the expression of BDNF and its related signaling pathways. Research indicates that it activates the BDNF–TrkB–CREB pathway, a molecular cascade known to enhance synaptic transmission, protect against neuronal injury, and improve cognitive performance.[49] This pathway is essential for forming new neural connections and for supporting long-term brain health. The researchers also found evidence that acupuncture may help regulate energy metabolism in the brain and reduce excitotoxicity, both of which contribute to neuroprotection and slower cognitive aging.[50]

Expanding on these findings, more recent research has described how acupuncture influences multiple BDNF-related pathways.[51] These include those involved in neurogenesis, synaptic plasticity, and mitochondrial energy regulation, which are all essential to maintaining both mental clarity and emotional resilience as we age. The review also noted that BDNF modulation by acupuncture appears to be highly adaptive and region-specific. This suggests that acupuncture may influence particular brain areas involved in trauma recovery, mood regulation, and cognitive decline.

Adding yet another layer, research has shown that acupuncture can affect BDNF through epigenetic mechanisms. It alters DNA methylation at key regulatory sites of the BDNF gene, effectively increasing its expression. This not only leads to an increase in BDNF levels in the short term but may also promote longer-lasting changes in how the brain supports emotional and cognitive resilience over time.[52]

From the lens of TCM, these findings mirror classical teachings. The mind, or Shen, is housed in the heart, rooted in the kidneys, and nourished by the liver. When these organs are balanced and supported, cognition is clear, emotions remain stable, and vitality is preserved. Recent studies on BDNF and acupuncture reflects this same principle. Healing, at its core, is not only about eliminating symptoms. It is about reawakening the brain's natural ability to adapt, grow, and restore itself. In this way, acupuncture supports longevity not just by relieving distress in the moment but by helping the entire system remember how to renew.

The Way of Inner Regulation

A foundational way in which TCM supports longevity is through practices that nourish the kidneys, preserve jing, and calm the Zhi. Breathwork, gentle movement, restorative sleep, warming seasonal foods, emotional regulation, and acupuncture are all traditional methods recommended to protect this essence and fortify inner strength. Recent studies shows that these same practices benefit the ANS, enhancing HRV supporting hormonal balance, and increasing the body's resilience to physical and emotional stress.[53]

Recent research on mind-body practices such as Tai Chi and Qigong has shown notable improvements in key indicators of autonomic function, including high-frequency power, which reflects vagal or parasympathetic activity, and SDNN, a measure of total HRV and overall adaptability. These changes indicate that consistent practice helps shift the body out of chronic sympathetic dominance and into a more resilient, restorative state. Notably, the effects were strongest in interventions that emphasized meditative attention, breath awareness, and slow, intentional movement, the very qualities emphasized in TCM for supporting kidney essence. The review also found reductions in perceived stress and improvements in emotional regulation, confirming that these ancient practices still hold therapeutic relevance today. When integrated consistently, they appear to restore harmony between the nervous system, endocrine system, and emotional core.

When the kidneys are nourished through these inner-centered rituals, the nervous system becomes more adaptable. When the nervous system is regulated, the Zhi has room to express willpower and purpose. In this way, essence, spirit, and neurobiology form an elegant triad, a living blueprint for a meaningful, grounded, and enduring life.

Jing, Zhi, and the Blueprint of Longevity

Longevity is not merely the extension of one's lifespan but the sustained expression of purpose, vitality, and adaptive strength throughout the years. In both TCM and integrative health models, true longevity encompasses more than physical endurance. It reflects a deep continuity of spirit, resilience, and alignment with one's inner nature. While genetics, environment, and lifestyle all contribute to how we age, TCM places special emphasis on preserving jing, or essence, stored in the kidneys. This essence serves as the foundation for growth, reproduction, regeneration, and mental clarity. When jing is conserved and nourished, the body ages with grace and the spirit remains rooted in will and clarity.

To nourish the Zhi is to reconnect with the deep current of will that flows beneath distraction, depletion, and fear. It asks us to listen inward, to sit in stillness long enough to remember what truly matters. In the season of Water, when nature draws its energy underground, we too are called to rest, restore, and reflect. The following practices are designed to help you align with this inner wisdom. Use them to strengthen your sense of purpose, deepen your resilience, and renew your connection to the quiet power within.

Stillness Breath - Anchoring the Deep Will

To calm the nervous system and reconnect with inner direction.

Sit comfortably with your spine supported and your hands resting gently on your lower back or just above your navel.

Inhale slowly. As you breathe in, direct the breath downward into the back body, imagining it filling the space of your kidneys.

Exhale softly allowing tension and scattered energy to release.

At the bottom of the breath, pause in stillness and feel yourself sink inward.

Repeat this cycle 3 times

With each inhale, feel yourself gathering inner strength from the depths. With each exhale, release fear, confusion, or urgency. This breath restores clarity and helps the Zhi root deeply into the wellspring of your being.

Winter Reflection Journal Prompt

Zhi is the spirit of long vision, memory, and resolve. These prompts reconnect you with your why:

1. What inner direction am I being called to remember or reclaim?
2. In what area of my life do I need more stillness before taking action?
3. What does my deepest inner will want me to commit to this season?
4. Write without editing. Let your truth rise like water from the well of your soul.

Kidney-Nourishing Foods for Zhi Resilience

Warm, salty, and mineral-rich foods in small amounts, help replenish essence and support the deep reserves of the kidneys. Black sesame seeds, walnuts, and goji berries nourish jing and promote vitality. Bone broth and miso soup strengthen the body's foundation and soothe the nervous system. Seaweed provides trace minerals that fortify the Water element, while black beans, lamb, and root vegetables offer grounding nourishment and deep energy.

17

The Ethereal Soul - Honoring the Hun for Vision, Flow, and Longevity

The Hun, the ethereal soul, is our inner dreamer, a quiet current of imagination and creativity that guides us toward our life's true direction. In the *Huang Di Nei Jing Suwen* it is said, *"The Liver is the basis of exhaustion to the utmost. It is the location of the hun-soul"*.[1] In TCM, the kidneys hold the deepest reserves of Life as yin and jing, the foundation of vitality and essence. Yet it is the liver that makes these reserves accessible. By storing and regulating blood and anchoring the Hun, the liver mobilizes the body's vitality under extreme stress. If the liver becomes depleted, the Hun loses its anchor, and even the deepest reserves in the kidneys become unreachable.

The liver stores blood, and through this blood the Hun is anchored. With its roots deep and steady, the Hun can hold a clear vision and a steady sense of purpose. When these reserves are plentiful, the Hun moves easily between sleep and waking, bringing back dreams and insights to guide our path. When the liver is depleted, the Hun becomes untethered, and our inner compass begins to lose its true north. The liver, then, is not only a physical organ. It is a source of renewal, a keeper of direction, and a vessel through which the soul's journey unfolds.[2]

In TCM, the liver governs the Wood element and is associated with springtime, renewal, and growth. While the Po anchors us in the body and in the instinct to survive, the Hun lifts us into realms of imagination, insight, and transcendence.[3] It allows us to dream of what could be, to plan for the future, and to navigate life with a sense of direction and meaning. As the *Suwen* teaches, *"The Liver is the official functioning as general. Planning and deliberation originate in it"*.[4] In the language of the classics, this image of the general reflects liver's role as strategist and visionary, the one who surveys the landscape, anticipates change, and coordinates the steps needed to move forward. Through its storage of blood and regulation of qi, the liver provides the clarity to see the path ahead and the flexibility to adapt when circumstances shift. In this way, it grants both the strategic foresight and the energetic momentum to act on one's vision, ensuring that inspiration has the grounding and timing it needs to become reality.

This classical image of the general is deepened in the *Ling Shu*, *"The Liver stores the blood. The blood hosts the hun-soul"*.[5] In the classical view, the Hun is a traveler, moving between the inner world of dreams and the outer world of action. Yet it must have a home to return to; blood is that home. When liver blood is full and flourishing, the Hun is rooted, allowing vision to remain steady, decisions to be clear, and the path ahead to feel attainable. From that rootedness comes the capacity to dream boldly and act with direction. But when liver blood is weak or depleted, the Hun becomes unanchored, like a ship without a mooring. Dreams may scatter, purpose may fade, and the inner compass may lose its true north, leaving a person adrift in restlessness, confusion, or aimlessness.[6]

The Hun is also intimately connected to the Shen, the spirit of the heart. In the *Suwen* it is written that *"the Liver stores the hun-soul,"* and the classical commentator Wang Bing adds, *"It supports the essence-spirit"*.[7] In this context, "essence-spirit" (*jing Shen*) refers to the union of our foundational vitality (*jing*) and our conscious awareness (*Shen*). By anchoring the Hun through its storage of blood, the liver provides stability for this essence-spirit, allowing vision and awareness to work together. The movement of the Hun mirrors the coming and going of the Shen, the conscious mind.[8] When these spirits move in harmony, we feel inspired, aligned, and able to translate our dreams into action.

The Hun is said to enter the body at birth and return to the stars at death. This is a poetic expression of its celestial origin and spiritual nature. It reflects our inner capacity to reach beyond the known, to envision what is possible, to hope, to dream, to plan, and to take inspired action. When the Hun is nourished and rooted, individuals tend to exhibit clarity of purpose, decisiveness, adaptability, and the ability to pursue meaningful goals with grace and resilience. They are not easily swayed by obstacles, and their creative energy flows with ease, unimpeded by internal stagnation.[9]

At night, the Hun returns to the liver to rest, supporting deep, nourishing sleep and coherent dreaming. When liver blood is deficient or liver qi becomes stagnant, the Hun loses its anchor and begins to drift. This can lead to restless sleep, vivid or disturbing dreams, and a racing mind that prevents true rest. Over time, it may also give rise to emotional instability, confusion, and a lack of direction, leaving individuals trapped in cycles of indecision, frustration, or impulsive action. These patterns suggest that the ethereal soul is unsettled, no longer grounded within its home.[10] And so, the dreamer within us, that quiet current of vision and imagination, depends upon the liver's deep reserves to stay rooted. When we tend to those reserves, the Hun can travel freely and return home again, carrying dreams that renew both heart and spirit. The broader role of sleep in health and longevity will be explored in Chapter 38.

While the ancient physicians spoke of the Hun's journey in the language of qi, blood, and the stars, modern science is mapping a similar journey in the language of nerves, microbes, and molecules. One such map is found in the gut–liver–brain axis, a network that mirrors the classical idea that the Hun's root in the liver depends on harmony throughout the body.

The Gut–Liver–Brain Axis and the Hun

Recent research has deepened our understanding of the gut–liver–brain axis, a finely tuned communication network linking the enteric nervous system, the liver's metabolic and detoxification processes, and the brain's regulatory centers. When this dialogue is healthy, each system supports the others, maintaining digestion, detoxification, emotional stability, and mental clarity. When the dialogue is disrupted, the effects ripple outward.

Studies link imbalances in this axis to mood disorders, cognitive decline, and altered stress responses. These are patterns that closely resemble the classical image of a Hun unmoored from its root.

Findings indicate that the trillions of microorganisms in the gut, known as the gut microbiota, influence this axis.[11] When the microbiota is balanced, it supports smooth communication between the gut, liver, and brain, promoting stable mood and clear thinking. But when this community becomes imbalanced, in a state called dysbiosis, the gut lining weakens. Harmful substances can then enter the bloodstream, sparking inflammation throughout the body and even in the brain. This inflammation impairs liver function, disrupts brain signaling, and unsettles emotional and cognitive states.

In TCM the spleen and stomach are the body's central processing hub, transforming food into energy (qi) and blood. When they function well, they produce clear qi that nourishes the entire system. When weakened by poor diet, chronic stress, or illness, dampness is generated. This is a form of internal stagnation. If this dampness lingers, it may mix with heat from diet, emotions, or infection to create damp heat.[11] In the Five Element framework, damp-heat can invade the liver, an organ system that thrives on the free flow of qi. Obstructed liver qi disturbs the Hun, the ethereal soul, making it restless and unfocused. This can appear as irritability, mood swings, poor sleep, or a loss of direction in life.[12]

From a modern perspective, this chain of events is significantly similar to how chronic gut inflammation disrupts liver metabolism and brain chemistry, resulting in mood instability and cognitive difficulties. Both systems describe the same phenomenon, one through the lens of physiology, the other through the language of qi and organ spirits.

Balancing the Gut–Liver–Brain Axis for Clarity of Mind

In both ancient medicine and modern science, the health of the digestive system is recognized as a foundation for mental clarity and emotional balance. The classics teach that the liver relies on nourishment from a well-functioning spleen and stomach to root the Hun and give it strength. In today's language, we might say that a healthy gut microbiome supports a healthy liver, which in turn sustains the brain.

Emerging research continues to show that the health of the gut is deeply intertwined with the health of the brain. In 2025, a systematic review and meta-analysis examined ten randomized controlled trials involving 778 people with cognitive impairment, ranging from mild cognitive impairment to Alzheimer's disease.[14] Across these studies, probiotic supplementation led to measurable improvements in memory, attention, and overall cognitive function. The strongest effects appeared when a single probiotic strain was used, the intervention lasted twelve weeks or less, and cognition was measured using the Mini-Mental State Examination. These findings point to a therapeutic sweet spot, a focused, time-limited course of probiotic support may offer the most benefit.

How probiotics support brain health comes down to the microbiota–gut–brain axis. The gut microbiome communicates with the nervous system through immune, endocrine, and neural pathways, including the vagus nerve. Balanced gut flora can lower inflammation, regulate neurotransmitters like serotonin and dopamine, and improve the way the brain processes and stores information.

In TCM, the gut–brain relationship echoes the harmony between the spleen and stomach (digestive health) and the Shen and Hun (mental and spiritual clarity). When digestion is supported, the mind can settle, focus sharpens, and emotions become more stable. Nourishing the gut is another way of nourishing the spirit. This web of connections reveals that the Hun's stability is as much a matter of physiology as poetry. When the gut, liver, and brain communicate smoothly, vision flows. When that dialogue is disrupted, the Hun grows restless. This is a state both TCM and neuroscience describe in distinctly similar ways.

The Restless Hun - Linking Ancient Wisdom and the Nervous System

When viewed through both TCM and modern neuroscience, parallels emerge between a "restless" or "unrooted" Hun, as described in TCM when liver qi is stagnant or liver blood is deficient.[15] In this lens, the unsettled Hun can be likened to patterns of sympathetic hyperarousal, where a person may push forward impulsively without clear direction, or to dorsal vagal withdrawal, where one retreats into emotional stagnation and despair.[16] While these frameworks arise from different traditions, both view emotional disorientation as deeply embodied. These experiences align with polyvagal-informed research, which describes how the nervous system encodes safety, threat, and shutdown through distinct autonomic states.

Healthy expression of the Hun depends on the foundation of a well-regulated nervous system. It is through a state of ventral vagal engagement, when the body feels safe, open, and connected, that true vision can arise.[17] In this parasympathetic state, the spirit is no longer in defense. The mind becomes receptive, and the Hun can offer clear direction. Just as fertile soil allows a seed to take root and grow, a calm and nourished internal environment creates the conditions for the Hun to flourish and guide us forward.[18]

When people lack direction or feel their vision has faded, it is not necessarily a failure of willpower or ambition. More often, it is the result of an overactive sympathetic nervous system or unresolved trauma that keeps the body locked in a defensive state. The Hun may continue to offer guidance, but when the body is in survival mode, that guidance cannot be followed. Practices that nourish the liver and calm the nervous system, help create internal safety and allow the Hun to return. As this happens, a renewed sense of purpose, possibility, and emotional clarity can emerge.[19]

To understand why this restlessness can so immensely affect health, we need to look closer at the liver's direct conversation with the nervous system itself, a network of "invisible wires" carrying signals that shape both emotion and metabolism.

The Liver's Invisible Wires

What ancient doctors described in the language of qi and organ spirits, modern neuroscience is now uncovering in the language of nerves and signaling. The nervous system has a direct influence on the liver. It is connected to the brain through a network of sympathetic and parasympathetic nerves. Both branches send messages to the liver through tiny nerve fibers that reach deep into the tissue. These fibers connect not only with liver cells (hepatocytes) but also with the immune cells and repair cells that live there, such as hepatic stellate cells (HSCs). Through these pathways, the ANS influences how the liver stores and releases energy, processes fats and sugars, manages inflammation, and repairs itself after injury.

When the sympathetic "accelerator" stays pressed for too long, as happens with prolonged stress or unresolved anger, the liver shifts into a state of overdrive. Studies show that high sympathetic activity can increase the production of sugar in the liver, encourage fat buildup, and activate repair cells in a way that creates more scar tissue rather than true healing. Over time, this can lead to a stiff, inflamed liver and make it harder for the Hun to rest and feel anchored.

The parasympathetic "brake" works in the opposite way. Vagus nerve stimulation, a key part of parasympathetic activity, has been shown to reduce liver inflammation, improve how the body uses sugar, and decrease the buildup of fat in the liver. This branch of the nervous system helps the liver recover and return to balance after stress. Some studies have found mixed effects when it comes to scar tissue, but overall, the parasympathetic system is linked to better healing conditions.[20]

From the perspective of Chinese medicine, these findings are another way of seeing the ancient teaching that anger injures the liver. Today we know that emotional stress often triggers the sympathetic system to stay active for too long. In doing so, it changes the liver's chemistry, fuels inflammation, and disrupts its natural rhythm. Whether described in the language of qi and blood or in the language of nerve fibers and cytokines, the message is the same: calming the nervous system is an act of protecting the liver, rooting the Hun, and restoring harmony to the whole being.

When the Liver's Nerves Wear Down

The brain and the liver are in constant quiet conversation. Through the ANS, signals pass back and forth to steady blood sugar, balance fats, and adjust energy use moment by moment. In health, this dialogue is seamless. The liver responds to the body's needs without strain, and the nervous system guides its rhythms like a trusted partner.

In the early stages of metabolic disease, this conversation begins to change. Studies show that in conditions such as obesity and type 2 diabetes, the liver can first be flooded with *too much* sympathetic input, the "fight or flight" branch of the nervous system. At first, this may be the body's way of trying to keep blood sugar from dropping too low. Over time, this overdrive can wear down the very nerve fibers that carry the messages. Scientists call this *hepatic diabetic neuropathy*, nerve damage within the liver itself.

The damage doesn't happen all at once. It tends to unfold in phases. First comes overactivation, which keeps the liver working at a pace it was never meant to sustain. Then, gradually, the nerves begin to fray, and the connection between brain and liver weakens. The result is a liver that is less able to respond to the body's needs, and a nervous system that has lost one of its key anchors in metabolism.

Scientist have traced this breakdown to three main processes:

- **Sugar overload in the nerves**: When blood sugar is high for long periods, excess glucose seeps into nerve cells. There it is converted to sorbitol, a sugar alcohol that builds up and creates oxidative stress, a kind of chemical "rust" that can damage nerve structure.
- **Sticky sugars and inflammation**: Glucose can also attach itself to proteins, forming advanced glycation end products (AGEs). These sticky compounds collect in tissues, including the liver, where they fuel inflammation and disrupt normal function.
- **Immune attack on the nerves**: Chronic, low-grade inflammation in the liver can directly strip away sympathetic fibers. In animal studies, blocking a single inflammatory signal, TNF-α, was enough to restore some of these nerves.

This pattern has been called the bimodal hypothesis of liver nerve control. In the first phase, sympathetic overactivity pushes the liver into constant alert, increasing blood sugar and fat output. In the second phase, the system burns out, leaving the liver partially disconnected from the brain's guidance.[22]

From a TCM perspective, this is not a foreign idea. The classics teach that when the liver is held in a state of prolonged tension, it first becomes overactive, then depleted. The Hun, which depends on the liver for its home, can lose its anchor. First swept up in agitation and then left without the strength to find direction.

Both ancient and modern wisdom offer the same counsel. Protect the liver from chronic overdrive. Ease the excess push of the sympathetic system, strengthen the calming influence of the parasympathetic, and nourish the body so the Hun can root again. In doing so, we safeguard not only the body's ability to metabolize and repair, but also our capacity for emotional steadiness, vision, and purpose.

These nerve pathways are not only shaped by physical demands. They are deeply influenced by our emotional states. Feelings like stress, frustration, and anger can tilt the balance between sympathetic "drive" and parasympathetic "calm," setting in motion a cascade of chemical and metabolic changes within the liver. In this way, emotions become both messengers and shapers of the liver's health.

Stress and the Physical Burden on the Liver

What the classical physicians described in metaphor, modern research is now mapping in physiology. Emotional strain, especially stress, leaves an imprint not only on the mind but on the tissues of the body. In a large population study of over 171,000 healthy adults, observers found that higher levels of perceived stress were independently associated with a greater likelihood of having non-alcoholic fatty liver disease (NAFLD), even after adjusting for lifestyle habits and metabolic risk factors.[23] Participants in the highest stress category had a 17% higher odds of NAFLD compared to those with the lowest stress levels.

This connection was present across all demographic groups but was strongest in men and in people with obesity, two groups known to have more intense sympathetic nervous system responses to stress. From a TCM perspective, this heightened reactivity parallels the classical teaching that the liver is particularly sensitive to "anger" and "constraint," leading first to overactivity and later to depletion.

As mentioned in the previous chapter, stress activates the body's primary stress pathways, including the sympathetic nervous system and the HPA axis. This response elevates cortisol, norepinephrine, and inflammatory cytokines, which in turn influence how the liver metabolizes fats and sugars.Over time, this can increase visceral fat, promote insulin resistance, and create inflammatory conditions that damage liver cells and encourage fat buildup.

Interestingly, even when accounting for behaviors often associated with stress, such as smoking, alcohol use, and reduced physical activity, the relationship between stress and NAFLD remained. This suggests that the effect of stress on the liver is not simply about unhealthy coping habits, but also about direct neuroendocrine and inflammatory pathways that strain the organ.[24]

From the lens of TCM, this study offers modern language for an old truth: prolonged emotional tension taxes the liver's reserves, weakens its ability to regulate qi and blood, and leaves the Hun without a stable home. Whether measured in cortisol and cytokines or in the shifting currents of qi, the outcome is the same. The liver loses its rhythm, and the whole being feels unmoored.

While stress alone can alter the liver's metabolism and structure, it rarely travels alone. In many people living with liver disease, stress is joined by deeper emotional burdens, depression, anxiety, and a quiet erosion of hope. These states are not just byproducts of illness; they can shape its course, influencing symptoms, treatment outcomes, and even survival.

Depression, Anxiety, and the Liver's Vitality

What Chinese medicine calls disturbances of the Hun and constraint of liver qi, modern medicine often names depression and anxiety. In people with chronic liver disease (CLD), these emotional burdens are far from rare. Depression affects about 16% of this population, and nearly half experience significant anxiety.[25]

The gut–liver–brain axis provides a direct biological pathway between emotional and physical health. In CLD, changes in gut bacteria, increased intestinal permeability, and inflammation ripple outward, altering the hypothalamic-pituitary-adrenal (HPA) axis and shifting the metabolism of key neurotransmitters like serotonin and glucocorticoids. These changes can leave a person more vulnerable to mood instability, fatigue, and brain fog.

Emotional health also shapes the course of the disease itself. Depression and anxiety can make it harder to follow treatment plans, increase the severity of symptoms such as fatigue and pain, and are linked with higher risks of opioid dependence, suicide, and even early death. TCM shows this is the lived reality of qi that has lost its smooth flow. This becomes a liver burdened by stagnation and depletion, unable to fully anchor the Hun.

The everyday experience of CLD is a constant dialogue between body and spirit. Muscle cramps, itching, restless nights, chronic pain, and the loss of familiar roles can quietly erode a person's energy and joy. These challenges don't just weigh on the heart, they shape the chemistry and rhythms of the liver itself.

Modern guidelines echo what the classics have long taught. Caring for the liver includes caring for the emotions. Regular screening for depression and anxiety is now recommended, using tools adapted to the unique needs of people with liver disease. First-line care often includes mindfulness practices and cognitive behavioral therapy. It may also involve gentle movement such as yoga or Tai Chi, along with building strong social support. All of these approaches resonate with the classical aim of regulating the emotions and harmonizing the liver. In more severe cases, medications can help restore balance, while avoiding drugs that may aggravate liver function.[26]

Ancient and modern wisdom align here, when we ease the grip of anxiety and depression, we give the liver room to breathe. Qi begins to move again. The Hun finds its anchor. And the body's capacity for healing, physical and emotional, grows stronger.

Just as sadness can quietly drain the liver's strength, anger can ignite it into a restless storm. Both are movements of qi, and both can loosen the Hun from its root. Where depression and anxiety may dim the inner horizon, anger can whip the winds of the spirit into turbulence, scattering vision and unsettling the heart. To understand the Hun, we must also understand how anger moves through the body, and how, when untempered, it can shift the course of both health and purpose.

How Anger Shapes the Hun

In the Five Element framework, the liver enables us to direct the soul toward a purposeful life. It gives us the vision we need to move forward and create. When the Hun and the liver are healthy, a person can easily manifest their purpose and hold a clear vision for their life's path. But when this vision and purpose are blocked or suppressed, frustration builds, and the energy of the Hun can turn toward rage and anger.[27] Over time, this unresolved anger can give rise to physical and emotional illness.

The Suwen teaches in Chapter 5, *"Among the depots it is the Liver... among the states of mind it is anger... If anger causes harm, it harms the Liver".*[28] This is a critical link in understanding how the Hun is affected. The liver is the home of the Hun. When anger injures the liver, the Hun's root is shaken. Without stability, the ethereal soul cannot rise in healthy ways toward vision, creativity, and purpose. Instead, it may scatter or become consumed by reactive emotion.

In TCM, anger causes qi to rise. This upward surge often shows itself as tension in the neck and head, dizziness, headaches, and tinnitus.[29] The *Huang Di Nei Jing* states in Chapter 39, *"When one is angry, then the qi rises."* The classical commentator Wang Bing elaborates, *"When anger excites, the Liver Qi rises in a reverse movement... when anger abounds and does not end, then it will harm the mind".*[30] This points to a twofold injury. Anger not only destabilizes the Hun by disrupting liver qi, but also agitates the Shen, the spirit of the heart.

The *Suwen* also notes, *"The Liver rules the sinews"*... Wang Bing comments, *"They keep the motive apparatus tied together. Their movement follows the spirit".*[31] When a person feels their destiny suppressed or their forward movement blocked, the sinews may tighten and contract. The body mirrors the mind, just as emotions become constrained, the physical form becomes tense and bound. This constriction reflects the Hun's inability to guide us forward.

If anger remains unresolved, it can transform into depression.[32] What begins as an outward, rising force may collapse inward, leaving a person feeling stagnant, hopeless, or disconnected from their sense of purpose. In this way, anger is not merely an emotion to be avoided, it is a signal. It points to where the Hun's vision has been obstructed, and to where the flow of liver qi needs to be restored so the soul can return to its natural course.

While anger may arise from the storms of daily life, the pressures of the modern world ensure that the liver's load rarely lifts. Even without open conflict or personal grievances, today's pace, diet, and environment act as constant irritants. In this way, the subtle injuries of unresolved emotion and the steady wear of external stressors meet in the same place, the liver, and through it, the Hun.

Modern Lifestyle Stressors - Rooting the Hun Amid Environmental Strain

In the classical world, the liver's health was shaped by the rhythms of nature, emotional balance, and simple dietary practices. In the twenty-first century, those same principles are challenged daily by the pace and pressures of modern life. In today's high-speed, convenience-driven culture, the liver, absorbs the brunt of constant demands: relentless stress, processed and refined foods, environmental toxins, and chemical pollutants.[33] Over time, these exposures erode the liver's vitality and unsettles the ethereal Hun from its grounding source, leaving vision and purpose adrift.

Ultra-Processed Foods and Liver Health

Ultra-processed foods (UPFs) are industrially manufactured products high in refined sugars, unhealthy fats, sodium, and chemical additives, but low in fiber, vitamins, and phytonutrients. From a biomedical perspective, these foods promote insulin resistance, disrupt gut microbiota, and create systemic low-grade inflammation, all of which strain the liver.[34] In TCM terms, the continuous metabolic burden weakens liver blood, impairs the smooth flow of liver qi, and deprives the Hun of the rootedness it requires for stability and clarity.

A 2023 systematic review and meta-analysis evaluated observational studies involving thousands of adults across multiple countries to determine the relationship between UPF intake and non-alcoholic fatty liver disease (NAFLD).[35] They found that individuals in the highest UPF consumption category had a 22% higher risk of NAFLD compared to those with the lowest intake. Importantly, for every 10% increase in UPF consumption, the risk of NAFLD rose by an additional 6%. This dose–response relationship suggests that even moderate reductions in UPF intake could meaningfully lower liver disease risk.

Another study from 2022 followed 5,867 older adults in Spain, all with overweight or obesity and metabolic syndrome, for one year as part of the PREDIMED-Plus trial.[36] Researchers tracked their food intake and assessed liver health using two validated measures. These measures were the Fatty Liver Index (FLI) and the Hepatic Steatosis Index (HSI).

The findings were significant. Even a 10% increase in daily ultra-processed foods such as sweets, processed meats, sugary drinks, or packaged meals was enough to raise liver scores noticeably. These changes held true even after adjusting body weight, waist size, diet quality, and other metabolic risk factors. While excess body fat, especially around the waist, explained much of the effect, the association persisted beyond weight alone. Lower adherence to the Mediterranean diet also played a role. This finding suggested that UPFs harm not only by what they contain but also by displacing nutrient-rich whole foods.

UPFs are typically high in saturated and trans fats, refined carbohydrates, and chemical additives. At the same time, they are stripped of fiber and protective plant compounds. The study showed that nutrient quality explained only part of the harm. This points toward other effects of ultra-processing, such as breakdown of the natural food structure and the impact of additives on gut and liver function.

From a TCM perspective, the ongoing metabolic burden created by UPFs disrupts the liver's role in ensuring the smooth flow of qi and emotions.

When this function is impaired, liver qi can stagnate and generate heat, which over time may overact on the spleen and stomach. This can weaken digestion, lead to dampness accumulation, and further burden the body's ability to transform and transport nutrients. The combination of modern findings and ancient theory suggests that reducing UPF intake not only lightens the liver's physiological workload but also protects its energetic function. Choosing fresh vegetables, whole grains, legumes, fish, and nuts supports the liver's harmony with the spleen, nourishes liver blood, and provides the stability the Hun needs for vision and clarity. In both modern science and classical teaching, these dietary choices help preserve metabolic balance, safeguard the liver, and sustain vitality with age.

When the Air We Breathe Reaches the Liver

The liver is not only sensitive to what we eat and drink. It is also shaped by the air that passes through our lungs. Modern medicine is now revealing what TCM has suggested for centuries. Environmental factors can burden the liver and disrupt its ability to regulate, cleanse, and nourish the body.

A large 20-year cohort study (2025) in Taiwan followed over 62,000 adults to explore the link between air quality and liver health.[37] Participants underwent regular health examinations between 1996 and 2016, including liver ultrasounds to screen for nonalcoholic fatty liver disease (NAFLD). This condition affects nearly one in three adults worldwide and can progress to scarring, cancer, and organ failure.

Each participant's long-term exposure to fine particulate matter (PM2.5), nitrogen dioxide (NO_2), and carbon monoxide (CO) was estimated based on where they lived. These are common pollutants from traffic emissions, industrial processes, and fossil fuel combustion. NAFLD occurred at a rate of 53 cases per 1,000 person-years. After adjusting for lifestyle and health factors, people living in areas with both high PM2.5 and NO_2 had a 25 percent higher risk of developing NAFLD compared to those in low-exposure areas. High PM2.5 combined with high CO carried an even greater burden, with a 28 percent higher risk.

Another large population-based study (2022) examined over 318,000 adults aged 65 years and older to see how long-term air pollution exposure affected liver function.[38] Analyst measured participants' exposure to PM2.5, PM10, sulfur dioxide (SO_2), nitrogen dioxide (NO_2), carbon monoxide (CO), and ozone (O_3), and tracked changes in their serum liver enzymes. Higher pollutant levels were linked to increased concentrations of alanine aminotransferase (ALT) and aspartate aminotransferase (AST), both markers of liver cell injury. For example, each interquartile increase in CO exposure was associated with a 6.2 percent increase in ALT and a 6.1 percent increase in AST, along with a 31 percent higher likelihood of elevated ALT and a 57 percent higher likelihood of elevated AST.

From a biomedical perspective, these pollutants may drive inflammation, oxidative stress, and metabolic changes that strain the liver's ability to process fats and sugars, while also causing direct hepatocellular injury. From a TCM perspective, chronic exposure to "turbid" or "dirty" qi from the environment can weaken liver blood, obstruct the smooth flow of liver qi, and unmoor the Hun. This can lead to both physical and emotional imbalance.

The message is clear. Protecting the liver is not only about food, alcohol, or stress. It is also about the quality of the air we breathe. Supporting liver health in a modern world may require as much attention to clean environments and restorative practices as it does to diet and exercise.

Why This Matters for the Hun

The Hun depends on a stable and well-nourished internal foundation to function as intended. In a healthy system, the liver filters toxins, regulates the smooth flow of qi, stores blood, and nourishes the ethereal soul. But when the liver is chronically burdened by poor diet, environmental pollutants, or systemic inflammation, the Hun's stability is compromised. Without sufficient liver blood to anchor it, the Hun may drift, leading to aimlessness, agitation, or an inability to envision a clear future.

When this drifting occurs alongside nervous system dysregulation, the effect is amplified. The individual may experience cycles of hyperarousal and collapse, a constant swinging between overextension and withdrawal. In these states, the Hun's guidance is muffled, not because it has disappeared, but because the body is too preoccupied with survival to act on its vision.

When the liver is weighed down by the strains of modern life, its ability to anchor the Hun weakens. Yet the same traditions that first described this connection also offer pathways to restore it. Acupuncture, refined through centuries of practice and now studied through the lens of modern science, has shown a unique ability to both protect and repair the liver's function.

Rebalancing the Liver and Rooting the Hun

Across thousands of years of practice, acupuncture has been used to restore the liver's strength, regulate qi, and steady the Hun. In modern research, these same treatments show measurable effects on liver function, inflammation, and tissue repair. A 2020 meta-analysis of fifteen randomized controlled trials involving over one thousand patients with liver cirrhosis found that acupuncture, when combined with standard care, significantly improved key measures of liver health, including reductions in ALT, AST, and total bilirubin, alongside increases in albumin levels.[39] These changes point to improved liver cell integrity, better protein synthesis, and reduced toxic load in the blood.

From the lens of TCM, these improvements reflect the clearing of stagnation, the enrichment of liver blood, and the harmonization of the liver's relationship with the other organs. Acupoints such as Liver 3, Stomach 36, Gallbladder 34, and Spleen 6 were most commonly used in the trials. These points have long been valued for their ability to regulate the flow of qi, nourish blood, and address both physical and emotional imbalances.

Modern biomedical perspectives suggest that acupuncture guides the liver's healing through a harmony of actions. It quiets inflammation, softening the surge of cytokines and settling the immune response. It slows the hardening of tissue by calming the stellate cells that weave scar into the organ's fabric. It steadies the rhythms of metabolism, allowing lipids, glucose, and proteins to be handled with greater ease. It also restores balance between nerve and immune pathways. In doing so, it shapes the release of neurotransmitters and gradually invites the ANS into a state where repair can take root.

For patients, these changes are not just numbers on a chart. They can translate into less fatigue, improved appetite, better sleep, and relief from symptoms such as abdominal distension. From the TCM perspective, this is the Hun regaining its home. This is seen as a liver no longer overburdened, qi that can move freely, and blood that can anchor vision and purpose.

Nonalcoholic Fatty Liver Disease - A Modern Challenge, An Ancient Approach

Nonalcoholic fatty liver disease (NAFLD) has quietly become one of the most common liver conditions worldwide. In Western medicine, it is linked to excess fat in the liver, often alongside weight gain, insulin resistance, and metabolic strain. Left unchecked, it can progress into more serious states such as liver fibrosis, cirrhosis, and even cancer.[40] In TCM, this picture can look like the liver's qi becoming heavy and stagnant. Its natural flow disrupted, its vitality weighed down. This heaviness doesn't stop at the physical. Over time, it can touch the emotions, dampening motivation, clouding vision, and leaving the Hun without its clear direction.

A 2020 systematic review protocol by Zang and colleagues set out to gather and evaluate all the clinical evidence for acupuncture in NAFLD.[41] Their goal was to examine randomized controlled trials comparing acupuncture, either alone or alongside conventional care, with other standard treatments. What makes this work stand out is its scope: they searched major medical databases in both English and Chinese, ensuring that studies from Western hospitals and TCM clinics were included.

The review builds on a growing body of earlier research showing that acupuncture may help the liver recover in multiple ways. Clinical trials had already reported improvements in imaging results, reductions in liver enzymes, and healthier lipid profiles. Patients receiving acupuncture often showed better blood sugar regulation and reduced insulin resistance. These are both key to slowing NAFLD's progression. Studies offered clues about why this might be happening. Acupuncture seemed to calm liver inflammation, lower oxidative stress, and help liver cells break down and release stored fats more effectively.

The choice of acupuncture points in these studies was no accident. Points like ST36, CV4, and KD1 have deep roots in classical practice. ST36 is known for strengthening the body's overall vitality and harmonizing digestion. CV4 supports the core reserves of energy that nourish all the organs. KD1, located on the sole of the foot, draws excess heat and agitation downward, helping the body find grounding. In modern studies, needling these points was shown to influence the expression of certain proteins in the small intestine, reducing lipid absorption and easing the liver's burden.

From a holistic perspective, these findings speak to something TCM has always emphasized. The liver's health is inseparable from the flow of qi through the entire body. NAFLD isn't just a liver problem. It is part of a wider pattern that touches digestion, metabolism, mood, and the body's ability to adapt to stress. By working on both physical and energetic levels, acupuncture offers a way to ease the liver's load, restore balance, and help the Hun reclaim its clear vision.

When the liver finds its flow again, changes often ripple outward. Energy returns in a steady, sustainable way. The mind feels lighter. Emotions no longer feel like weights to be carried but currents that can move through and out. This is the kind of renewal TCM has sought for thousands of years.

Acupuncture, Anger, and the Frontal Lobes

In recent years, researchers have begun to explore not just how acupuncture shifts the body's physiology, but also how it may alter the brain's patterns during strong emotions. A 2023 pilot study examined what happens when anger is intentionally triggered and then soothed with acupuncture.[42]

Thirty-four participants, each with high scores on the Novaco Anger Scale, underwent a sequence designed to evoke anger, while brain activity was monitored through electroencephalogram (EEG). The focuses was on a specific neural marker called *frontal lobe alpha band asymmetry* (FAA), a difference in brainwave activity between the left and right frontal lobes. Elevated left-sided FAA has been linked to approach-related anger and difficulties with emotional regulation.

After anger induction, FAA levels rose sharply, especially in the left hemisphere. Acupuncture was then applied to GB20 and GB21, points on the gallbladder channel that course near the base of the skull and the upper shoulders. These regions are traditionally used to clear excess yang, calm the spirit, and relieve tension in the head and neck. During acupuncture, FAA levels significantly decreased, reversing the left-sided dominance. While the effect softened after needle removal, the change suggested that acupuncture could immediately modulate the brain's electrical patterns associated with anger.

The findings echo what TCM has long described about the liver and Hun. When anger is excessive or constrained, the qi rises toward the head, distorting vision and judgment. Calming the uprising, whether through point selection that opens the channels around the head or by restoring the nervous system's balance, can help return the mind to clarity.

While this was a small study without a control group, it offers compelling preliminary evidence that acupuncture not only shifts emotional state subjectively but can also be tracked in the language of modern neuroscience. The brain, like the body, can return toward harmony when the pathways between stimulus and reaction are softened.

The Hun, the Liver, and the Roots of Longevity

From the earliest pages of this chapter, we have followed the Hun, the ethereal soul, in its journey between vision and action, rest and movement. The classics teach that the Hun depends on the liver's blood for its root. When that root is strong, we have a clear sense of direction, the ability to plan for the future, and the resilience to adapt when life changes. When the root is weakened, the Hun wanders, leaving us restless, indecisive, or disconnected from purpose.

This is not only a matter of spirit, but of long-term health. In TCM, the liver governs the smooth flow of qi, stores the blood, and nourishes the sinews. Its vitality is linked to clarity of mind, adaptability of body, and steadiness of spirit. These are qualities that allow us to live well throughout many seasons. Modern science affirms this in its own way. The liver plays a central role in metabolism, detoxification, immune balance, and brain function. When it is healthy, it can regenerate and repair itself. When it is injured or depleted, the entire body feels the strain.

Throughout this chapter, several themes have emerged that connect directly to longevity. Emotional regulation is one of them. Unresolved anger, prolonged stress, and emotional stagnation can injure the liver. Classical texts remind us that "anger injures the liver," and modern studies confirm the same pattern, showing that chronic stress and anger are linked to inflammation, fat accumulation, and reduced regenerative capacity. Protecting emotional balance is therefore an act of protecting the organ that roots the Hun and sustains vitality over time.

Another theme is the gut–liver–brain axis. Ancient physicians saw the body as an interconnected whole, and modern medicine echoes this view. Imbalances in digestion can inflame the liver and alter mood, cognition, and resilience. Supporting digestion through seasonal foods, mindful eating, and gentle movement helps stabilize this axis and with it the foundation of the Hun.

Environmental and dietary influences also play a critical role. Just as dampness, heat, and toxins can obstruct the liver in Chinese medicine, modern studies show that processed foods, poor-quality fats, and airborne pollutants damage liver tissue, disrupt metabolism, and impair emotional regulation. Choosing clean, whole foods and seasonal greens becomes a direct investment in longevity.

Nervous system balance is another thread that runs through this discussion. The liver's health is deeply tied to the ANS. Excess sympathetic drive, often fueled by stress and unresolved emotion, accelerates liver injury. Parasympathetic activation promotes repair, lowers inflammation, and supports regeneration. Practices such as breathwork, meditation, Tai Chi, and acupuncture invite the ventral vagal state and, in doing so, help protect both emotional stability and liver vitality.

Finally, acupuncture itself emerges as a longevity practice. Studies show that it can calm anger-related brain activity, improve liver enzyme profiles, reduce inflammation, and support tissue repair. In the language of TCM, these are the signs of qi flowing freely, blood being nourished, and the Hun being well anchored. When a therapy protects and restores the liver, it also helps preserve the roots of long life.

When we step back, the message is simple but profound. Longevity is not just a matter of the years we live, but of the strength and harmony of the systems that sustain us. The liver is one of those central systems, that is a bridge between body and spirit, metabolism and mood, vision and action. Each time we nourish it with seasonal foods, protect it from emotional strain, or restore it with acupuncture and mindful living, we are planting seeds for a life that is not only longer, but richer, clearer, and more aligned with our deepest purpose.

Rooting the Ethereal - A Breath, Touch, and Nourishment Ritual for the Hun

The Hun is light, mobile, and expansive by nature. It travels between the realms of sleep and waking life, carrying vision, purpose, and creativity. But like any traveler, it needs a safe home to return to. That home is found in the liver and in the blood it stores.

When we are overstimulated, chronically stressed, or disconnected from our bodies, the Hun can become unmoored. This leaves us scattered, emotionally fragile, and unsure of our direction. The following ritual combines breathwork, acupressure, gua sha, and seasonal nourishment to anchor the Hun, regulate the nervous system, and restore the liver's vitality.

The Return to Center Breath

1. Sit in a comfortable position with feet grounded on the earth.
2. Inhale gently through expanding the ribs and belly.
3. Visualize a gentle green mist surrounding the liver beneath the right rib cage.
4. Exhale slowly through the mouth, releasing tension and wandering thoughts.
5. At the bottom of the breath, pause and whisper inwardly: *I return to myself.*

When to practice: Before sleep for deeper rest and dream clarity, or anytime you feel scattered or unanchored.

These points help regulate liver qi, nourish liver blood, and calm the Shen. Apply gentle pressure or slow massage for 30 seconds - 1 minute each while breathing evenly.

- **Liver 3 (Taichong)** – On the top of the foot, in the depression between the first and second toes. Smooths liver qi, eases irritability, and clears the mind.
- **Liver 4 (Zhongfeng)** – On the inner ankle, anterior to the medial malleolus, in the depression just medial to the tendon. Helps release emotional constraint, addresses self-esteem, reduces inflammation, and supports flexibility and growth, both physical and emotional.

Nourishing the Hun Through Food

In TCM, the Hun's vitality mirrors the state of liver blood. Deeply pigmented, slightly sour, and nutrient-rich foods nourish blood, move qi, and anchor the ethereal soul.

Blood-Nourishing Foods:

- Dark leafy greens (dandelion, kale, nettles, spinach)
- Beets, carrots, black sesame seeds, goji berries, red dates
- Blueberries, plums, cherries, mulberries
- Bone broth and organic liver (if consuming animal products)

Liver-Soothing & Qi-Moving Foods:

- Lemon or apple cider vinegar (sparingly)
- Mung beans, artichokes, radish
- Fresh herbs like mint, basil, and cilantro

Longevity-Linked Additions:

- Cruciferous vegetables (broccoli, Brussels sprouts, bok choy)
- Omega-3 rich seeds (flax, chia)
- Fermented vegetables

Rhythm and Ritual

The Hun thrives in environments of flow, not chaos. Keep regular mealtimes, honor the body's need for rest, and create evening rituals to signal the return home.

Nighttime example:

- A small cup of goji-berry and chamomile tea
- Gentle gua sha along the liver meridian
- Three rounds of the Return to Center Breath
- A few minutes of dream journaling before sleep

These small, consistent acts are part of how we root the Hun, restore the liver's vitality, and plant the seeds for long life.

18

Emotional Harmony and the Nervous System - A Lifelong Key to Vitality

Over the last several chapters, we have walked with the Five Spirits: The Shen, Hun, Po, Yi, and Zhi. Each one is a unique facet of the human experience. We have explored how grief, vision, instinct, thought, and will shape the way we meet the world. We have seen how the nervous system holds the imprint of each emotion. Now, we return to see the whole picture.

Longevity is not simply the result of diet, exercise, or genetics. It is also the quiet accumulation of moments when we restore emotional balance, release the grip of stress, and allow the nervous system to return to its natural rhythm. Emotional regulation is more than a skill. It is a biological strategy for survival and renewal. When the Five Spirits are in harmony, the ANS shifts from states of protection to states of growth. The body receives the message that it is safe.

When the spirits become disconnected, the inner world may lose coherence. The *Ling Shu* describes this vividly. *"When the spirit essence is disturbed and fails to rotate... the essence spirit, the Hun and Po will dissipate and no longer stay with each other. Hence one speaks of confusion."*[1] In this state, the soul becomes scattered. The body may remain, but the guiding spark of direction, insight, and clarity drifts away.

To live a life of meaning, all the spirits must move together. The Shen, Hun, Po, Yi, and Zhi are like a constellation. Each star must remain in relation to the others for the whole pattern to shine. In both ancient and modern understanding, this coherence is not only the foundation of emotional well-being. It is also a key to health, vitality, and long life.

Shen - The Spirit of the Heart and the Rhythm of Renewal

In the classical view, the heart is the sovereign of the five Zang. It is the residence of the Shen. If the sovereign is bright, the body will be at peace. When the Shen is calm and rooted in the heart, there is clarity of mind, steadiness of emotion, and harmony in the body. This balance is not only the foundation for emotional well-being. It is also essential for preserving vitality over time.

In the pages you have just read, we traced how both ancient and modern perspectives agree that a disturbed Shen mirrors a dysregulated nervous system. In TCM, this disturbance can arise from trauma, overwork, or emotional strain that consumes heart blood, stagnates liver qi, and weakens kidney essence. In modern terms, it is reflected in chronic sympathetic activation, disrupted sleep, and diminished vagal tone.

We have seen how acupuncture and other calming practices restore parasympathetic balance, improve HRV, and create the conditions for the Shen to return to stillness. Whether described as anchoring the spirit, nourishing the heart, or re-establishing vagal regulation, the message is the same. Presence, breath, and rhythm are the roots of renewal. In tending the Shen, we tend the life force itself.

Po - The Breath of Release and the Rhythm of Letting Go

Longevity is nourished not only by physical health, but also by steady breath and emotional balance. When grief is honored and the lungs are free to move qi, the body regains its natural pace. Breath becomes steady, emotions begin to settle, and the nervous system shifts from vigilance into rest. Earlier we explored how unresolved sorrow can burden immunity, strain the heart, and disrupt sleep, all patterns that weaken resilience and shorten lifespan.

We also saw that conscious breathing, acupuncture, and gentle ritual invite the parasympathetic system to return, restoring both emotional steadiness and physiological repair. Every slow exhale becomes a quiet act of renewal. It is a reminder that letting go is not an end, but a sacred transformation.

To tend the Po is to tend the breath of the soul. In that tending, the body remembers its rhythm, the spirit softens, and the foundation for longevity is restored.

Yi - The Mind of Intention and the Nourishment of the Center

The Yi, rooted in the spleen, is the quiet intelligence that transforms both food and thought into energy. When the spleen is strong, the mind is clear, digestion is smooth, and energy is steady. When overthinking or worry takes hold, qi knots and the body's rhythm falters.

In this section of the book, we explored how this inner stillness, or its absence, shapes the course of aging. Chronic pensiveness, like a meal never digested, can weaken immunity, disturb sleep, and slow the body's repair. Modern research mirrors this truth, showing that ongoing psychological strain accelerates biological aging, while optimism and emotional steadiness protect resilience.

We have also seen that tending the spleen supports both the gut and the mind. Nourishing meals, mindful pauses, breathwork, and acupuncture all help release the weight of rumination. In this return to rhythm, digestion strengthens, thoughts lighten, and the nervous system reclaims its balance.

Longevity through the Yi is not built on constant striving. It rests in the quiet power of a nourished center. In every meal taken with presence, in every moment of pause, we protect the harmony that sustains life.

Zhi The Deep Current of Will and the Preservation of Essence

The Zhi is the spirit of will, endurance, and quiet strength. Earlier we saw how its vitality depends on the preservation of jing. This is our essence that underlies growth, regeneration, and clarity of mind.

When chronic stress or depletion overactivates the stress response, the body stays on high alert, wearing down the very reserves it needs to endure. Both classical and modern perspectives agree: restoring regulation is essential for long life. Acupuncture, slow breathwork, restorative movement, and mindful rest all help shift the nervous system out of survival mode, conserving essence and renewing inner steadiness.

We have also seen how these practices strengthen adaptability, improve HRV, and align the mind with its deeper purpose. In this harmony, the Zhi can guide life with intention rather than reactivity.

Longevity, through the lens of the Zhi, is not only measured in years. It is the sustained capacity to move forward with clarity, to adapt without losing direction, and to live in rhythm with one's nature. In tending the Zhi, we tend the quiet blueprint for a grounded and enduring life.

Hun – The Spirit of Vision and the Flow of Direction

The Hun, rooted in the Liver, carries the soul's capacity for vision, movement, and renewal. It is the spark that dreams forward, guiding us toward possibility and purpose. When the Liver qi flows freely, the Hun provides clarity of direction, resilience in times of change, and a sense of inner spaciousness.

When this spirit becomes unsettled, the inner compass drifts. Anger, frustration, or unexpressed emotions may stagnate the Liver, clouding foresight and scattering purpose. Modern science reflects this view, showing how chronic stress and disrupted circadian rhythms impair both mood and adaptability. The nervous system, caught in vigilance, loses its ability to rest into creativity and renewal.

Restoring the Hun means restoring flow. Practices that smooth Liver qi, such as acupuncture, mindful movement, breathwork, and periods of deep rest, help re-establish both physiological and emotional rhythm. In this return, vision clears and direction is regained.

Longevity, through the Hun, is not only about the span of years. It is about living with purpose and fluidity. To tend the Hun is to keep the pathways of imagination and renewal open, ensuring that the journey of life remains guided by clarity, movement, and a deeper sense of connection.

The Constellation Within

Each return to balance strengthens the nervous system's adaptability. In TCM, this adaptability is called harmony. In modern science, it is known as homeostasis.

True health is not the absence of emotion. It is the ability to move with it. Anger protects boundaries. Grief teaches release. Fear sharpens awareness. Joy expands connection. Worry invites trust. In the Five Element view, each emotion belongs to a season, an organ, and a spirit. When they flow, they renew us. When they stagnate, they burden us.

The nervous system is the bridge between the visible and invisible, holding the memory of life. When we treat it as sacred, we honor its signals. This is where physiology meets spirit. Tending the Shen, Hun, Po, Yi, and Zhi becomes both a biological and spiritual act of preservation.

Longevity is not the sum of isolated habits. It is the living rhythm that emerges when all Five Spirits move together. In tending this inner constellation, we preserve not only years, but the depth and vitality within them.

Practice: The Inner Constellation Ritual with Acupressure

1. Settle In

Find a quiet space. Sit or lie down comfortably. Let your hands rest gently on your belly or over your heart. Feel the weight of your body supported.

2. Coherence Breath

Inhale slowly through the nose.
Exhale gently through the mouth.
Let your shoulders soften.
Repeat for five rounds.
This helps activates the parasympathetic system and signals safety.

3. Acupressure for the Five Spirits

As you breathe, you may stimulate the following points — holding each for 30 seconds - 1 minute with gentle pressure.

- Shen (Heart) – HT7 Shenmen ("Spirit Gate") – On the wrist crease, in line with the little finger tendon. Calms the mind and anchors the

Shen.
- Hun (Liver) – LIV3 Taichong ("Great Surge") – On the top of the foot, between the first and second toes. Smooths liver qi and restores vision and purpose.
- Po (Lungs) – LU9 Taiyuan ("Great Abyss") – On the wrist crease, in line with the thumb tendon. Strengthens lung qi and supports release.
- Yi (Spleen) – SP3 Taibai ("Great White") On the inside of the foot, just behind the bump of the big toe joint. You will feel a natural hollow before the arch begins. Press here to strengthen digestion, support energy, and calm overthinking.
- Zhi (Kidneys) – KI3 Taixi ("Great Stream") – In the depression between the inner ankle bone and Achilles tendon. Strengthens kidney essence and willpower.

You can work through all five points in sequence or choose the one that resonates most with your current state.

4. Soften the Inner Dialogue
    As you breathe and hold each point, repeat silently:
    "I am safe now."
    "I trust my body to restore balance."
    "Longevity begins in peace."

5. Touchpoint Grounding (Reflective Practice)
    Many people find that bringing awareness to certain areas of the body offers a sense of grounding and calm. You might gently tap or massage:

    - The upper chest, just beneath the collarbones
    - The sides of the neck where you feel tension

6. Journal Prompt (Optional)

    - What signals me that I am in balance?

- How can I create a daily rhythm that supports emotional steadiness?
- What practices help me return to calm when life becomes overwhelming?

Repeat this practice anytime your body feels tense, reactive, or fatigued. Each time you engage in emotional regulation, you are not only calming the mind. You are also making an investment in your future health and longevity.

19

Integration – The Healing Rhythm of Balance

Healing is rarely a straight line. It moves like breath. We inhale, exhale, pause, and return. The path toward health and longevity begins with learning to move in harmony with the body's natural rhythms. The ANS sits at the heart of this process. It helps us shift between safety, stress, and restoration. When cared for, it can become a steady ally in creating both long life and emotional freedom.

Throughout this book, we have seen how emotions take root in the body. They shape breath, posture, muscle tone, and organ function, all of which are regulated by the ANS. In TCM, these changes are described through the Zang-Fu, where each organ carries both a physical role and an emotional one. Grief may settle in the lungs, constricting breath and shifting respiratory rhythms. Fear can disturb the kidneys, weakening the will and altering stress-response patterns. Anger often disrupts the liver's smooth flow, creating tension in muscles and fascia. Worry can weigh down the spleen, slowing digestion and affecting gut motility. Even joy, when unbalanced, may overstimulate the heart, altering heart rate and circulation. Modern trauma research mirrors these ancient insights, showing that unresolved emotions can create long-term changes in both the ANS and the body's physiological systems, leaving imprints that shape health and longevity.

The Rhythm of Safety and Repair

We have seen that the ANS is remarkably adaptable. Practices such as acupuncture, breathwork, meditation, and somatic awareness can soften long-held patterns of stress and guide the system back toward balance. As parasympathetic tone grows, sleep becomes deeper, digestion steadier, hormones more stable, and immunity stronger.

HRV offers a clear way to see this adaptability in action. HRV measures how fluidly the body moves between rest and alertness. Higher HRV often signals emotional stability, lower inflammation, stronger immunity, and ultimately longer health span. Lower HRV tends to appear during periods of chronic stress. Slow breathing, mindful movement, and vagal-toning practices can help restore this flexibility and strengthen resilience.

Lasting vitality also depends on something more subtle. A steady sense of safety within the body allows the nervous system to shift into repair mode. In this state, tissues mend, inflammation lowers, hormones rebalance, and energy can be used for growth instead of constant defense. Without it, the body remains guarded, and over time this constant vigilance drains reserves and speeds the aging process. Daily rhythms that nurture the ANS, such as deep breathing, restorative rest, meaningful connection, acupuncture, and gentle movement, help the body feel secure enough to restore and regenerate.

The Living Harmony of Healing

The Five Element framework has shown us that health is not a fixed point but a living harmony. It changes with the seasons and responds to the circumstances of life. Emotions are part of this movement. They are not flaws to be eliminated but essential forms of energy. Anger can help protect. Grief can help release. Fear can help guard. Joy can help expand. Even worry can guide us toward trust when it is understood and processed.

From the earliest chapters, we have held the nervous system as something more than a biological system. It is a meeting place between body and spirit. When we care for the Po, open the Shen, and steady the Zhi, the threads of body, emotion, and spirit come together in a more unified rhythm.

If there is one thread that runs through all we have explored, it is that healing begins in presence. Each time we return to the breath, notice the body, and soften our defenses, we step back into safety. Over time, this return becomes a steady rhythm that builds resilience, steadies the heart, calms the mind, and supports repair on every level.

Practice This: The Rhythm of Return

This simple practice gathers many of the skills we have explored and puts them into a form you can return to whenever you need to restore balance.

1. Create a Quiet Space

Find a place where you will not be disturbed. Light a candle or rest your hand over your heart. Let this signal to your body that it is safe to rest.

2. Breathe for Coherence

Inhale through the nose for a count of four.
Exhale slowly through the mouth for a count of six.
Release tension from the jaw, shoulders, and chest.
Repeat for five rounds with eyes softly closed.

3. Affirm Your Rhythm

With each exhale, silently repeat:
"I return to balance."
"My body remembers peace."
"This moment is enough."
Allow these words to settle in your body.

4. Anchor with Touch

Place one hand on the chest and the other on the lower belly.
Feel the breath rise and fall.

Notice the steadiness beneath your skin.
Whisper, "I trust the wisdom within me."

5. Journal Prompt (Optional)

- What does balance feel like in my body today?
- What helps me return to regulation when life feels overwhelming?
- How can I honor my nervous system as part of my healing journey?

Acupressure for Nervous System Regulation

These points help calm the mind, balance the ANS, and create a grounded sense of safety. You can use them alongside the above breathing practice or on their own.

How to Use This Sequence

- Move through the points in the order listed, spending 30 seconds - 1 minute at each point
- Keep your breath slow and steady.
- Notice the sensations in your body as you work.
- End by placing your palms over your lower belly, feeling the warmth of your hands, and resting for a few moments in stillness.

1. Yintang (Hall of Impression)

- Location: Between the eyebrows.
- How: Use your index or middle finger to apply gentle pressure while breathing slowly.
- Benefit: Calms the Shen (spirit), eases anxiety, and helps shift the body toward parasympathetic rest.

2. Anmian (Peaceful Sleep)

- Location: Behind the ear, in the depression just before the hairline.
- How: Massage gently in small circles for on each side.
- Benefit: Soothes restlessness, supports deep sleep, and quiets an overactive mind.

3. Pericardium 6 (Neiguan – Inner Gate)

- Location: On the inner forearm, about three finger-widths above the wrist crease, between the tendons.
- How: Press with your thumb gently with comfortable pressure, while breathing evenly.
- Benefit: Opens the chest, calms the heart, and relieves nervous tension.

4. Stomach 36 (Zusanli – Leg Three Miles)

- Location: On the outer side of the shin, about four finger-widths below the kneecap and one finger-width to the outside of the shinbone.
- How: Apply firm but comfortable pressure with your thumb on each leg.
- Benefit: Strengthens overall vitality, supports digestion, boosts immune function, and helps regulate the nervous system.

5. Liver 3 (Taichong – Great Rushing)

- Location: On the top of the foot, in the webbing between the big toe and the second toe, about two finger-widths back from the margin of the skin.
- How: Press with your thumb, gently while making small circles on each foot.
- Benefit: Smooths the flow of liver qi, relieves irritability and stress, and restores emotional balance.

6. Lung 9 (Taiyuan – Supreme Abyss)

- Location: On the wrist crease, in the depression on the radial side of the pulse.
- How: Use your thumb to apply gentle pressure on each wrist while focusing on deep, slow breaths.
- Benefit: Strengthens lung qi, supports healthy breathing, and deepens the calming effects of breathwork.

7. Kidney 1 (Yongquan – Bubbling Spring)

- Location: On the sole of the foot, about one-third down from the base of the toes in the center.
- How: Use your thumb to apply gentle pressure or make small circles on each foot.
- Benefit: Grounds scattered energy, relieves fear, and draws the mind back into the body.

Return to this practice as often as you need. Every choice to regulate is an investment in the long and beautiful rhythm of your life.

Ancient Insights, Modern Proof

The journey we have taken so far has been one of connection. We have explored how the body, mind, and spirit communicate through the rhythms of the nervous system, and how daily practices can bring those rhythms back into harmony. These insights are rooted in ancient wisdom and supported by lived experience. Yet they are also increasingly validated by modern science. In the next section, we will turn to the research itself, examining the growing body of evidence that shows how acupuncture and related practices influence the nervous system, support emotional health, and help the body restore its natural balance. The wisdom is old, but the data is now catching up.

V

Tracing the Currents of Balance

Mapping the Healing - What Modern Research Reveals About Acupuncture and the Nervous System

"The sages did not treat those already ill, but treated those not yet ill, they did not put in order what was already in disorder, but put in order what was not yet in disorder"
— *Haung Di*
"Only the sages follow the Way; hence, their bodies have no strange disease"
— *Haung Di*

20

How Modern Science Validates Acupuncture's Ancient Wisdom

In the previous chapters, we explored how emotional states and traditional concepts like the Po, Shen, and Zhi interact with the nervous system, drawing from both classical Chinese medicine and emerging findings on trauma, breath, and vagal tone. These insights help us understand the emotional expressions of the ANS.

Now, we turn to the physiological mechanisms themselves, the deeper circuitry of the ANS. This includes the anatomical pathways, brain-body feedback loops, and the emerging science of acupuncture's regulatory effects on inflammation, pain, and HRV. In doing so, we move from the *felt experience* of dysregulation to the *measurable physiology* behind it.

The Evidence for Balance

Throughout history, acupuncture has been rooted in observation, rhythm, and resonance. Ancient physicians mapped the body not with dissection, but with insight, following the tides of pain and healing, pulse and breath, emotion and energy. What they discovered became the foundation of TCM, a living, dynamic network of relationships governed by yin and yang, blood and qi, spirit and sensation.

In today's world, we use different tools to trace the same truths. We measure neurotransmitters and inflammatory markers, record HRV, and monitor shifts in parasympathetic tone. And yet, the story remains remarkably similar. Acupuncture brings balance. It calms the overactive, nourishes the depleted, and restores communication between the systems that make us whole.

This section brings together peer-reviewed research spanning over four decades, drawing from studies in neuroscience, cardiology, pain management, and integrative medicine. These articles reflect a growing consensus: acupuncture can influence the ANS in measurable, reproducible ways.

From regulating blood pressure and digestive function to reducing anxiety and chronic pain, the research reveals a powerful pattern. Acupuncture supports homeostasis. It modulates both the sympathetic and parasympathetic branches of the ANS, reduces markers of stress and inflammation, and improves the body's capacity to self-regulate.

This research not only supports the clinical insights of TCM but also invites a new generation of healers, researchers, and patients into the conversation. Acupuncture is no longer just ancient wisdom. It is modern medicine in motion, and the data confirms what the pulse has always known.

Research Scope & Methods

To fully appreciate the power of acupuncture in regulating the nervous system, it's helpful to turn to the growing body of clinical research that supports what practitioners have observed for centuries: acupuncture restores balance.

As part of my doctoral research, I conducted an in-depth review of peer-reviewed studies from the last 40 years, drawn from PubMed-indexed databases using MESH terms such as *ANS, acupuncture therapy, pain, inflammation*, and *psychosomatic disorders*. The aim of this review was to examine how specific acupuncture points and protocols influence various branches and functions of the ANS.

Out of more than 850 articles screened, several studies were selected for detailed review based on their relevance, quality, and clear reporting of acupuncture's effect on the nervous system. Exclusion criteria included studies not focused on the ANS, or studies involving children, pregnancy, or cholinergic-specific systems unrelated to autonomic function.

These studies were categorized into six core domains:

- Cardiovascular regulation (e.g., heart rate, blood pressure, vasodilation)
- Vagal nerve activity and parasympathetic tone
- Respiratory system modulation
- Digestive system regulation (e.g., IBS, dyspepsia)
- Pain and inflammation control

Together, these findings recognize what both ancient medicine and modern physiology describe. Acupuncture has the ability to modulate the nervous system. It helps restore yin-yang balance and supports self-regulation, not just as a theory, but as a biological reality.

21

The Science of Balance - What Research Reveals About Acupuncture and the ANS

Acupuncture has long been recognized for its ability to influence the nervous system in order to promote healing, regulate internal balance, and restore function.[1] More specifically, modern studies show that acupuncture exerts many of its effects by modulating the ANS. It helps correct dysfunction in both the sympathetic and parasympathetic branches. As a result, it supports improvements in physiological and emotional health outcomes.[2]

The ANS, as reviewed in Chapter 3, influences nearly every bodily system. It plays a key role in cardiovascular function, digestion, respiration, immune activity, and emotional regulation. This broad influence helps explain why acupuncture holds such a wide therapeutic scope. When used strategically, it can help restore homeostasis. It also eases chronic pain and supports the treatment of many conditions linked to nervous system dysregulation.[3]

The following section highlights key research studies that explore acupuncture's regulatory effect on the ANS, organized by clinical focus. These studies further confirm what has been understood in TCM for centuries: when we balance the nervous system, the body remembers how to heal.

How Acupuncture Affects the ANS

As mentioned in previous chapters, the ANS governs the body's involuntary physiological functions. These include blood pressure, heart rate, HRV, skin temperature, pupil dilation, gastrointestinal activity, and muscle nerve response. It acts as the body's internal regulator, helping us adapt to changes in both our external environment and emotional states.[4]

In a comprehensive review (2022), acupuncture research was complied from a wide range of clinical and experimental studies, supporting acupuncture's ability to influence the ANS. This research highlighted that acupuncture does more than offer temporary relief. It exerts significant measurable and biologically effect on autonomic regulation.

The findings reveal that acupuncture modulates key autonomic markers, including skin conductance, HRV, blood pressure, and muscle activation. These physiological shifts indicate changes in sympathetic and parasympathetic tone, reflecting real-time nervous system adjustments in response to treatment. Importantly, these effects are not limited to laboratory measurements, they translate into meaningful clinical outcomes.

The review further identifies a wide range of conditions that benefit from acupuncture's regulatory effects on the ANS, particularly those rooted in imbalance or dysregulation. These include chronic and acute pain disorders, depression and anxiety, mood disturbances, cardiovascular conditions such as hypertension, arrhythmia, and palpitations, as well as digestive challenges including nausea, functional dyspepsia, and impaired gastric motility. Taken together, this body of research illustrates that acupuncture works beyond surface-level symptom relief, addressing the deeper rhythms of regulation within the body. It engages the body's core regulatory systems, helping to re-establish balance and restore homeostasis. By directly modulating the ANS, acupuncture offers a powerful therapeutic approach to conditions that are often resistant to conventional treatments, bridging ancient practice with modern physiological insight.

Acupuncture, HRV, and the Vagal Response

As previously discussed, one of the primary indicators of ANS regulation is HRV. This measure reflects the subtle fluctuations between heartbeats and serves as a window into the balance between sympathetic and parasympathetic tone. Higher HRV is typically linked to greater resilience, adaptability, and healthy vagal function.

In a comprehensive review (2021) scientist looked into the influence of acupuncture on ANS regulation was explored through the biomarker of HRV.[6] Drawing from several clinical and experimental studies, the authors systematically analyzed how acupuncture impacts HRV, a widely accepted, non-invasive indicator of autonomic balance and vagal tone.

Their findings revealed consistent evidence that acupuncture can enhance parasympathetic activity, reflected in improved HRV outcomes across a wide range of patient populations and clinical conditions. Among the hundreds of acupuncture points examined, four emerged as the most frequently used for modulating the ANS:

- **Neiguan (PC6)** – commonly used for calming the heart and regulating emotional states.
- **Zusanli (ST36)** – a potent point for digestive and immune support, also known to influence vagal tone.
- **Fengchi (GB20)** – often applied in the treatment of headaches, dizziness, and hypertension, suggesting its role in sympathetic down-regulation.
- **Hegu (LI4)** – a powerful point for pain modulation and stress reduction, with measurable autonomic effects.

These points were not only among the most studied, but also consistently associated with statistically significant improvements in HRV parameters. These findings also indicated enhanced parasympathetic activation and greater vagal modulation.

HRV is recognized as a direct and reliable measure of autonomic tone, especially in relation to parasympathetic (vagal) input. When acupuncture enhances HRV, it signals a physiological shift toward greater balance, regulation, and resilience. These are fundamental principles upheld in both TCM and modern neurobiology.[7]

Together, these findings reinforce the idea that acupuncture can access deep regulatory systems through specific and strategic point selection, supporting its ability to treat not just symptoms, but the autonomic roots of chronic illness

Neuroimaging Confirms Acupuncture's Effect on the Central Nervous System

Advancements in neuroimaging have opened new pathways for understanding how acupuncture affects not only peripheral nerve signaling but also central nervous system function and autonomic regulation. In a pivotal 2013 study, Takamoto and colleagues utilized both positron emission tomography (PET) and functional magnetic resonance imaging (fMRI) to investigate the central mechanisms of acupuncture's effects on the human brain.[8]

Their research involved stimulating specific acupuncture points while monitoring real-time changes in cerebral blood flow and brain activity. The imaging data revealed a consistent pattern. Acupuncture led to the *deactivation* of several key brain regions associated with cognitive control, motor planning, and sensory integration. Notably, these included the prefrontal cortex (PFC), the pre-supplementary motor area (pre-SMA), and the supplementary motor area (SMA). These brain structures are critical for regulating conscious attention, voluntary movement, and the processing of sensory stimuli. These functions are often heightened in stress-related states.

The deactivation of these regions was found to correlate with a measurable shift in autonomic tone. Specifically, participants demonstrated a reduction in sympathetic nervous system activity. This is the hallmark of the fight-or-flight response. At the same time, there was an increase in parasympathetic activation, which governs rest, digestion, and internal repair mechanisms. Physiological measures such as heart rate and respiration rate supported this shift, confirming a move toward a more regulated, restorative state.

What makes this study particularly significant is its ability to trace acupuncture's effects from the surface of the body (meridian stimulation)

all the way to the central command centers of the brain. This central-peripheral linkage provides a neurobiological explanation for acupuncture's far-reaching therapeutic effects, from reducing anxiety and pain to improving digestion and cardiovascular function. It also reinforces the TCM perspective that balance is not merely localized, it is orchestrated throughout the entire mind-body system.

By illuminating the brain's response to acupuncture, Takamoto et al. (2013) contribute valuable evidence to a growing body of research that positions acupuncture as a scientifically grounded method of influencing both peripheral and central autonomic regulation.

Acupuncture, Skin Conductance, and Sympathetic Activation

In a 2012 study, experts Krista Lynne Paulson and Barbara L. Shay explored how acupuncture affects the ANS by measuring changes in skin conductance and temperature.[9] These are two key markers of sympathetic nervous system activity.

This single-blind, randomized controlled trial included 36 healthy adults who had not participated in forearm strength training or any repetitive upper body exercise. All participants were asked to perform a fatiguing wrist extension protocol to induce delayed onset muscle soreness (DOMS). They were then randomly assigned to one of three groups:

- **Group 1**: No treatment
- **Group 2**: Acupuncture treatment
- **Group 3**: Sham acupuncture (placebo-controlled)

Skin conductance and temperature were measured 20 minutes prior to treatment, during the 25-minute intervention, and again 10 minutes afterward.

The ANS regulates both skin perfusion and temperature.[10] This study aimed to determine if acupuncture would elicit a physiological shift. The results were clear. The acupuncture group experienced a significant increase in skin perfusion and electrical conductance. They also showed a decrease in skin temperature. These markers are consistent with sympathetic nervous system activation.[11]

These findings add to the growing body of evidence that acupuncture influences internal organ systems. It also creates measurable changes at the surface level of the body. These surface changes reflect deeper shifts within the ANS. By stimulating specific points, acupuncture appears to activate neurovascular responses and alter thermoregulation, supporting its role as a precise tool for restoring nervous system function.

Acupuncture, Norepinephrine, and Sympathetic Nervous System Modulation in Humans

Our nervous system is always adjusting, rising to meet challenges and settling back toward rest. In some conditions, that balance leans too heavily in one direction, leaving the body less able to find ease. Researchers have been looking into how acupuncture might help restore a calmer rhythm. A clinical study with patients living with heart failure explored this question, looking at how acupuncture could influence the signals of the sympathetic nervous system during mild stress.[12]

In this investigation, experts examined how acupuncture influenced autonomic activity in patients with heart failure. These individuals are known to exhibit elevated sympathetic tone and reduced parasympathetic function.

Participants were subjected to mild mental stress, a condition that typically provokes a measurable increase in sympathetic nervous system activity. The researchers then administered acupuncture and monitored changes in key physiological markers, including plasma norepinephrine (NE) levels and muscle sympathetic nerve activity (MSNA). Both NE and MSNA serve as direct indicators of sympathetic arousal.

Remarkably, acupuncture was found to significantly suppress sympathetic outflow. Plasma norepinephrine levels dropped, and muscle sympathetic nerve activity decreased, indicating a calming shift in autonomic tone. This evidence supports the idea that acupuncture can rebalance the ANS by down regulating sympathetic activity. This is the very system involved in our stress response, pain perception, and cardiovascular health.

These findings contribute to the growing body of evidence demonstrating that acupuncture does more than just stimulate nerves locally. It exerts system-wide effects, including the regulation of neurotransmitters and neurohormones that govern emotional and physiological balance. Lower norepinephrine levels may explain why many patients experience not only reduced pain, but also a sense of calm and improved emotional resilience after treatment.

22

From Systemic Balance to the Wandering Nerve

Emerging research aligns with foundational principles of TCM. Through pulse assessment, channel theory, and clinical experience, it has long recognized acupuncture's ability to initiate deep physiological regulation. Acupuncture initiates these changes by engaging the body's core regulatory systems. From modulating neurotransmitters like norepinephrine to shifting HRV and inflammatory markers, the ANS emerges as a central player in how the body responds to needling.

Among the many components of the ANS, the vagus nerve has received increasing scientific attention for its role in healing, maintaining homeostasis, and regulating emotions.

In this chapter, we will explore how this remarkable nerve, sometimes referred to as the "wandering healer," serves as a key interface between acupuncture, the brain, and the body's inner terrain of safety and restoration.

The Wandering Healer - Understanding the Vagus Nerve

As discussed in earlier chapters, the vagus nerve, also called the tenth cranial nerve, originates from the medulla oblongata and travels through the neck, chest, and abdomen. Along the way, it connects with several major organs, including the heart, lungs, and digestive system.[1] Its name, which means "wandering" in Latin, reflects its broad influence throughout the body. About 80 percent of its fibers are sensory afferents that carry information from the organs to the brain, while the remaining 20 percent are motor efferents that send signals from the brain to the body. This two-way communication helps regulate vital autonomic functions such as heart rate, breathing, and digestion.[2]

From Nerve to Immunity - The Science Behind Acupuncture's Healing Potential

For centuries, healers have observed that when the mind calms, the body follows. In TCM, this is spoken of as harmony between the Shen and the body's vital currents. In science, the same truth is traced through the vagus nerve. It is here, along this wandering pathway, that the nervous system communicates directly to the immune system. In a detailed review by clinicians Kavoussi and colleagues (2007), research highlighted the crucial role of the vagus nerve in mediating parasympathetic-driven anti-inflammatory effects.[3] Specifically, the review highlighted that stimulating the efferent (motor) branches of the vagus nerve activates the cholinergic anti-inflammatory pathway."

This is a neural mechanism through which the nervous system directly regulates immune activity. The pathway operates by signaling immune cells to reduce the production of pro-inflammatory cytokines. In doing so, it helps limit systemic inflammation.

These findings were further supported by controlled experiments in which electrical stimulation was applied to the vagus nerve of the subjects. This led to a measurable reduction in both localized swelling and systemic inflammatory markers. The results provided strong evidence that activating vagal pathways can suppress inflammation at both the cellular and tissue levels. These insights have important implications for understanding how nervous system regulation influences immune function, particularly in conditions marked by chronic inflammation.

This research provides important insight into the biological mechanisms behind systemic healing by showing that targeted vagus nerve stimulation can directly influence inflammatory processes. This offers a possible explanation for how interventions like acupuncture exert their effects.

Acupuncture can influence vagal tone, and these findings help connect Eastern medical traditions with Western biomedical research. They illustrate how neuroimmunological mechanisms support the long-held view of acupuncture as a means of restoring balance and promoting homeostasis.

Ear to the Heart - Auricular Acupuncture and Vagal Regulation

Research has shown that auricular (ear) acupuncture can directly stimulate the auricular branch of the vagus nerve, activating its afferent pathways and producing significant parasympathetic effects. Because the vagus nerve influences cardiovascular, respiratory, and gastrointestinal functions, its modulation through the ear offers a targeted approach for restoring internal balance. In a comprehensive study He et al. (2012), conducted several experimental trials examining the effects of auricular acupuncture on vagus nerve activity and autonomic regulation.[4] The following sections break down each branch of their findings by participant group and treatment approach."

In one of these trials, experts examined the effects of auricular acupuncture.[5] The technique used involved stimulating specific points on the ear that are believed to correspond to various bodily systems. The study focused on trained basketball players who received auricular acupuncture treatment after intense physical exertion. Results showed a significant reduction in heart rate within 30 to 60 minutes post-exercise. This suggests that auricular stimulation may support faster autonomic recovery and promote a shift toward parasympathetic dominance following sympathetic over activation during exercise.

In a separate arm of the same study, a second group of healthy participants was examined to assess changes in respiratory sinus arrhythmia (RSA), a reliable indicator of vagal tone. This is a non-invasive biomarker of vagal tone and parasympathetic nervous system activity. RSA reflects the natural variation in heart rate during the breathing cycle and is widely regarded as a key indicator of autonomic flexibility and resilience. The study found that auricular acupuncture led to significant improvements in

RSA, indicating an enhancement in parasympathetic modulation via the vagus nerve.

Together, these findings suggest that auricular acupuncture may support autonomic recovery, vagal activation, and cardiovascular regulation in both athletic and non-athletic populations. They also reinforce the broader understanding that acupuncture, especially when applied to auricular points with known vagal innervation, can produce systemic regulatory effects on the ANS. This contributes to homeostasis and supports the body's ability to recover from stress.

Parasympathetic Activation Through Auricular Electroacupuncture

As part of this multifaceted clinical study, He et al. examined the effects of electroacupuncture at the auricular points Erjian and Shenmen.[6] These points are traditionally associated with calming the mind, regulating cardiovascular function, and influencing systemic balance.

The study measured physiological markers before and after treatment and found a significant reduction in both blood pressure and heart rate following stimulation. These measurable changes reflect a shift in autonomic tone and suggest increased activation of the parasympathetic nervous system. The parasympathetic branch is responsible for promoting rest, relaxation, and internal regulation. Its activation is associated with reduced cardiovascular strain and improved recovery from stress.

These insights support the broader conclusion that auricular electroacupuncture has the potential to influence cardiovascular function through vagal pathways. It offers additional evidence that acupuncture does not merely affect local tissues but can exert systemic effects on core regulatory systems, such as heart rate modulation and blood pressure control. These findings also underscore the value of auricular points like Erjian and Shenmen in therapeutic strategies aimed at nervous system regulation and cardiovascular health.

The Healing Power of the Heart Point - Acupuncture's Impact on Stress and Blood Pressure

Among the most notable findings in auricular acupuncture research is the consistent and measurable impact of the heart point on the ear. This point is located within the auricular concha. It is innervated in part by the auricular branch of the vagus nerve. In TCM, it is traditionally used to regulate emotional states, calm the Shen or spirit, and support cardiovascular function.

In another arm of the same study, He et al. explored the impact of stimulating the heart Point in healthy volunteers, focusing on heart rate and autonomic balance.[7] The results showed a significant decrease in heart rate following stimulation. This indicates a shift toward parasympathetic dominance and reflects a calming effect on the ANS. It supports the traditional use of this point to regulate both emotional and cardiac activity.

A follow-up study within the same research body focused on a group of 30 individuals diagnosed with hypertension. Participants received repeated stimulation of the heart point over a defined treatment period. The study reported both immediate reductions in blood pressure after each session and sustained improvements over time. This suggests that regular auricular acupuncture targeting the heart point may offer a cumulative therapeutic effect for cardiovascular regulation.

These findings add to the growing evidence that auricular acupuncture can influence autonomic functions such as heart rate, blood pressure, and emotional regulation. The heart point, located on the ear, appears to be a key site for engaging vagal pathways that promote parasympathetic activity and cardiovascular balance. This research supports the traditional Chinese medical view that the ear reflects the entire body, and that stimulating specific points can lead to measurable shifts in nervous system function. Auricular acupuncture offers a non-invasive and clinically effective method for enhancing vagal tone, reducing stress, and supporting overall autonomic regulation.

The Concha Gateway - Surface Access to the Vagus Nerve

The auricular concha is a small, curved hollow near the ear canal. It is considered one of the most accessible areas on the body where stimulation may directly influence the vagus nerve. This region is innervated by the auricular branch of the vagus nerve (ABVN), which connects to the nucleus of the solitary tract in the brainstem. This brain region plays a central role in autonomic regulation. Because of this anatomical relationship, the concha is often targeted in auricular acupuncture and vagus nerve stimulation techniques that aim to support parasympathetic activity and systemic balance.[8]

Further supporting this anatomical insight, findings from the previously discussed study by He et al.[9] emphasize that the auricular concha is richly innervated by the auricular branch of the vagus nerve (ABVN). This peripheral branch connects directly to the nucleus of the solitary tract (NTS), a vital center in the brainstem responsible for regulating cardiovascular function, digestion, mood, and metabolic balance.

The ability of surface-level stimulation at the concha to modulate core autonomic pathways underscores the therapeutic potential of acupuncture as a non-invasive intervention for influencing internal physiological function. When applied to this zone, auricular acupuncture may help harmonize the ANS. It can reduce stress and promote systemic healing by activating vagus-mediated feedback loops.

Measuring the Shift - Auricular EA and Vagal Tone in Clinical Trials

The concha of the ear is a quiet hollow, often chosen in acupuncture for its calming influence. Modern anatomy reveals that this small space is directly linked to the auricular branch of the vagus nerve, a pathway that helps guide the body toward balance. Because of this connection, researchers have begun to study whether gentle stimulation here can shift the nervous system toward greater ease. One such investigation was led by experts La Marca and colleagues (2010). In a randomized three-arm clinical trial, they investigated the effects of auricular electroacupuncture (EA) on vagal activity in healthy male participants.[10] The study focused on the concha region of the ear, which is innervated by the auricular branch of the vagus nerve (ABVN) and is recognized as a key site for accessing the parasympathetic nervous system. To evaluate vagal tone, they measured respiratory sinus arrhythmia (RSA), a widely accepted marker of parasympathetic activity. RSA values were adjusted for tidal volume to ensure that the results reflected genuine autonomic changes rather than differences in breathing depth.

The participants were divided into three groups. One group received EA at vagally innervated points on the concha. The second received sham stimulation, and the third served as a no-intervention control. The group that received real EA showed a significant increase in RSA, while the sham and control groups did not. This outcome confirmed that stimulation of the concha produced measurable vagal activation. The study offered strong physiological evidence that auricular acupuncture can influence core autonomic functions through the vagus nerve.

Sishen Cong and the Heart-Brain Axis

Some points open not through muscle or skin, but through spirit and mind. Sishen Cong, a crown of four points at the top of the head, has been used for centuries to clear the mind and lift consciousness. Modern studies now reveal another dimension. These points also nudge the heart and nervous system back into balance, bridging heaven and body through the vagus nerve. In a 2002 study, Wang et al. explored the effects of Sishen Cong, a group of four acupuncture points located at the vertex of the head, on ANS balance.[11] The study involved nine healthy male participants, and the team recorded electrocardiograms (ECGs) over a 40-minute period. These measurements were taken before, during, and after stimulation of the Sishen Cong points.

The results were significant. Stimulation of Sishen Cong led to enhanced cardiac vagal activity. This is a key marker of parasympathetic function. At the same time, there was a suppression of sympathetic output.

This dual modulation suggests that Sishen Cong may influence the central-autonomic interface. This supports the idea that certain acupuncture points on the head affect not only consciousness and clarity, but also core physiological regulation.

This study adds to the growing body of evidence that acupuncture can shift cardiac autonomic balance, not only through auricular or abdominal points, but also through cranial point groups like Sishen Cong.

Scientific Evidence of Acupuncture's Effect on the Vagus Nerve

A growing body of clinical research now confirms what TCM has observed for millennia. Acupuncture can influence the body's internal balance through specific nerve pathways. Among these, the vagus nerve plays a central role. Often called the "wandering nerve," it links the brain with vital organs and regulates key autonomic functions such as heart rate, blood pressure, digestion, and inflammation.

From Regulation to Relief - The Next Layer of Autonomic Healing

The studies reviewed in this chapter underscore the vast role the vagus nerve plays in mediating the effects of acupuncture on autonomic regulation. Auricular points like Shenmen and the heart point. Cranial points such as Sishen Cong. Across these studies, we see consistent evidence that acupuncture can enhance vagal tone. It can suppress sympathetic activity. It supports the body's return to physiological homeostasis.

Vagal stimulation is just one branch of acupuncture's broader interaction with the ANS. In the next chapter, we will explore how acupuncture's ability to shift sympathetic-parasympathetic balance also makes it a powerful tool for treating chronic and acute pain conditions. With insights from neuroimaging, HRV analysis, and patient-reported outcomes, we will examine the mechanisms by which acupuncture reduces pain, not only by treating symptoms, but by restoring the internal communication that governs healing.

23

When Pain Signals a System Out of Balance

Pain is not only a symptom. It is a signal of imbalance. In cases of chronic low back pain, this imbalance often extends beyond the muscles and joints. It reaches into the deeper terrain of the ANS. Mounting research suggests that dysregulation within the ANS, marked by elevated sympathetic activity and diminished vagal tone, plays a central role in the persistence of pain.[1] Acupuncture has long been valued in TCM for its ability to restore balance. It is now being recognized in scientific literature as a neuromodulatory intervention.[2] Acupuncture not only influences local tissues, but also affects central autonomic networks that regulate stress, inflammation, and healing.[3] This chapter examines the growing body of clinical evidence showing how acupuncture, especially electroacupuncture, modulates the nervous system to relieve chronic pain and support systemic recovery.

Restoring Balance in the Back and the Nervous System

Chronic low back pain is one of the most common and debilitating conditions worldwide.[4] Increasingly, it is being recognized not only as a musculoskeletal issue but as a disorder with systemic effects, particularly on the ANS. The body's stress response, pain signaling, and regulation of cardiovascular function are all closely tied to autonomic balance. In a randomized controlled trial, Shankar and colleagues (2011) explored how electroacupuncture might influence both pain and autonomic function in patients with chronic low back pain.[5]

The study enrolled 60 patients with longstanding low back pain and 30 healthy volunteers who served as a baseline comparison. The patient group was randomly assigned to one of two treatment protocols. Group A received 10 sessions of electroacupuncture therapy over the course of several weeks, targeting acupoints traditionally used for back pain and autonomic modulation. Group B received standard care, which included pharmaceutical management and physiotherapy.

To evaluate the impact of each intervention, experts conducted a non-invasive battery of cardiovascular autonomic function tests. These included heart rate response to deep breathing, the Valsalva ratio, and postural changes in blood pressure, key indicators of parasympathetic and sympathetic tone. These measurements were taken before and after the treatment period to assess changes in autonomic activity.

The results were significant. At baseline, participants with chronic low back pain showed significantly reduced vagal tone and increased sympathetic activity compared to the healthy control group. This confirmed the presence of autonomic dysregulation associated with their pain condition. Following treatment, the electroacupuncture group demonstrated meaningful improvements in both pain scores and autonomic measures. The standard care group also showed minor improvements in pain. It should be noted that improvement in autonomic status appeared in both groups, but pain reduction was greater for electroacupuncture. These findings suggest that electroacupuncture may positively influence both pain and some measures of autonomic function in people with chronic low back pain, supporting its potential role as an adjunct to standard care.

This study offers compelling support that acupuncture can do more than relieve symptoms. It may also help target the deeper regulatory systems that perpetuate chronic pain. By engaging the body's internal rhythms, electroacupuncture may help restore physiological balance.

The Brainstem Connection - Acupuncture and Sympathetic Regulation

The power of acupuncture to regulate the body's internal environment extends well beyond the physical site of needling. While local effects such as muscle relaxation and improved circulation are valuable, acupuncture's deeper therapeutic potential lies in its ability to influence the central nervous system. At the core of this influence is the brainstem, a vital structure that controls essential autonomic functions like heart rate, respiration, blood pressure, and thermoregulation.

In a 1995 study, clinicians Andersson and Lundeberg explored how acupuncture affects the sympathetic branch of the ANS through its action on the brainstem and hypothalamus.[6] These areas serve as key command centers, constantly processing internal and external sensory input to fine-tune the body's physiological responses.

Their research suggests that both acupuncture and physical exercise generate rhythmic discharges in peripheral nerve fibers. These signals travel inward toward central autonomic structures, particularly within the spinal cord, brainstem, and hypothalamus. This rhythmic neural activity was strongly associated with modulations in autonomic output, influencing pain perception, vascular tone, and body temperature regulation.

In this research, acupuncture was found to affect specific hypothalamic nuclei involved in homeostasis. The hypothalamus is a master regulator that bridges the nervous and endocrine systems, controlling hormonal balance through its influence on the pituitary gland. Through this pathway, acupuncture may help recalibrate the body's response to stress, modulate inflammation, and restore physiological stability.

These ideas are especially relevant for individuals living with chronic pain or stress-related illness. In such conditions, the sympathetic nervous system is often in a state of overdrive, contributing to systemic dysregulation. By accessing central control hubs within the brain, acupuncture may help calm this heightened state and promote a shift toward parasympathetic restoration.

This theoretical framework laid the groundwork for understanding acupuncture not just as a local intervention but as a method of engaging the body's internal control systems. Anderson and Lundeberg's work supports the idea that acupuncture initiates a top-down cascade of effects that support healing, balance, and resilience throughout the entire system.

Rewiring Pain - Electroacupuncture and the Body's Inner Pharmacy

A closer look at how electroacupuncture affects chronic pain comes from a collaborative review by Zhang et al (2014).[7] Their study synthesized findings from a wide range of clinical and experimental research. The goal was to explore the mechanisms through which electroacupuncture (EA) helps alleviate persistent musculoskeletal pain in various subjects. This review reinforced the idea that EA is not simply a passive modality for pain relief. It is an active stimulus that reorganizes how the nervous system responds to stress, inflammation, and injury.

In both preclinical and clinical trials, repeated sessions of electroacupuncture led to meaningful reductions in pain intensity. Patients with chronic musculoskeletal pain who received EA reported significantly less pain over time. Some studies suggest electroacupuncture may reduce the need for pharmaceutical analgesics in certain patient populations, but this effect is not universally observed across all trials. In many cases, they also reduced their reliance on pharmaceutical opioids. These findings indicate that electroacupuncture helps activate the body's endogenous pain-relief systems, allowing for a gradual restoration of physiological balance from within.

A key focus of the review was the role of the endogenous opioid system. EA has been shown to promote the release of naturally occurring peptides such as endorphins, enkephalins, and dynorphins. These molecules bind to opioid receptors in the brain and spinal cord, helping to dampen pain signals and promote a sense of calm. Unlike external opioids, these internal chemicals work in concert with the body's existing feedback systems and do not produce the same risks of tolerance or dependence.

However, the therapeutic scope of EA does not end with opioid release. Zhang and colleagues also highlighted the impact of electroacupuncture on the sympathetic nervous system, which plays a critical role in the body's stress response. In states of chronic pain, the sympathetic system is often overactive. This leads to constricted blood vessels, reduced oxygenation, impaired tissue repair, and increased inflammation. EA helps counteract these effects by calming sympathetic output and improving blood flow to affected tissues. This shift supports both structural repair and neurological reset.

Moreover, electroacupuncture was found to modulate inflammatory pathways. It downregulates the release of pro-inflammatory cytokines while promoting anti-inflammatory signaling. This dual action helps reduce tissue sensitivity and prevents the escalation of pain into a chronic, system-wide problem.

The findings presented by Zhang et al. offer a powerful case for the integration of electroacupuncture into chronic pain care. The treatment does not merely target the physical site of discomfort. It engages the broader healing networks of the nervous and immune systems. Electroacupuncture's targeted stimulation of specific acupoints is associated with neurochemical and immunological changes that may influence the body's stress and pain response mechanisms.

Frequency, Endorphins, and the Inner Pharmacy

Scientist have long sought to understand how acupuncture communicates with the body's internal systems. In a 2004 study, Dr. Ji-Sheng Han observed how electroacupuncture (EA) stimulates the central nervous system to release a spectrum of endogenous opioids.[8] These are chemicals the body naturally produces to reduce pain and restore balance. Among them are β-endorphin, enkephalin, endomorphin, and dynorphin, each playing distinct roles in modulating pain, mood, stress, and inflammation.

What makes Han's research especially important is the discovery that different frequencies of EA trigger different neurochemical responses. Low-frequency stimulation, such as 2 Hz, increases the release of β-endorphin, enkephalin, and endomorphin, all known for their calming and pain-relieving effects. High-frequency stimulation, such as 100 Hz, boosts the release of dynorphin, a peptide associated with a more complex modulation of pain and the stress response. By alternating between these frequencies, practitioners can engage a wider range of therapeutic mechanisms.

To confirm this pathway, Han used naloxone, a drug that blocks opioid receptors. When naloxone was administered, it reversed the pain-relieving effects of EA. This confirmed that the changes were not simply mechanical or suggestive, but chemical in nature. Interestingly, higher frequencies of stimulation required larger doses of naloxone to block the effect. This demonstrated a clear, dose-responsive relationship between stimulation frequency, opioid release, and therapeutic impact.

This study provides a biological explanation for how acupuncture helps reduce pain, regulate emotions, and promote healing. It shows that acupuncture can activate central autonomic networks involved in inflammation, cardiovascular balance, and emotional regulation. Han's research supports what TCM has long understood. The body holds its own inner pharmacy. With the right input, it knows how to heal.

Calming the Circuits of Pain - Brain Rhythms and Acupuncture's Subtle Power

Modern neuroscience is beginning to uncover mechanisms that help explain acupuncture's effects on pain. Pain is not simply a message from the body. It is a full-body state involving neural rhythms, emotional responses, and patterns of internal defense. In a 2017 study, Hauck and colleagues explored how acupuncture changes brain activity in response to pain.[9] Their findings offer insight into how this gentle intervention may help quiet overactive systems and guide the body back to balance.

The researchers focused on gamma oscillations, a type of high-frequency brainwave linked to heightened pain sensitivity, sensory overload, and emotional reactivity. These oscillations tend to spike when the nervous system is in a state of arousal. During the study, participants were exposed to painful stimuli while their brain activity was monitored. Those who received acupuncture showed a significant reduction in gamma power. This suggests that acupuncture helped calm the brain's response to pain.

The study also revealed changes in functional connectivity between brain regions that regulate pain and stress. Acupuncture shifted the communication patterns between the somatosensory cortex, the prefrontal cortex, and parts of the limbic system. These regions play a role in sensation, emotional regulation, and autonomic function. The changes observed pointed to a quieting of neural pathways associated with distress and hypervigilance.

Although the observers did not directly measure autonomic markers like HRV, the decrease in gamma activity is closely associated with reduced sympathetic activation. As the brain quiets, breath slows. Blood flow improves. The nervous system begins to shift toward a more regulated, parasympathetic state. Clinically, this mirrors what many patients describe after acupuncture, a sense of relief, clarity, and internal stillness.

This study reinforces the idea that acupuncture does not simply block pain at the site. Acupuncture helps reorganize how the nervous system processes pain altogether. Through subtle, targeted stimulation, it supports a deeper re-patterning of stress, sensation, and emotion. These findings suggest that acupuncture influences how the nervous system processes pain, potentially supporting broader regulation of stress and sensation

Restoring the Rhythm: Acupuncture, Migraine, and the Brain's Balance Centers

Migraines are more than just severe headaches. They reflect deeper imbalances in the brain's sensory and regulatory systems. Many individuals who suffer from migraine without aura experience not only pain, but also sensitivity to light and sound, nausea, and a persistent sense of overwhelm. These symptoms point to widespread dysregulation involving both the sensory cortex and the ANS. A 2021 study by Tian and colleagues investigated how acupuncture affects functional connectivity within brain networks in individuals with migraine.[10]

Published in *Frontiers in Neuroscience*, the study examined resting-state brain activity in individuals with migraine, both before and after acupuncture treatment. Scholars focused on changes in functional connectivity, which refers to how different areas of the brain communicate and synchronize with one another. In migraine patients, they observed disrupted connectivity in key regions involved in pain regulation, emotional processing, and internal awareness. These included the insula, cingulate cortex, and inferior parietal lobule.

After a course of acupuncture treatments, participants showed more balanced and coordinated communication between these brain regions. This change in connectivity was associated with reductions in both migraine frequency and intensity, indicating that acupuncture may contribute to symptomatic improvement through alterations in brain network function.

While the researchers did not directly measure markers of autonomic activity such as HRV, the areas affected by acupuncture are known to influence autonomic tone. The insula plays a central role in interoception. It helps the brain monitor internal signals like heart rate, breath rhythm, and the stress response. When connectivity in this region is impaired, the nervous system tends to stay in a hypervigilant, sympathetic state. By restoring communication in this area, acupuncture may help the body shift out of reactivity and return to a more stable, regulated rhythm.

This study supports the view that acupuncture is not only a tool for managing symptoms. It is a gentle yet powerful way to reorganize the brain's internal communication. By encouraging healthy connectivity between the networks that govern pain, emotion, and internal regulation, acupuncture supports a return to coherence. It helps the nervous system remember its own rhythm and find its way back to balance.

Acupuncture's ability to relieve pain is more than a matter of muscle relaxation or endorphin release. It is a regulatory response rooted in the body's nervous system.

Together, these studies explore how acupuncture, and specifically electroacupuncture, modulates autonomic function to reduce chronic and inflammatory pain.

24

The Heart Remembers - Acupuncture, Autonomic Rhythm, and the Return to Flow

In Chapter 13, we explored the heart as both a physiological organ and an emotional-spiritual center. It is known as the "Emperor" in TCM and serves as a mirror of our inner world in modern neurocardiology. We examined how the heart reflects emotional states, trauma, and autonomic tone, bridging the ancient concept of *Shen* with the modern understanding of HRV and vagal influence.

Here, we return to the heart not to revisit its symbolic meaning, but to examine its regulation through the lens of autonomic balance and acupuncture. While the earlier chapter focused on the emotional and spiritual expressions of the heart, this chapter explores the measurable cardiovascular outcomes of autonomic intervention, particularly in patients with hypertension or at risk for cardiovascular complications.

Ancient Wisdom, Modern Frequency - TEAS and the Regulation of the Heart

The heart responds to more than pressure and flow. It also listens to the quiet signals of the nervous system and the subtle influences of touch. Acupuncture has long been viewed as a way to soften tension and restore balance within this delicate rhythm. Building on this understanding, a randomized controlled trial conducted by Ling-Hui Ma and colleagues in 2024 explored how transcutaneous electrical acupoint stimulation (TEAS), a needle-free form of electroacupuncture, might support individuals with mild hypertension.[1]

The aim was not only to reduce blood pressure, but also to explore how TEAS might influence the deeper regulatory mechanisms of the ANS. Participants received TEAS at either 2 Hertz or 10 Hertz, applied three times per week over the course of treatment. The study tracked changes in both systolic and diastolic blood pressure, along with HRV, a sensitive measure of autonomic balance that reflects the interaction between sympathetic and parasympathetic activity.

Hypertension is not only a matter of numbers on a chart. It reflects how the body's rhythms, vessels, and nerves interact under pressure. The analyst looked to see whether gentle electrical stimulation at acupoints could help ease that load.

In this trial, patients continued their usual medication while some also received TEAS several times a week. After four weeks, both groups who received TEAS showed lower systolic blood pressure compared with those who received only standard care. The 10 Hz frequency was associated with a greater reduction than the 2 Hz frequency. Alongside blood pressure improvements, the TEAS groups also demonstrated shifts in nervous system markers, including lowered heart rate and changes in HRV that suggested a move toward greater parasympathetic activity. Quality-of-life scores did not change, yet the physiological shifts hinted at the body finding a slightly more balanced state. The authors concluded that TEAS at 10 Hz may be a useful complement to conventional care, though longer and larger studies are needed to confirm its role.

This research echoes the core of TCM, where healing is seen as the restoration of rhythm and harmony. TEAS, though modern in its delivery, reflects ancient principles. It supports the body's natural intelligence and capacity for self-regulation. As the heart steadies and sympathetic tension recedes, the body remembers balance. It remembers how to regulate itself so healing can happen.

Holding the Pulse - How Electroacupuncture Supports the Heart in Surgery

The heart carries us through moments of crisis with a rhythm both fragile and resilient. When a blocked artery is reopened, blood does not always return to the smallest vessels as it should. This slow or absent flow can hinder recovery and place the heart at risk. To explore a gentler path of support, researchers in Shanghai have begun a single-center, pilot randomized controlled trial that is still ongoing. They are asking whether electroacupuncture, applied during surgery itself, might help restore microcirculation and bring steadier balance to the heart.

A study led by Yanbin Peng and colleagues explored whether electroacupuncture (EA), applied during surgery, could reduce the risk of the slow-flow or no-reflow phenomenon in patients with acute myocardial infarction (2024).[2] This complication arises when, despite reopening the blocked coronary artery, the smaller vessels fail to deliver blood to the heart muscle. It is associated with poorer recovery and a higher risk of complications after surgery. The researchers set out to see whether EA might offer protection by improving microcirculation and supporting autonomic balance during the procedure.

Sixty patients undergoing percutaneous coronary intervention (PCI) were randomly assigned to receive either standard care or PCI combined with intraoperative electroacupuncture. Treatment was given at two well-known pericardium points, Neiguan (PC6) and Ximen (PC4), chosen for their traditional role in calming the heart and improving circulation. Needles were placed with sterile technique, and low-frequency electrical stimulation was applied continuously throughout the procedure.

The main outcome was whether EA reduced the incidence of slow or no reflow, measured by angiographic assessment of coronary blood flow. The study also monitored cardiac biomarkers, markers of inflammation, electrocardiogram recovery, patient reports of chest pain and anxiety, and overall safety. Patients were followed for one month after surgery to assess recovery and any adverse events.

Even at this early stage, the trial points to an important question. Could acupuncture serve as a safe and supportive companion to modern cardiac intervention, helping the heart recover more fully after a crisis? By linking traditional points known for calming and regulating flow with one of the most advanced procedures in modern cardiology, this research opens a new space of possibility.

Healing the Heart Through the Brain - Acupuncture's Effect on Angina and Neural Balance

Acupuncture is well known for its ability to relieve chest discomfort in people with chronic stable angina, but how it works deep within the body has remained a mystery. A recent clinical study by Lei Lan and colleagues (2022) set out to explore what happens inside the brain when acupuncture is used to treat this condition.[3] Their goal was to better understand the relationship between the brain, the heart, and the specific acupoints used in TCM.

The researchers worked with patients diagnosed with chronic stable angina pectoris and compared their brain scans to those of healthy individuals. They also divided patients into two treatment groups. One group received acupuncture at points directly associated with the heart meridian. The other group was treated at points related to the heart only indirectly. The study used resting-state functional MRI to observe changes in brain activity before and after treatment.

What they found was compelling. Before treatment, patients with angina showed unusually high activity in areas of the brain linked to visual processing, pain perception, and emotional regulation. After acupuncture, these regions calmed down. In particular, a region known as the calcarine cortex became significantly less active. This part of the brain, though involved in vision, is also connected to how we interpret pain and regulate stress.

The real breakthrough came when researchers studied how this brain region communicated with others. Patients who received acupuncture on heart meridian points showed increased connectivity between the calcarine cortex and areas like the hippocampus, thalamus, and middle cingulate cortex. These are brain regions involved in regulating pain, memory, emotional stress, and, importantly, ANS function. Strengthening these connections suggests that acupuncture may help restore communication between the brain and heart, calming the nervous system from the top down.

The study also confirmed a long-held belief in Chinese medicine: the choice of acupoints matters. Those treated with heart-specific points experienced deeper and more widespread changes in their brain function. This supports the traditional view that the heart meridian plays a central role in both emotional and cardiovascular regulation.

This research offers modern evidence for a timeless idea. The heart is not just a physical organ. It is a vessel of feeling, perception, and connection. Acupuncture appears to influence this system by quieting overactive brain circuits and strengthening the neural pathways that link the brain to the heart. In doing so, it offers a path not just for symptom relief, but for deeper healing and restored balance.

Restoring Rhythms - Acupuncture and the Intelligence of the Heart

The human heart does more than circulate blood. It reflects our inner world, responding to stress, safety, emotion, and environment. Scientist study this connection by examining HRV, which measures the slight changes in time between each heartbeat. A well-regulated nervous system allows the heart to respond flexibly, adjusting to the body's needs in each moment. When this balance is disrupted, HRV can become erratic or rigid, often signaling chronic stress or dysfunction.

In a clinical study led by Ole Bernt Fasmer and colleagues (2012), explored how acupuncture influences this subtle rhythm of the heart.[4] Forty patients with a variety of conditions, including insomnia, back pain, and digestive concerns, received individualized acupuncture treatments. Their heart rhythms were recorded before, during, and after the sessions using advanced HRV analysis.

The results revealed a fascinating pattern. Acupuncture did not simply stimulate or sedate the heart. Instead, it brought about a sense of order. The overall variability in heart rhythms decreased, suggesting a calming effect on scattered or chaotic fluctuations. At the same time, the measure known as sample entropy increased. This indicates that the heart rhythm became more complex and adaptive, a sign of improved nervous system resilience. Rather than suppressing the system, acupuncture appeared to refine it, allowing the heart to beat with greater coherence and intelligence.

Notably, the balance between sympathetic and parasympathetic input remained stable. This shows that acupuncture does not force the body into one extreme or another. Instead, it helps the system reorganize itself from within, encouraging a more harmonious and integrated response.

This study supports the core idea found in both TCM and modern neurocardiology: healing occurs when the body remembers how to regulate itself. Acupuncture may serve as a gentle signal that helps the heart and nervous system return to their natural rhythm, restoring flow and balance where it was once disturbed.

A Lasting Shift - How Electroacupuncture Helps Regulate Blood Pressure

High blood pressure is often called the silent killer. It strains the heart and blood vessels, increasing the risk of stroke, heart attack, and chronic disease. While medication can help manage it, clinicians have long been curious about how acupuncture might offer a deeper, more systemic solution.

A clinical trial conducted by Peng Li et al (2015) offered compelling insight.[5] In this randomized controlled study, patients with mild to moderate hypertension received a series of electroacupuncture treatments over the course of eight weeks. Electroacupuncture uses a gentle electrical current applied to traditional acupuncture needles. The treatment focused on points such as Pericardium 5 and 6 and Stomach 36, which are traditionally known to calm the heart, regulate qi, and strengthen overall circulation.

The study revealed meaningful improvements. Patients who received electroacupuncture experienced a significant drop in both systolic and diastolic blood pressure. Even more remarkable, these improvements lasted for up to a month after the treatments had ended. This suggests that acupuncture's effects were not just immediate but enduring.

What made this study especially important was its exploration of how acupuncture achieved these results. Experts found that electroacupuncture helped calm overactivity in the sympathetic nervous system. This is the part of the ANS that governs the body's stress response. When it is too active, blood vessels constrict, and blood pressure rises. By quieting this system, acupuncture helped open the vessels and reduce the heart's workload. The treatment also appeared to influence the renin-angiotensin system, a hormone pathway closely tied to blood pressure regulation.

This trial offers modern confirmation of what TCM has long taught. The body holds an innate ability to return to balance when gently guided. Acupuncture does not force change. It invites the nervous system to settle and remember its rhythm. In doing so, it helps the heartbeat with more ease and the vessels relax into flow. This is not only healing, it is regulation at its deepest level.

Returning to Rhythm

Together, these studies illuminate a shared truth. Whether we observe the body through the lens of TCM or modern neurocardiology, the message is the same. The heart thrives in rhythm. It is shaped not only by anatomy and blood flow, but by emotion, perception, and the dynamic balance of the ANS. Acupuncture, as shown across diverse clinical settings such as hypertension, surgery, angina, and anxiety, helps restore this rhythm. It calms excessive drive without dulling vitality. It strengthens flow without forcing direction. The needles may be fine, the currents gentle, but the effects are profound. They remind the body how to regulate, not through control, but through resonance. In this quiet recalibration, the heart begins to remember its nature.

25

Regulating the Gut - Acupuncture, Autonomic Balance, and Digestive Health

The foundational view on digestion in TCM was explored in depth in Chapter 15. There, we examined the roles of the stomach, spleen, and the Yi, the spirit associated with thought, and how they contribute to both physical and mental digestion. These organs are responsible not only for transforming food into usable energy but also for integrating thought and emotion. We also discussed how chronic worry, overthinking, and emotional stress can disrupt the middle jiao and lead to a range of digestive symptoms.

This chapter builds on that foundation by shifting the focus toward the physiological regulation of digestion through the ANS. While TCM uses terms like qi stagnation, dampness, and spleen deficiency, modern medicine speaks of altered motility, vagal dysfunction, and sympathetic overactivity. Both systems recognize that the gut is highly sensitive to internal imbalance, particularly under chronic emotional strain.

Acupuncture has long been used to support digestion, ease gastrointestinal discomfort, and restore appetite. Its effects are now being confirmed by scientific research, which shows that acupuncture influences the ANS in meaningful ways. Studies have documented improvements in vagal tone, reductions in visceral hypersensitivity, and positive changes in gut-brain communication in conditions such as irritable bowel syndrome and functional dyspepsia.

What emerges is a unified view. Acupuncture does not act on the gut alone. It affects how the nervous system modulates digestion, responds to stress, and restores internal balance. In the sections ahead, we explore the clinical research behind these effects and consider how acupuncture serves as both a therapeutic and regulatory tool for digestive health.

The Middle Path - How Acupuncture Balances the Gut

Digestion is a mechanical process, and it is also a reflection of balance between body, mind, and spirit. When the rhythms of nourishment are disrupted, the entire system can feel unsettled. Acupuncture has long been used to restore this inner harmony, and modern research is beginning to reveal how its influence extends into the subtle networks that regulate the gut. A review by Toku Takahashi (2011), offers a broad perspective on how acupuncture can support digestive health.[1] The study highlights acupuncture's therapeutic potential across a wide range of gastrointestinal disorders, including functional dyspepsia, irritable bowel syndrome (IBS), diabetic gastroparesis, constipation, diarrhea, postoperative ileus, and visceral hypersensitivity.

Rather than addressing symptoms in isolation, acupuncture appears to influence the deeper regulatory systems that govern digestive function. Takahashi explains how acupuncture modulates both central and peripheral pathways, promoting healthy gut motility, calming visceral pain, and supporting the natural rhythm of peristalsis. These effects are understood to occur through shifts in ANS activity, particularly through enhanced vagal tone and changes in neurochemical signaling.

What makes this review especially valuable is its integration of traditional and modern views. It connects the classical wisdom of TCM, which emphasizes harmony and flow in the digestive organs, with contemporary research on the brain-gut axis and autonomic regulation. The findings affirm that acupuncture offers more than symptom relief. It helps restore the dynamic balance that underlies healthy digestion.

Acupuncture, Autonomic Flow, and Digestive Renewal

The gut is often called our second brain, a place where emotion and physiology meet. Within its quiet rhythms lies a conversation between the nervous system, the immune system, and the ancient patterns of nourishment. Acupuncture has been used for centuries to ease digestive distress, yet only recently has science begun to uncover the pathways that connect the needle to the body's deepest regulatory networks. A significant study on acupuncture and autonomic regulation comes from Yu-Wei Li and colleagues (2022), who published a comprehensive review in *Frontiers in Neuroscience*.[2] The authors explored how the ANS may serve as a key mediator of acupuncture's therapeutic effects, particularly in digestive and visceral regulation.

According to their findings, stimulation at points such as ST36, ST37, and ST25 was frequently associated with measurable improvements in gastrointestinal function. These acupoints were shown to influence vagal activity, enhance parasympathetic tone, and support the regulation of intestinal permeability. The researchers proposed that acupuncture acts through a brain–gut–nerve circuit, involving both afferent and efferent vagal pathways as well as key brainstem centers that modulate digestive and immune responses.

Although many of the studies reviewed were preclinical in design, the authors emphasized that the mechanisms uncovered through controlled experimentation provide valuable insights into how acupuncture may restore homeostasis. These mechanisms included improvements in motility, suppression of inflammation, and regulation of sympathetic and parasympathetic balance.

The review also highlights the broader concept that the ANS is not simply a passive responder, but a dynamic interface through which acupuncture communicates with the body's internal environment. By targeting specific points, practitioners may be influencing both neural and immunological systems that contribute to healing, especially in the digestive tract.

This synthesis of neuroanatomy, physiology, and TCM theory reinforces the long-held belief that acupuncture supports the body's innate capacity to rebalance and repair. It provides a compelling modern framework for understanding why points like ST36 are repeatedly used across conditions involving the gut, stress, and systemic inflammation.

The Nervous System in Motion - Acupuncture and Gastrointestinal Rhythm

Digestion is shaped by rhythms of movement that are easily disrupted by stress, illness, or emotional strain. When these rhythms falter, the nervous system often holds the key. Acupuncture, with its precise selection of points, has been observed to influence these patterns in ways that align the gut with a state of greater ease. Modern research is now beginning to map how stimulation at different regions of the body communicates through autonomic pathways to either calm or enliven digestive function. In a comprehensive review by, Zhi Yu (2020) examined how acupuncture influences gastrointestinal motility through its effects on the ANS.[3] The study revealed that acupuncture points located on different regions of the body produce distinct responses, depending on how they interact with either sympathetic or parasympathetic pathways.

Stimulation of abdominal acupuncture points was found to inhibit the movement of the stomach, duodenum, and jejunum. This response was linked to the activation of sympathetic efferent nerves, which are typically associated with slowing digestive function during times of stress or heightened alertness. In contrast, acupuncture points located on the limbs, particularly the lower extremities, were found to facilitate gut motility. These effects appeared to occur through stimulation of vagal efferent nerves, which support digestion, repair, and restoration.

Yu's review also noted that specific lower limb points, such as ST36 and ST37, are capable of activating sympathetic responses under certain conditions. When electroacupuncture was applied at these points in healthy individuals, researchers observed an increase in sympathetic nervous system activity. This was measured using HRV and a technique called microneurography, which records nerve signals in real time from the peroneal nerve.

The study emphasizes that acupuncture does not produce a single, uniform response. Its effects are shaped by the selection of points, the method of stimulation, and the individual's baseline nervous system tone. These findings help clarify how acupuncture can be used to either stimulate or calm gastrointestinal activity, depending on the therapeutic need.

Unlocking Motility - How ST36 and Auricular Points Stimulate Digestion

The digestive system does not move on its own. Its rhythm is guided by an ongoing dialogue between nerves, muscles, and the subtle signals of the parasympathetic branch of the ANS. When this dialogue is disrupted, digestion may slow or become irregular. Acupuncture has been shown to reawaken these rhythms, inviting the gut to return to its natural flow. Research, Han Li and Yin-Ping Wang (2013) explored the effects of acupuncture on gastrointestinal motility by stimulating specific auricular and body acupuncture points.[4] The research involved stimulation at points corresponding to the stomach and small intestine, as well as the well-known point ST36.

The results showed that stimulation at these points significantly increased gastrointestinal motility (as assessed by GI transit rate), suggesting an association between acupuncture and enhanced digestive function. The researchers observed that both auricular acupuncture and body acupuncture (ST36) produced similar improvements in gastrointestinal motility.

When the team introduced atropine, a substance known to block parasympathetic (vagal) activity. When atropine was administered, the pro-motility effects of the acupuncture stimulation were no longer present. This finding strongly suggested that the observed improvements in gastrointestinal function were mediated through the vagus nerve, a central player in the parasympathetic nervous system.

The study supports that acupuncture at certain points can enhance gastrointestinal motility via vagal pathways, though no significant change in HRV (a vagal activity marker) was observed

Vagal Pathways to Relief - TEA for Constipation in Stroke Recovery

Constipation after serious illness is more than discomfort. It is a sign that the body's inner rhythms have been disrupted, often reflecting the strain placed on both the nervous system and the gut. When the natural flow of elimination slows, healing can feel stalled. Acupuncture-inspired approaches, even in their modern adaptations, are being explored as ways to restore this flow by working with the body's regulatory networks rather than against them. A clinical study conducted by Liu and colleagues (2018) examined the use of transcutaneous electrical acustimulation, or TEA, in addressing constipation following ischemic stroke.[5] This type of constipation is a common complication that can significantly affect recovery and quality of life, yet it is often difficult to treat with standard approaches. The experts set out to explore whether TEA could support bowel function by influencing the ANS.

The study enrolled 86 individuals recovering from ischemic stroke. Participants were randomly assigned to receive either active TEA or a sham treatment for comparison. TEA involves the application of gentle electrical stimulation to acupuncture points using surface electrodes, making it a noninvasive technique modeled after traditional acupuncture.

Over a two-week period, participants tracked their bowel movements using daily diaries and the Bristol Stool Form Scale, a clinical tool used to assess stool consistency and frequency. In addition, electrocardiogram recordings were used to evaluate ANS activity through HRV, providing insight into changes in sympathetic and parasympathetic function.

The results showed clear benefits for those who received TEA. Participants experienced more frequent bowel movements, less straining during elimination, and a reduced need for laxatives. Physiologically, the TEA group showed signs of increased vagal activity and decreased sympathetic nervous system tone, which suggested that improvements in bowel function were closely tied to shifts in autonomic regulation.

These findings suggest that TEA, by modulating ANS activity through increased vagal tone, may help improve bowel function in patients with disrupted nervous system regulation after ischemic stroke. It also suggests that TEA may help regulate the ANS, which plays a key role in digestive health, in patients with post-stroke constipation.

Restoring Autonomic Balance - Electroacupuncture for Acute Pancreatitis

Inflammation is often the body's first language of distress. When it rises beyond measure, it can overwhelm organs and unsettle the delicate balance that keeps us alive. Acupuncture has long been seen as a method to calm internal storms, and modern research is beginning to show how this may occur through the body's own regulatory networks. By engaging the vagus nerve, acupuncture appears to quiet inflammation at its roots, offering new possibilities for conditions once thought to be beyond its reach. Research led by Zhang and colleagues (2021) explored the effects of electroacupuncture (EA) in the treatment of acute pancreatitis.[6] Pancreatitis is a serious inflammatory condition that can lead to organ failure and widespread systemic complications. The analyst aimed to understand how EA might influence inflammation through autonomic pathways, particularly by engaging the vagus nerve.

To do this, they used two well-established experimental models of acute pancreatitis. EA was applied at the acupuncture point ST36, a point commonly used in both clinical and research settings for its systemic regulatory effects. Following treatment, the researchers observed a significant increase in vagus nerve activity along with a reduction in systemic inflammation. This was accompanied by improvements in pancreatic tissue health, including fewer signs of cellular damage and a decrease in leukocyte infiltration, which is a marker of immune system overactivation.

One of the strengths of the study was its use of HRV to assess changes in ANS balance. Electrocardiographic signals were recorded immediately after treatment, and the ratio of low-frequency to high-frequency (LF/HF) components was analyzed. This ratio is commonly used as an indicator of sympatho-vagal balance. A higher LF/HF ratio indicates sympathetic nervous system dominance, whereas a lower LF/HF ratio reflects increased parasympathetic (vagal) activity.

Following EA at ST36, the LF/HF ratio shifted in favor of parasympathetic tone, suggesting that acupuncture promoted a calming, anti-inflammatory response through vagal activation. This supported the conclusion that EA exerts protective effects in acute pancreatitis by activating the cholinergic anti-inflammatory pathway mediated by the vagus nerve.

This research adds to the growing body of research showing that acupuncture can have far-reaching effects on inflammation, not by targeting the affected organ directly, but by regulating the nervous system that governs immune response and internal balance. In the context of acute pancreatitis, these findings offer hope for non-invasive approaches that support healing by restoring autonomic and immune harmony.

From Points to Pathways - Modulating Pain Through Autonomic Regulation

Pain can be one of the most overwhelming aspects of illness, often eclipsing every other part of the healing journey. In conditions like acute pancreatitis, pain is not only a symptom but a reflection of deep internal inflammation and nervous system strain. Acupuncture has been used for centuries to ease suffering, and modern research is beginning to ask whether its benefits can extend even into the most severe clinical settings. A clinical trial designed by Jang and colleagues (2018) set out to evaluate the effectiveness of electroacupuncture for managing pain in patients with acute pancreatitis.[7] While previous studies had shown that electroacupuncture could reduce the severity of pancreatitis in experimental settings, its ability to relieve pain in human patients had not yet been formally assessed.

The trial was conducted as a randomized, controlled, three-arm, multi-center study. Patients diagnosed with acute pancreatitis were randomly assigned to one of three groups: a control group that received standard medical care alone, a group that received local electroacupuncture, and a third group that received both local and distal electroacupuncture. All participants received conventional treatments such as fasting, intravenous fluids, and pain management, which reflect the current standard of care.

In the local electroacupuncture group, stimulation was applied to two abdominal acupuncture points, (CV12) and (CV13), which are commonly used to address digestive discomfort and abdominal pain. The group receiving both local and distal treatment also received stimulation at twelve additional points on the limbs and extremities. These included well-known points such as LI4, PC6, SP6, GB39, ST36, and ST37, which are believed to support systemic regulation and relieve internal organ pain.

Electroacupuncture was administered once daily for up to four days or until the patient's pain resolved. The primary outcome was pain intensity, measured on the fifth day using the Visual Analog Scale. Secondary outcomes included daily pain scores, the amount of analgesic medication used, time to pain relief, changes in inflammatory markers, and overall length of hospital stay.

The aim of the trial was to determine whether electroacupuncture, especially when applied to both local and distal points, could enhance pain relief beyond what standard care could achieve. The researchers proposed that electroacupuncture might influence pain and inflammation by modulating the ANS. They suggested that point stimulation may enhance parasympathetic activity through vagal pathways while reducing the sympathetic nervous system's role in driving inflammation and pain.

If shown to be effective in the completed study, electroacupuncture could become a valuable integrative option for reducing abdominal pain in patients with acute pancreatitis and supporting the body's healing response through autonomic regulation.

Tuning the Gut - Vagal Stimulation for Functional Dyspepsia

Sometimes discomfort arises not from what can be seen, but from subtle disruptions in rhythm. Functional dyspepsia is one such condition, where the stomach struggles to move with ease despite appearing structurally normal. For many, this imbalance carries not only physical discomfort but also emotional strain. Modern therapies inspired by acupuncture are now being explored for their ability to calm these hidden disturbances by working through the vagus nerve, the body's quiet messenger of balance. A 2021 study conducted by Zhu and colleagues investigated whether a noninvasive therapy called transcutaneous auricular vagus nerve stimulation (taVNS) could improve physiological dysfunction in patients with functional dyspepsia.[8] This common condition is marked by symptoms such as upper abdominal discomfort, bloating, early fullness, and nausea. While it does not involve structural abnormalities, functional dyspepsia is often linked to disrupted gastric motility and ANS imbalance, particularly reduced vagal tone.

To explore whether taVNS could offer therapeutic benefits, a two-part clinical study was conducted. In the first phase, 36 individuals with functional dyspepsia received two types of treatment on separate occasions. One session involved active taVNS applied to specific regions of the outer ear that correspond to branches of the vagus nerve. The other session involved a sham stimulation for comparison. During both sessions, participants underwent detailed testing to assess gastric function and ANS activity.

Measurements included gastric accommodation, the stomach's capacity to relax and expand after a meal, and gastric slow wave rhythms, which regulate the contractions that move food through the digestive system. These were recorded using an electrogastrogram. Autonomic function was assessed through HRV, derived from electrocardiogram readings, to evaluate sympathetic and parasympathetic activity.

The results of the active stimulation session showed improvements in all key areas. Gastric accommodation increased, the rhythm of slow gastric waves became more regular, and signs of vagal activation were observed. These outcomes suggested that taVNS had a direct impact on parasympathetic nervous system function and digestive coordination.

In the second phase of the study, the same group of participants was randomized to receive either daily taVNS or sham stimulation over a two-week period. By the end of the treatment course, those who had received taVNS reported significant improvements in dyspeptic symptoms. They also showed reductions in anxiety and depression scores. Physiological testing revealed further enhancements in gastric function and increases in vagal efferent activity. These improvements were not seen in the group receiving sham stimulation.

Compared to healthy controls, individuals with functional dyspepsia had lower vagal tone, poorer gastric motility, and higher emotional distress. The results of this study confirmed that taVNS could help restore autonomic and digestive function by enhancing parasympathetic output.

This research highlights the broader potential of therapies that target the vagus nerve. Although taVNS does not use acupuncture needles, it operates through similar neurological mechanisms. Like auricular acupuncture, it engages vagal pathways to support digestion and emotional regulation. The findings support a more integrative understanding of functional gastrointestinal disorders. These conditions may arise not solely from local dysfunction in the gut, but from deeper disturbances in autonomic rhythms. By restoring vagal tone and improving coordination between the brain and digestive system, interventions like taVNS may offer lasting relief and whole-body balance.

The Middle Path to Balance - Restoring Digestive Harmony

Acupuncture is not simply a tool for symptom relief. It is a method of restoring relationship between brain and body, organ and spirit, thought and digestion. Whether described through the language of qi and the middle jiao or the physiology of vagal tone and motility, both ancient insight and modern science affirm a shared understanding. The digestive system is highly sensitive to internal balance.

When this balance is disrupted, symptoms appear. When balance is restored, healing becomes possible. The research reviewed in this chapter demonstrates that acupuncture and related therapies influence the nervous system in ways that re-establish digestive rhythm, calm inflammation, and support the body's return to harmony. As we move forward, we will continue exploring the role of the vagus nerve, the gut-brain connection, and how restoring regulation within the nervous system creates a foundation for deep and lasting nourishment.

26

Breath and Balance - Acupuncture's Autonomic Influence on Respiratory Function

Breathing is far more than a mechanical exchange of gases. It is a dynamic and intelligent process, intimately linked to emotional states, autonomic regulation, and the internal rhythm of life. In Chapter 14, we explored the Po, the corporeal soul, and its association with the lungs, delving into the emotional and spiritual dimensions of grief, release, and embodied awareness. Here, we return to the lungs not through the lens of spirit, but through their physiological regulation and clinical relevance. TCM recognizes the lungs as the master of qi, governing respiration, dispersing wei qi (defensive qi), and establishing the body's rhythmic order.[1]

This foundational view finds meaningful parallels in modern neuroscience, where respiratory function is understood as a direct reflection of autonomic balance. Breathing patterns are now recognized as both shaped by and shaping the ANS, particularly through parasympathetic pathways and vagal tone. Emerging research confirms that changes in respiration can influence HRV, inflammation, and emotional reactivity. In this chapter, we will examine how acupuncture and breath-centered interventions regulate the nervous system, enhance lung function, and support both physical health and emotional equilibrium through the shared terrain of the breath.

Awakening the Breath Within - Vagal Access through the Auricular Lung Point

Breath is more than air moving in and out of the lungs. It is the bridge between body and spirit, shaping how we feel and how we connect with the world around us. In TCM, the lung is seen as the keeper of rhythm, dispersing qi and opening the chest so that life can move freely. Modern anatomy adds another layer, showing that the auricular lung point lies in a region of the ear touched by the vagus nerve, a key pathway of autonomic regulation.[2] In the auricular microsystem, the lung point is found in the concha of the ear. This region is not only energetically linked to respiration. It is also anatomically innervated by a branch of the vagus nerve.[3]

In a single-blind study conducted by Tanaka and Mukaiano in 1981, experts examined the neurological effects of stimulating this lung point in healthy individuals.[4] The study involved twenty-three participants and focused on a specific outcome: changes in olfactory recognition threshold. Although olfactory function might at first appear independent from respiratory processes, research indicates that olfactory pathways are connected to regions of the brainstem involved in autonomic regulation. Some of these areas participate in modulating vagal tone and other aspects of the parasympathetic nervous system, though this connection was not directly assessed in the present study.

They found that auricular acupuncture at the lung point led to a measurable reduction in olfactory recognition threshold. In other words, the participants became more sensitive to scent following treatment. This change suggests increased activity within the central nervous system. Because the lung point is innervated by branches of the vagus nerve, these results raise the possibility that stimulation of this site might activate vagal afferent pathways. However, the study did not directly test for vagal or brainstem activity, so any influence on these systems remains hypothetical.

Although the primary focus was on olfactory sensitivity, the use of a vagally innervated auricular point suggests potential broader effects on autonomic function. It is conceivable that stimulating the lung point could influence central nervous pathways beyond olfaction, such as those involved in respiratory or chest regulation, but this has yet to be explored in future research.

Breathing touches every level of our being. It reflects the nervous system, carries our emotions, and moves with the subtle currents of energy within us. Some practitioners suggest that auricular acupuncture at the lung point may help ease tension and support the natural flow of breath. While this study does not fully confirm those interpretations, it offers a glimpse into how ancient understandings of breath may intersect with emerging insights from modern neurophysiology.

Restoring Breath After Surgery - Electroacupuncture and Lung Recovery

Surgery unsettles the body's inner balance. Pain, inflammation, and stress spread beyond the site of incision, echoing through the ANS. In the aftermath of an operation, the body often shifts into sympathetic dominance. Breathing becomes shallow. The chest feels restricted. The vagus nerve quiets. These changes can impair respiratory function at a time when oxygen and calm are most needed for healing.

In a 1981 clinical study, Facco and colleagues compared the effects of electroacupuncture with the opioid analgesic pentazocine in patients recovering from hysterectomy performed through a subumbilical midline incision.[6] Electroacupuncture was administered for 40 minutes using bilateral stimulation at GB26, ST36, SP6, and auricular Shen Men.

The outcomes were carefully measured. Acupuncture provided pain relief equivalent to 30 mg of pentazocine. Yet its most distinctive effect was seen in respiratory function. Patients who received electroacupuncture experienced a significant increase in vital capacity—the volume of air moved with each full breath. This improvement was evident during the period of acupuncture analgesia and lasted for three to four hours after treatment. By contrast, pentazocine did not increase vital capacity, and lung function remained at pre-treatment levels.

These findings suggest that acupuncture does more than manage pain. By shifting autonomic tone, it supports deeper breathing and restores the rhythm of the lungs. Points like ST36 and SP6 are associated with parasympathetic activation, while Shen Men is often chosen to ease tension and regulate the stress response. Together, their stimulation may have reduced sympathetic resistance in the chest, engaged the diaphragm more fully, and enhanced oxygen exchange.

Findings from this research demonstrates that acupuncture has the potential to bridge pain relief with functional recovery. It not only soothes discomfort but also strengthens breath, creating conditions for rest, resilience, and repair in the vulnerable hours following surgery.

Rewiring Breath - Electroacupuncture and the Cervical Ganglion

Breath is more than airflow. It is a reflection of the nervous system. When sympathetic dominance constricts the airways, the body struggles to take in what it needs. But when parasympathetic tone is restored, breath deepens.

In a 2021 clinical trial, Takahashi and researchers investigated how low-frequency electroacupuncture at 2 Hz could influence respiratory function.[7] The intervention targeted a region near the cervical sympathetic ganglion, an area that helps regulate both cardiac and respiratory autonomic output.

Twenty-four healthy adults participated in the study. Each was randomly assigned to one of three conditions: no treatment, needle insertion alone, or electroacupuncture delivered at the level of the sixth cervical vertebra. Acupuncture was applied for five minutes, with respiratory function assessed before and after each session.

The results were specific. Electroacupuncture produced significant increases in peak expiratory flow (PEF) and vital capacity (VC) compared to baseline and to the no-treatment group. By contrast, forced expiratory volume in one second (FEV_1) and forced vital capacity (FVC) did not change significantly.

These findings found that stimulation near the cervical sympathetic region may improve certain aspects of airflow, possibly by influencing autonomic pathways involved in bronchial dilation.

Although this trial was conducted in healthy adults, it offers a window into how acupuncture may affect breath through its interaction with the nervous system. The results invite further exploration in clinical conditions where autonomic imbalance contributes to respiratory difficulty.

The Auriculovagal Reflex - Bridging Ear Stimulation and Systemic Healing

The ear is more than an organ of hearing. Within its curves lie pathways that reach deeply into the nervous system. The auricular branch of the vagus nerve, found in the concha of the ear, connects this outer landscape to the brainstem centers that regulate breath, heart rhythm, and digestion. For centuries, auricular acupuncture has been used to ease tension and restore balance. Contemporary science is now beginning to map the precise mechanisms behind these effects. A review by He and colleagues in 2012 examined both experimental and clinical trials that explored this connection.[8] The ABVN, located primarily in the concha region of the ear, provides a direct route for affecting central autonomic pathways through targeted external stimulation.

According to the findings reviewed, auricular acupuncture at ABVN sites was shown to increase parasympathetic tone. This was measured through indicators such as HRV, respiratory sinus arrhythmia, and changes in respiratory performance. Notably, several trials demonstrated clear improvements in olfactory sensitivity and vital capacity following auricular stimulation, suggesting a measurable impact on respiratory function.

In one controlled, single-blind analyses, stimulation of the auricular lung point led to a significant decrease in the olfactory recognition threshold among healthy volunteers. Another investigation showed that bilateral stimulation of the auricular point TF4, when combined with body points GB26, ST36, and SP6, resulted in a marked increase in vital capacity. These improvements lasted for several hours following treatment, during a period of acupuncture-induced analgesia.

Further evidence showed that auricular electrical stimulation had a positive effect on respiratory sinus arrhythmia when adjusted for tidal volume. This result was observed in healthy men and is considered a reliable indicator of increased vagal activity. These findings suggest that ear stimulation affects not only sensory and motor responses but also the core autonomic circuits responsible for regulating breath and respiratory balance.

To explain these observations, He and colleagues proposed a mechanism called the auriculovagal afferent pathway. This model suggests that stimulation of the ABVN sends signals to the nucleus of the solitary tract, a key brainstem center involved in autonomic integration. From there, these signals influence respiratory centers that control breath rate, airway tone, and pulmonary reflexes. This network may help explain how auricular acupuncture can promote bronchial dilation, improve airflow, and restore coherence between the breath and the nervous system.

While the review also noted positive effects in cardiovascular and digestive systems, the respiratory findings are particularly relevant to understanding the lungs' role in autonomic regulation. In TCM, the lungs are said to govern qi, oversee respiration, and establish rhythm throughout the body. The modern research on the ABVN reflects this classical view, offering insight into how auricular acupuncture can help regulate breath, reduce respiratory distress, and support vagal tone.

Regular stimulation of the ABVN may assist in respiratory recovery, ease tension in the breath, and contribute to emotional calm. These effects may be particularly useful in conditions like post-operative healing, asthma, or anxiety-related breath restriction. Although the early results are promising, further clinical trials are needed to clarify treatment protocols and the long-term impact on respiratory disorders.

Acupuncture and the Breath - Supporting Respiratory Recovery in the ICU

Breath becomes especially fragile in times of critical illness. When patients remain on mechanical ventilation for long periods, the body's natural rhythm of respiration can be difficult to restore. Acupuncture has been explored as a way to support this process, not only by easing strain but also by helping the nervous system find its way back toward balance.

In a 2018 retrospective observational study, Matsumoto-Miyazaki and colleagues examined patients who had been mechanically ventilated for more than 14 days in intensive care.[9] Sixteen patients were included. Half received conventional care alone, while the others received conventional care with acupuncture as an additional therapy.

The results showed that patients in the acupuncture group were more likely to be successfully weaned from the ventilator. Although this study did not measure changes in arterial blood gases such as PaO_2 or $PaCO_2$, the improved outcomes suggest that acupuncture may have helped stabilize breathing enough to support recovery.

Treatments followed a standardized protocol using points along the lung and kidney meridians. In TCM, these channels are understood to anchor breath, support fluid balance, and replenish the body's foundational reserves. The researchers proposed that their effects may also extend into autonomic regulation, calming sympathetic overdrive while encouraging parasympathetic tone.

Because this was a small retrospective analyses, its conclusions are limited. The research itself focused on respiratory outcomes and did not explore broader emotional dimensions. Still, within the larger body of acupuncture literature, breath and emotion are often seen as inseparable. The possibility that acupuncture may ease both physical and emotional restriction invites further study. These findings suggest that acupuncture has potential as a supportive therapy in critical care. It may not only relieve discomfort but also help restore rhythm to the breath, guiding the body gently toward healing.

Returning to the Breath - Rhythm, Regulation, and Repair

Throughout this chapter, we have explored the breath not merely as a physical act but as a vital expression of the body's inner regulation. From the subtle stimulation of the auricular lung point to the direct modulation of cervical and systemic pathways, the evidence reveals a clear pattern. Acupuncture reaches into the autonomic landscape and restores the natural rhythm that breathes life into the lungs and calm into the nervous system. Whether easing the shallow breath of post-operative stress, enhancing airflow in healthy individuals, or supporting critically ill patients through the strain of mechanical ventilation, acupuncture demonstrates a consistent capacity to restore coherence. This coherence is not limited to lung capacity or carbon dioxide clearance. It is a full body memory. A return to balance through the parasympathetic pulse. TCM has long viewed the lungs as the regulators of rhythm and qi. Modern research shows that intentional stimulation of the ear, the limbs, or the neck can influence the pathways that shape breath. Through these connections, the breath may be guided back into rhythm, steadied, and renewed. In this process, it is not only the lungs that find ease. The spirit softens, the mind grows quiet, and the body remembers its original cadence, the sacred rise and fall of life itself.

27

Final Reflections - A Unified Path of Healing

The research reviewed throughout this section reveals a consistent and powerful theme. Acupuncture fosters balance across every system touched by the ANS. Whether influencing heart rate, modulating inflammation, or improving digestive function, acupuncture does not force the body into submission. Instead, it invites a return to internal rhythm through the gentle regulation of sympathetic and parasympathetic pathways.

These effects are not random, nor are they limited to one domain. Classical points such as ST36 have demonstrated the ability to enhance gastric motility, support immune responsiveness, and even improve emotional resilience. PC6 and HT7, frequently used to calm the spirit, also exert measurable effects on vagal tone and cardiac coherence. This cross-system functionality reflects the foundational principle in TCM: the body is not a collection of parts, but an interconnected field of energy, constantly seeking balance.

Even in areas where modern research remains in its infancy, the emerging evidence points toward a unifying truth. Acupuncture does not merely suppress symptoms. It does not isolate the problem. It harmonizes the whole.

As science continues to explore the physiology behind these changes, new studies may further illuminate the pathways that link the vagus nerve, HRV, immune modulation, and psychosomatic healing. Even now, the message is clear. Healing begins when the body feels safe. It unfolds when the nervous system remembers its original intelligence. It restores itself when we stop pushing and start listening.

Acupuncture, in its essence, does just that. It listens. It asks the body to remember. In that remembering, balance returns.

From Healing to Longevity

As we close our exploration of the nervous system and its role in regulating physiology and supporting repair, we arrive at a deeper question. What allows the body not only to recover in the moment, but to endure across the years?

In both TCM and Contemporary science, longevity is not simply a matter of time. It is the ability to adapt, to heal, and to return to balance after disruption. The ANS is essential in this process, yet it is only one part of a larger picture.

The following section turns to other foundations that sustain vitality. By examining inflammation, vascular health, and cellular repair through classical teachings and contemporary science, we can see how acupuncture supports the inner conditions that make a long and vibrant life possible.

VI

From Regulation to Renewal

Acupuncture's Role in Healthy Aging

"Hence, they were one with the Way. That by which all of them were able to exceed a lifespan of one hundred years, while their movements and activities did not weaken."
— *Huang Di*
"Those who follow the Way are able to dispel old age and preserve their physical form."
— *Huang Di*

28

Acupuncture and Longevity - Restoring the Rhythms of Vital Aging

Longevity has never been just about living longer. Across cultures and eras, it has pointed toward something deeper. In TCM, to live long is to live in balance. This means maintaining clear qi flow, preserving jing, and keeping the spirit, or Shen, centered and luminous. These three treasures, qi, jing, and Shen, have long been regarded as the foundation of vitality and endurance.[1] As Wang Bing wrote in his commentary on the *Huang Di Nei Jing*, "When physical appearance and spirit are kept together, this is identical with an endowment of utmost longevity."[2]

Modern science echoes these insights through the study of the ANS. The ANS is the body's master regulator of stress, repair, and internal balance. As explored throughout this book, a well-regulated nervous system supports resilience. High HRV, strong vagal tone, and steady inflammatory signaling all reflect a system that knows how to recover and maintain order. This kind of flexibility is not just a physical strength. It is one of the clearest indicators of health over time.

You've seen these effects in earlier chapters on trauma, pain, digestion, and emotion. Now, these threads come together in a larger picture. Acupuncture's influence on the nervous system creates a foundation for aging that is not only longer but also more balanced, clear, and graceful.

The Wisdom of the Ancients, the Tools of Today

The *Huang Di Nei Jing* offers a meaningful observation. *"I have heard that the people of high antiquity, in the sequence of spring and autumn, all exceeded one hundred years. But in their movements and activities there was no weakening. As for the people of today, after one half of a hundred years, the movements and activities are weakened."*[3]

This ancient reflection reminds us that longevity is not just about extending time. It is about preserving coherence, strength, and adaptability throughout life. Recent research supports this idea. As the ANS becomes dysregulated with age, resilience fades. Recovery slows. Systems begin to break down. In TCM this loss of balance reflects a disruption between yin and yang. Yang is the active, outward force. Yin is the inward, restorative energy. When yang overpowers yin, the body's internal systems begin to unravel.

Acupuncture helps restore this balance. By stimulating specific points, it supports vagal tone and tempers excessive sympathetic activity. This shift is often reflected in higher HRV, a known marker of nervous system adaptability and lower mortality risk. The body becomes more capable of adjusting, healing, and responding to change

Bridging Traditions - The Roots of Longevity in Science and Spirit

The idea that vitality can be extended through internal regulation is not new. TCM has long emphasized harmony between organ systems, the movement of qi, and the balance of yin and yang as the foundation for a long and meaningful life. Current research, focus on nervous system balance, stress adaptation, and physiological resilience, affirms this view through a different language. Both perspectives recognize that longevity is not just the absence of disease. It is the presence of dynamic balance.

In the chapters that follow, we will explore how ancient texts and emerging research converge on shared principles of health and aging. From the classic teachings of the *Huang Di Nei Jing* to the latest studies in vagal modulation, inflammation, and cellular repair, acupuncture emerges as a powerful connector. It bridges time, culture, and method. And it offers us a map for aging not only longer, but with vitality, presence, and grace.

29

Key Research on Acupuncture, the ANS, and Longevity

As our scientific understanding of longevity continues to evolve, acupuncture is gaining renewed attention. It is no longer viewed only as a traditional healing practice but is increasingly recognized as a systems-level intervention that engages the body's deepest regulatory networks. Recent research suggests that the ANS is not merely a passive responder to disease or aging but an active determinant of long-term health. As explored throughout this book, the ANS serves as a core regulator of the body's internal landscape. It maintains equilibrium across vital functions such as heart rate, digestion, immunity, breath rate, and inflammation. Coordinated by the central autonomic network, this system continually responds to shifts in both the external environment and the body's internal state. Its role in supporting health, adaptability, and resilience has already been well established. Now we turn our attention to how this regulatory system intersects with the science of aging and the therapeutic effects of acupuncture.

Emerging research highlights the ANS as both a marker and a modulator of biological aging.[1] Modern preventive medicine often overlooks how subtle imbalances in this system contribute to age-related vascular decline. Standard assessments tend to focus on blood pressure, cholesterol, and glucose levels, yet HRV offers a deeper window into physiological resilience. Low HRV, a sign of reduced parasympathetic tone and limited adaptability, is consistently linked with higher risk of stroke, cardiovascular disease, and other chronic conditions associated with aging.

Rather than viewing autonomic dysfunction as a result of disease, current findings suggest it often develops earlier and actively drives degenerative change. People with stronger autonomic profiles, characterized by higher vagal tone and greater flexibility, show slower vascular deterioration, lower levels of inflammation, and greater overall vitality. These insights point to the importance of including autonomic markers such as HRV in longevity and wellness assessments, allowing for earlier detection of imbalance before it manifests as disease. Interventions that enhance parasympathetic activity appear especially beneficial for slowing biological aging and supporting long-term health. Practices that cultivate calm, regulate breath, and balance the nervous system help restore the body's natural rhythms of repair. Viewed through this lens, the ANS is not simply a background regulator but an early-warning system, reflecting how gracefully the body adapts to life's ongoing demands.

Acupuncture offers one of the clearest examples of how this system can be influenced toward balance. Stimulation of specific acupoints activates peripheral nerves that communicate with key regions of the brain involved in autonomic control. This network regulates functions such as heart rate, digestion, inflammation, and emotion. By modulating these pathways, acupuncture enhances parasympathetic tone, improves circulation, and supports the body's capacity to heal. At the cellular level, it influences neurotransmitters, immune signaling, and receptor sensitivity. These are mechanisms that together reinforce systemic harmony and resilience across the lifespan.

This understanding is further supported by research synthesizing more than two decades of studies on the autonomic mechanisms underlying acupuncture's therapeutic effects. The findings show that stimulation of specific acupoints activates peripheral nerves that relay signals through the spinal cord to brain regions such as the insular cortex, anterior cingulate cortex, hypothalamus, and nucleus tractus solitarius. These regions form part of the central autonomic network, which regulates both sympathetic and parasympathetic output to target organs. Through this mechanism, acupuncture has been shown to influence cardiovascular function, digestion, inflammation, emotional states, and pain signaling. At the molecular level, it modulates neurotransmitters, immune pathways, and receptor sensitivity, offering further support for acupuncture's role in restoring systemic balance through the dynamic networks of the ANS.[2]

Further evidence for this systems-based view comes from recent research examining acupuncture's role in regulating tumor metabolism and supporting the body during cancer treatment. Findings show that acupuncture influences both the central nervous system and the immune microenvironment, helping to ease pain, fatigue, depression, and digestive discomfort. These effects are not isolated or surface-level. They arise from acupuncture's ability to regulate the body's core physiological systems, including the autonomic, endocrine, and immune networks. By working with the body's internal terrain rather than targeting disease in isolation, acupuncture supports systemic resilience and recovery, both of which are key elements in the pursuit of healthy aging.[3]

Together, these findings present a unified perspective. Acupuncture is not merely a symptomatic therapy but a holistic approach that restores balance across neuroimmune, endocrine, and autonomic pathways. By reawakening the body's innate capacity for regulation and repair, it enhances adaptability and resilience. These qualities, now recognized as foundations of longevity, reflect a deeper truth acknowledged by both ancient medicine and modern science. The path to lasting vitality begins with restoring the rhythms that sustain life.

HRV and the Markers of Exceptional Longevity

Longevity is deeply tied to internal balance. One of the most promising physiological markers of this balance as we well know by now is HRV. This measure reflects the moment-to-moment changes in heartbeat and offers insight into the flexibility and health of the ANS.

In a study published in *Frontiers in Physiology* in 2020, Hernández-

Vicente and colleagues examined resting HRV in three age groups.[4] These included young adults, individuals in their eighties, and centenarians. Each participant was observed at rest, with key measurements such as SDNN (the standard deviation of normal heartbeats) used to assess autonomic function.

Their findings revealed a clear pattern. HRV tends to decline with age, reflecting the natural aging of autonomic processes. However, among centenarians, HRV still held predictive power. Those with SDNN values below 19 milliseconds had a higher likelihood of early death, while those with higher HRV scores were more likely to live longer. This suggests that a resilient parasympathetic nervous system remains essential well into extreme old age.

This research mirrors principles found in Chinese medicine. The Nei Jing teaches that longevity arises when the spirit is rooted and the breath flows without obstruction. HRV provides a modern biological lens into this ancient truth.

Research published in *The American Journal of Cardiology* in 2010 by Zulfiqar and Jurivich offers additional insight.[5] Drawing on 24-hour Holter monitor data from 344 healthy individuals aged 10 to 99, the researchers assessed four measures of HRV. These included indices that reflect both parasympathetic and sympathetic activity.

The results showed that parasympathetic HRV decreased sharply during early and midlife. However, among healthy older adults, especially those in their eighties and nineties, there was a surprising rebound. Those who maintained high HRV into advanced age were more likely to experience healthy longevity. This upward shift in vagal tone, observed in some individuals past their seventies, may serve as a key marker for long life.

These studies affirm that long life is not only about surviving. It is about adapting. A flexible nervous system, steady internal rhythms, and the ability to shift between rest and activity are all signals of vitality. Ancient medicine and modern science both point to the same truth. Longevity lives in rhythm. It lives in flow.

Acupuncture, Sleep, and the Parasympathetic Pathway of Renewal

KEY RESEARCH ON ACUPUNCTURE, THE ANS, AND LONGEVITY

Healthy aging is not just about how we live during the day. It is also deeply shaped by how we restore ourselves at night. Sleep is a time when the ANS recalibrates. It is during non-REM stages that the parasympathetic nervous system reaches its peak activity. This nocturnal shift into vagal dominance is crucial for cellular repair, hormonal balance, and long-term vitality.

A pivotal analysis by Umetani and colleagues (1998) helps establish the importance of this parasympathetic shift.[6] The analysts measured resting HRV in young adults, octogenarians, and centenarians. Their findings showed that while HRV naturally declines with age, individuals with higher HRV, especially those with a standard deviation of normal-to-normal intervals (SDNN) above 19 milliseconds, had significantly greater longevity. Those below that threshold had a hazard ratio for early death more than five times higher. This supports the concept that parasympathetic resilience plays a key role in healthy aging and survival.

Building on this foundation, a 2022 crossover trial by Akita and colleagues examined how acupuncture influences autonomic function during sleep.[7] Ten healthy adult males received both true acupuncture and sham-point stimulation across separate lab-monitored sleep sessions. Each subject served as his own control, allowing for a precise comparison of physiological changes.

Throughout the night, electrocardiography was used to track heart rate and HRV. The results were compelling. True acupuncture significantly lowered average heart rate across the full sleep period compared to sham stimulation. During non-REM sleep, both high-frequency and low-frequency components of HRV increased, indicating enhanced parasympathetic activity and autonomic adaptability. While REM sleep did not show significant HRV changes, heart rate still remained lower following acupuncture, suggesting a sustained calming effect.

These findings confirm that acupuncture modulates the ANS even during sleep. It promotes vagal activation, supports circadian rhythm stability, and reinforces the body's ability to repair and renew. This research adds further weight to a central theme of this book. Acupuncture is not simply a daytime treatment for stress or discomfort. It is a rhythm regulator that supports the body's capacity for resilience across both waking and sleeping states. By enhancing HRV and promoting restorative sleep physiology, acupuncture becomes a valuable ally in the pursuit of healthy aging.

Acupuncture and Survival - Cardiovascular Resilience in Chronic Illness

Longevity is not only influenced by cellular repair and nervous system regulation. It also depends on how the body sustains its vital functions through chronic disease. Among aging populations, heart failure remains one of the leading causes of mortality worldwide. While conventional treatments have improved over time, integrative therapies such as acupuncture are emerging as supportive tools that may enhance resilience and long-term outcomes.

A large-scale cohort study expanded on how acupuncture supports healthy ageing. Clinicians Hyungsun Jun et al (2025), analyzed data from over 95,000 adults with disabilities who were newly diagnosed with heart failure between 2014 and 2016.[8] Patients were divided into two groups: those who received at least two acupuncture sessions within the first year after diagnosis and those who received none. After adjusting for baseline characteristics using propensity score matching, each group included 21,001 patients with comparable clinical profiles.

Over a three-year follow-up period, the results revealed a distinctive pattern. Patients who received acupuncture had a 20 percent lower risk of death from all causes compared to those who did not receive it. Even more notable was the dose–response relationship. Those who received the highest number of acupuncture sessions experienced a 36 percent reduction in mortality risk. This protective effect was consistent across most subgroups, including older adults, women, higher-income individuals, and those with more severe disabilities. The benefits were less pronounced in younger men and individuals with mild impairment.

These findings reinforce a central idea explored throughout this book. Acupuncture is not just about symptom relief. It is a regulatory therapy that may influence deep physiological patterns, including cardiovascular adaptation, autonomic balance, and immune modulation. When integrated early in chronic care, acupuncture has the potential to support long-term survival and strengthen the body's capacity to endure.

Rather than targeting disease alone, this approach supports the terrain of the body. It promotes regulation, renewal, and resilience. These are principles that lie at the heart of both TCM and modern longevity science.

The Rhythm of Resilience and the Path to Longevity

In both ancient Chinese medicine and current science, longevity is defined by balance, adaptability, and inner rhythm. This chapter illuminates how the ANS, especially through HRV, serves as both a mirror and a mechanism of biological aging. Traditional texts like the *Huang Di Nei Jing* spoke of preserving appearance and vitality through the cultivation of internal harmony. Today, research reveals that individuals with higher HRV, greater vagal tone, and stronger parasympathetic resilience are more likely to enjoy healthy, extended lifespans.

Acupuncture emerges as a powerful tool in this context, not only by reducing symptoms but by recalibrating deep regulatory systems that govern repair, sleep, immune response, and cardiovascular stability. From improving sleep-stage HRV to reducing mortality risk in heart failure patients, acupuncture's systemic effects highlight its potential as a cornerstone of longevity medicine. It renews the rhythms that sustain life. It strengthens the body's capacity to adapt. And in doing so, it helps restore the very flow through which vitality is preserved.

30

The Pulse of Longevity - How Vessels Carry Time

Aging is not simply the passage of time. It is the gradual erosion of physiological resilience. From the biomedical perspective, this decline is driven by persistent low-grade inflammation, vascular rigidity, oxidative damage, and the progressive weakening of cellular repair mechanisms. In the framework of TCM, aging is described as the depletion of jing, the weakening of yin and yang, and the stagnation or deficiency of qi. Though the languages differ, both perspectives converge on the same truth. The pace and quality of aging depends not only on ANS function but also on the integrity of the body's regulatory systems. These systems govern circulation, immune balance, and repair. When these rhythms falter, vitality diminishes. When they are restored, longevity is nourished.

Circulation and Vascular Longevity

The classics remind us that the vessels are more than mere pathways for blood. They are *"the palaces of the blood"*.[1] Circulation is described as the basis of life itself. *"When man lies down the blood returns to the Liver. When the Liver receives blood one can see. When the feet receive blood one can walk. When the palms receive blood, they can grasp. When the fingers receive blood they can hold".*[2]

In these teachings, the liver appears as a reservoir that regulates blood flow to the senses and limbs, while the heart rules the system as a whole. As the *Suwen* states, *"The Heart rules the body's blood and vessels"*.[3] The condition of the heart is reflected in the state of the channels. When the heart is balanced, circulation flows freely, and when it is disturbed, the vessels falter.

Current clinical research now supports this vision in its own language. Vascular health is one of the clearest markers of longevity. Findings show that arterial stiffness plays a central role in overall health and survival, with age emerging as the strongest determinant of large artery stiffening.[4] Age is the single greatest determinant of large artery stiffening. Over time, the aorta and other central arteries lose elasticity, even in healthy individuals. Smaller muscular arteries retain more resilience. The central arteries that cushion and distribute the pulse, however, grow progressively rigid.

This stiffening alters the very shape of the blood pressure wave. Instead of moving fluidly and returning with ease, the pulse reflects back prematurely, creating higher systolic pressure and widening pulse pressure. In simple terms, the vessels lose their flexibility and the heart must pump against greater resistance. Research has shown that this shift is not benign. Increased aortic stiffness is strongly linked with cardiovascular morbidity and mortality. Those with greater stiffness and elevated pulse pressure face a significantly higher risk of stroke, heart failure, and death. The process is steady, advancing by roughly ten to fifteen percent each decade, and is accelerated by conditions such as hypertension and diabetes. Women tend to experience slightly less stiffness than men at the same age, yet the trajectory is shared across both sexes.

From a TCM perspective, this progression reflects the interplay of several patterns. The liver, charged with ensuring the smooth coursing of qi, loses its regulating power, allowing stagnation to form. The spleen, which governs the transformation and transport of qi and blood, weakens, leading to phlegm and dampness that obstruct circulation. Together, these imbalances manifest as rigidity in the channels, just as modern science observes in the arterial walls.

What emerges from the modern day research is a simple yet profound truth. The stiffening of the great vessels is not an isolated problem. It is a sign of the body's diminishing adaptability, a loss of rhythm and flexibility that resonates with the classical warning against stagnation. When the channels flow and the vessels remain supple, qi and blood can continue to nourish the whole body, and vitality is sustained deep into later years.

The Silent Stiffening of Time

As the years pass, the great vessels of the body inevitably change. Their once supple walls lose elasticity, and the steady rhythm of expansion and recoil that cushions the pulse grows less resilient. This decline in arterial compliance as one of the most notable signs of vascular aging.[5] In healthy adults, the compliance of the large elastic arteries such as the aorta and carotids can be reduced by nearly half between the ages of twenty-five and seventy-five.

This transformation arises from both structural and functional changes in the arterial wall. Elastin, the protein that provides stretch, begins to fray and fragment, while collagen increases, cross-links, and leaves the arteries stiffer and more brittle. Advanced glycation end products, fueled by oxidative stress and inflammation, further bind and harden the vessel wall. Smooth muscle cells within the artery multiply and migrate, thickening the intima-media layer and reducing pliancy.

Endothelial function also declines with age. The cells lining the arteries produce less nitric oxide, a natural vasodilator, while vasoconstrictor signals become more dominant. The sympathetic nervous system grows more active, stress molecules rise, and the balance between relaxation and tension in the vessels shifts toward rigidity.

The result is a steady loss of the body's ability to buffer the force of each heartbeat. Pulse waves return with greater force, systolic pressure rises, and the heart is left to work against increased resistance. Microscopic changes in elastin and collagen appear first. Over decades, these changes build. They become one of the most visible signatures of aging. Arteries stiffen. The change reverberates through every organ they nourish.

The March of Stiffness

Arteries do not all age in the same way. The large central vessels, like the aorta and carotids, gradually stiffen as the years pass, while the smaller muscular arteries of the periphery remain relatively unchanged. This stiffening alters the natural wave of blood through the body. Reflections return to the heart earlier, blood pressure rises, and the once-supple contour of the pulse grows more rigid.[6]

Clinical research highlights that this gradual stiffening is not a minor detail of aging but a direct risk factor for cardiovascular disease and mortality.[7] As arterial walls lose their elasticity, systolic blood pressure and pulse pressure climb steadily higher, placing greater stress on both the heart and the organs it serves.

The process unfolds slowly but persistently. Studies show that aortic and carotid stiffness, measured by pulse wave velocity, increases by roughly ten to fifteen percent over each passing decade. Women consistently show slightly lower stiffness than men, yet the trajectory is the same for both.

While aging is the most powerful determinant, other conditions accelerate the decline. Hypertension quickens the stiffening, particularly in older adults. Diabetes, both type 1 and type 2, exerts a strong effect, hastening the loss of vascular compliance. Patients with renal disease, heart failure, or atherosclerosis often present with marked stiffness as well, their vessels thickened, calcified, and less able to yield to the flow of life.

What begins as a gradual narrowing of resilience in the great vessels becomes, over time, one of the clearest signatures of biological aging. This presents as central arteries that harden and resist, shaping the rhythm of blood and the pace of longevity.

Acupuncture and Vascular Flexibility

While vascular stiffening has long been viewed as an inevitable part of aging, modern science shows that interventions such as acupuncture can help preserve the suppleness of the vessels. A clinical trial conducted by analysts Bentos et al (2002) explored this effect in middle-aged adults with hypertension.[8] Fifty participants were randomly assigned to receive either eight weeks of acupuncture therapy or serve as controls. They measured not just brachial blood pressure, but also more sensitive indicators of vascular function: aortic pressure, arterial stiffness (stiffness index, SI), and wave reflection (augmentation index, AIx).

After eight weeks, those receiving acupuncture showed significant reductions in brachial and aortic blood pressure, as well as measurable improvements in wave reflection and arterial stiffness. In contrast, the control group experienced no meaningful change. The findings suggest that acupuncture does more than simply lower surface blood pressure readings. It appears to act directly on the vascular system, improving the ability of the arteries to expand and recoil with each heartbeat.

From a physiological perspective, acupuncture may achieve this through several mechanisms. By modulating the ANS, acupuncture reduces sympathetic overdrive and enhances parasympathetic tone, allowing vessels to dilate more freely. It also influences the release of nitric oxide, a key vasodilator produced by endothelial cells, which supports smoother blood flow and reduces vascular tension. Together, these effects help restore the rhythm of expansion and relaxation that characterizes healthy vessels.

From a TCM perspective, these findings mirror classical teachings that acupuncture promotes the free flow of qi and blood through the channels. When stagnation is released and circulation is harmonized, the vessels remain pliant and the spirit remains well nourished. Just as the *Suwen* declared that *"the Heart rules the body's blood and vessels,"* acupuncture supports the sovereign heart by ensuring its pathways remain open and resilient.

This study shows that vascular health is not only preserved by lifestyle changes and medication, but also by restoring balance through acupuncture. The protection of vessel elasticity may be one of the key ways acupuncture contributes to healthy aging and the prevention of disease.

When the Vessels Listen

The language of acupuncture is subtle, yet the vessels listen quickly. At the crown of the head lies Baihui (GV20), a point long regarded in Chinese medicine as a meeting place of circulation and spirit. Modern research suggests that its influence reaches into the very rhythm of the arteries.[9]

In one clinical study, researcher Hiroyasu Satoh (2009) focused on needling Baihui produced an immediate shift in vascular tone.[10] During treatment, diastolic pressure and heart rate rose slightly, but the more important change came after the needles were removed. Wave reflection, a marker of arterial tension, dropped significantly and remained lower for up to forty minutes. This suggested that the vessels had been reminded how to release their grip, allowing blood to flow with less resistance.

A second pilot study conducted by Gerhard Litscher, Lu Wang, Ingrid Gaischek, and Xin-Yan Gao (2011), explored violet laser acupuncture at the same point. Researchers observed early signs of reduced arterial stiffness, measured by pulse wave velocity, along with changes in wave reflection. Though preliminary, these findings carry weight. They point to the possibility that acupuncture, even delivered by light, can influence the pliancy of vessels that typically harden with age.[11]

These studies hint at something remarkable. A gentle touch at the crown can send ripples through the cardiovascular system, softening the body's most resilient tissues. Ancient physicians taught that Baihui harmonizes the flow of qi through all channels. Science is now beginning to show that this harmony is not only energetic but also vascular, inviting the heart to work with less strain and the body to move in greater ease.

When Needles Move the Blood

For centuries, TCM has spoken of acupuncture as a way to move blood and restore balance. The classics remind us that points like Taichong (LR3) on the liver channel "regulate the blood" and "open into the eyes," while Zusanli (ST36) on the stomach channel strengthens digestion and circulation. Current findings have now given us a way to see these effects directly, allowing researchers to watch in real time as needles influence the flow of blood through the body's vessels.[12]

Researchers Shin Takayama et al (2012) used color Doppler ultrasound, a noninvasive imaging technique, to study how acupuncture alters circulation in both healthy volunteers and patients with glaucoma.[13] Their findings show that stimulation of LR3 on the foot and ST36 on the lower leg can shift blood flow in distant regions of the body in ways that reflect the classical functions of these points.

Needling LR3 produced immediate changes in the arms: blood flow in the radial artery decreased during needle stimulation, then rebounded to a higher level once the needle was removed. Even more notable was its effect on the vessels behind the eye. The short posterior ciliary arteries, which nourish the tissues essential for vision, showed a reduction in vascular resistance after LR3 acupuncture. This allowed blood to move more freely into the delicate structures of the eye. In traditional language, the liver "opens to the eyes," and here modern imaging confirms that activating the liver channel can enhance ocular circulation.

Stimulation of ST36, a point known for strengthening the stomach and spleen, increased blood flow in the superior mesenteric artery that supplies the small intestine and colon. This finding aligns with its traditional function of promoting digestion and nourishment.

The same study also included patients with open-angle glaucoma, a condition linked to impaired circulation in the eye. After acupuncture at a combination of points including LR3, ST36, and SP6, resistance in both the central retinal artery and the short posterior ciliary arteries dropped significantly. Acupuncture improved blood supply to the very tissues most at risk of damage, even in patients already receiving standard medical treatment.

The implications of these findings reach beyond the measurements of a Doppler screen. Acupuncture can directly reshape the dynamics of circulation in targeted areas: opening flow where it is sluggish, reducing resistance where vessels have tightened, and harmonizing supply to the organs.

In the language of TCM, this is the free coursing of liver qi, the strengthening of the spleen and stomach, and the replenishing of the channels that carry nourishment to the eyes and the gut. In biomedical terms, it is a modulation of vascular tone and resistance, guided by the ANS and local vascular regulators. Both perspectives converge on the same truth. Acupuncture moves blood. And when blood moves, life is supported.

Closing Reflection

Aging is the slow hardening of rhythm, the loss of flexibility in both body and spirit. Contemporary science names this process in terms of arterial stiffness, oxidative stress, and inflammation. TCM describes it as the depletion of jing, the exhaustion of yin and yang, and the stagnation of qi. Though the languages diverge, the truth they describe is the same. Longevity depends on whether circulation remains supple or grows rigid.

The vessels are more than conduits of blood. They are the palaces of vitality, the rivers through which life flows. When they constrict, the heart strains, the spirit dims, and the organs falter. When they open and move freely, resilience is restored, and years are carried more lightly.

The research we have explored makes clear that the stiffening of the arteries is not inevitable. Acupuncture demonstrates that even subtle interventions can remind the vessels how to breathe again, how to expand, release, and carry nourishment to the farthest reaches of the body. It is a therapy that speaks in the language of balance, harmonizing qi and blood in ways that modern imaging now confirms.

To preserve the pulse of longevity is to preserve flow. In every needle that loosens tension, in every vessel that rediscovers its rhythm, we see the possibility of aging not as decline, but as sustained vitality. The heart governs the vessels, but it is balance that governs time.

31

Inflammaging and Lingering Heat - The Slow Fire of Aging

In TCM, chronic inflammation can be seen as lingering Heat that smolders within the body. Sometimes it flares openly as redness, swelling, or pain. Other times it hides quietly, wearing away at strength and clarity over the years. This unresolved fire consumes yin fluids, agitates the blood, and blocks the free flow of qi. Over time, the balance between yin and yang weakens, leaving the tissues vulnerable and the spirit unsettled.[1]

Short bursts of Heat are part of the body's natural defense. When the fire does not disperse, it becomes a burden. This is what modern science calls chronic inflammation and what the ancient texts describe as pathological Heat and stagnation. The art of healing lies not in extinguishing fire altogether, but in guiding it toward resolution. In this way, the body may return to harmony and the work of repair may continue.

Lingering Heat and the Slow Fire of Aging

For centuries, physicians of TCM recognized this state as pathological heat, a concept now echoed in the biomedical idea of chronic inflammation. Rather than molecules or signaling pathways, the ancient doctors spoke of pathogenic factors that disrupt harmony when left unresolved.

Heat is one of the most corrosive of these factors. It consumes yin fluids, agitates the blood, and unsettles the Shen. For a short time, Heat serves a protective role, clearing pathogens to support healing. If it persists, it becomes a slow internal fire, smoldering beneath the surface and gradually eroding vitality.

Often this Heat binds with Dampness to form Damp-Heat, a heavy and turbid influence that obstructs the free flow of qi. These lingering patterns resemble what we now see in metabolic disease, when inflammation persists in the gut, the liver, and the vessels. Instead of cleansing, Damp-Heat stagnates and drains strength.

Both traditions converge on the same truth. Inflammation is not the enemy. It is a natural process that must run its course. Trouble arises when it is not resolved. The work of healing is to guide the fire back to balance, clear what is excessive, disperse stagnation, and replenish what is consumed. In this way, harmony can be restored and longevity supported across the years.[2]

Inflammation Across the Organs

The body carries within it both fire and water. When harmony is kept, fire rises to protect and water cools to restore. Yet when the balance falters, what was once a healing flame can turn into a slow burn that lingers within tissues and unsettles the mind. Ancient texts speak of this as heat that does not disperse. This is known as chronic inflammation in modern science. Both describe the same story. A signal meant to defend becomes a burden when it refuses to resolve.

Inflammation affects almost every organ in the body.[3] Inflammation is not always harmful. In fact, it is the body's natural defense system. When we get injured, sick, or exposed to toxins, inflammation acts like the body's emergency crew, rushing in to clean up damage and fight off invaders. When this response is short and controlled, it helps us heal and return to balance.

The trouble begins when inflammation does not turn off. Instead of protecting us, it becomes a constant low-level fire that slowly damages tissues. Over time, this ongoing stress contributes to heart disease, diabetes, arthritis, kidney and liver problems, digestive issues, reproductive disorders, and even brain conditions like Alzheimer's disease.

Scientists have found that this process is controlled by three main "switches" inside the body. The NF-κB pathway turns on genes that trigger immune responses. The MAPK pathway helps cells decide how to react to stress and injury. The JAK-STAT pathway carries messages from outside the cell directly into its command center, changing how the cell works. Together, these systems release chemicals called cytokines that summon immune cells to sites of damage. For a short time this is helpful. When these switches stay on too long, they keep fueling inflammation and prevent tissues from fully repairing.

As we have learned throughout this chapter, healing does not happen by simply suppressing inflammation. The body has to actively resolve it. This means that immune cells need to complete their job and then step back, while other cells step in to repair tissues and restore balance. If this "resolution phase" does not happen, inflammation lingers and becomes chronic. This state of long-term, low-grade inflammation is what scientists call "inflammaging."

From the perspective of TCM, these findings mirror what the classics describe as "lingering heat" and "stagnation." Heat that does not clear continues to burn up fluids, disturb the blood, and block the flow of qi. Over time, this weakens the body's foundation and unsettles the spirit. Just as modern medicine sees the danger of unresolved inflammation, TCM warns of the exhaustion that follows when internal fire is not properly guided.

Both perspectives point to the same conclusion. Inflammation itself is not the enemy. It is a natural process designed to protect and restore. The real problem arises when it does not resolve. Healing comes from helping the fire settle, clearing what is excessive, and nourishing what has been consumed. When this balance is restored, tissues repair, clarity of mind is preserved, and longevity can be supported across the lifespan.

Aging and Inflammation

The story of aging is written not only in our years but in the quiet exchanges within our cells. Signals of defense rise, repair begins, and harmony is restored. Yet over time, these rhythms can grow less steady.

What once healed with ease may now leave traces behind. In this slowing of renewal, inflammation can linger, reshaping the body's path toward health or decline.

Aging is a delicate balance between the damage that accumulates over time and the resilience mechanisms that repair it.[4]

When resilience falters, chronic diseases begin to appear. At the center of this decline is the immune system. Many have begun to hear more about the term inflammaging, which describes a persistent, low-grade activation of the immune system. It appears as elevated inflammatory markers in the blood and overactive immune cells in tissues. This state of unresolved inflammation increases the risk of nearly every age-related condition. It contributes to cardiovascular disease, diabetes, dementia, and physical decline.

Research has highlighted several root mechanisms that drive inflammaging. These include the overactivation of NF-κB and other inflammatory switches. Also noted is the weakening of immune regulation with age, known as immunosenescence. Additional factors are disruptions in the gut microbiome and maladapted stress responses in the body. Together, these processes create a cycle where damage feeds inflammation, and inflammation fuels more damage.

Inflammation is not only a marker of aging but also a target for intervention. Clinical trials show that diet, exercise, and other lifestyle practices can reduce chronic inflammation and extend the years of healthy life. This view aligns with Chinese medicine's teaching that longevity depends on nourishing balance throughout the life course. In both systems, harmony must be cultivated daily, not only through medicine but through the way one lives.

Acupuncture and the Resolution of Inflammation

Healing often begins in places too small to see. Within each cell, signals decide whether to defend or to repair, whether to inflame or to restore. Acupuncture enters this conversation quietly, yet its influence can ripple outward, touching not only the site of need but the whole landscape of the body. Recent research has highlighted on how acupuncture reduces inflammation across nearly every system of the body.[5] From the lungs and gut to the brain, joints, and circulation, studies reveal that acupuncture does more than ease symptoms. It actively shifts the body's immune response toward repair and balance.

At the local level, acupuncture changes the way immune cells behave. It helps macrophages move from a destructive, pro-inflammatory state into one that promotes healing. It quiets mast cells and regulates T cell activity, calming the storm of cytokines that drive chronic disease. It also reduces oxidative stress by increasing the body's natural antioxidants, preventing damage caused by free radicals.

Beyond the needle site, acupuncture activates a web of neuro-immune pathways that link the body and brain. Signals from acupoints travel through sensory nerves to the spinal cord and brainstem, where they stimulate the vagus nerve, the sympathetic system, and the hypothalamus-pituitary-adrenal axis. These pathways act like communication lines, releasing neurotransmitters and hormones that tell immune cells throughout the body to settle inflammation and restore equilibrium.

In TCM, this wide-reaching influence reflects the principle that treating the channels restores balance in the whole system. What the classics describe as clearing Heat and resolving stagnation, emerging research identifies as regulating inflammatory switches such as NF-κB and MAPK. Both views converge on the same insight. Acupuncture does not suppress inflammation the way drugs often do. Instead, it guides the body to resolve it naturally. This allows tissues to repair and vitality to be renewed.

ST36 and the Pathways of Healing

Known in Chinese medicine as Zusanli, ST36 has long been considered a major point for strengthening vitality and supporting immunity. Current findings now show that its influence reaches into multiple systems, from the gut and nervous system to the blood and organs. Recent research examining acupuncture at the point ST36 has revealed consistent evidence of its ability to regulate inflammation throughout the body.[6]

Acupuncture at ST36 has consistently been shown to reduce inflammation by calming overactive immune pathways. research shows that ST36 activates the vagus nerve and the body's cholinergic anti-inflammatory reflex. This reaction tells which immune cells to stand down once their work is complete. It also shifted macrophages, the immune system's cleanup crew, from a destructive state into a healing one. In addition, it quieted toll-like receptor 4 (TLR4) and NF-κB signaling. These are two molecular switches that drive chronic inflammation. Other mechanisms included balancing MAPK pathways and restoring harmony across different tissues.

From the perspective of TCM, these effects echo the traditional use of ST36 to "tonify qi and blood," strengthen the body against illness, and clear lingering pathogenic factors. What the classics recognized through clinical observation, modern studies now describe through molecular detail. Both reveal the same principle. Stimulating ST36 helps resolve inflammation. It supports the body's capacity for repair and protects vitality across the lifespan.

Acupuncture, Movement, and the Renewal of Vitality

Knee osteoarthritis is one of the most common challenges of aging, bringing both pain and limitation to daily life. In 2023, Chen and colleagues reviewed eleven high-quality trials with more than seven hundred participants to explore what happens when acupuncture is paired with active exercise.[7]

Their findings showed a clear pattern. When the two therapies were combined, people reported less pain, greater ease of movement, and stronger function in the joints. Scores on measures of pain, mobility, and range of motion all improved more in the combined groups than with acupuncture or exercise alone. Acupuncture appears to quiet the inflammatory signals that disturb the joint, while exercise supports circulation, strength, and renewal. Together, they form a partnership that helps the body move with greater freedom.

The authors cautioned that some of the measures used in these studies are subjective and that more research is needed. Yet the overall picture is encouraging. Integrating acupuncture with movement practices may offer a gentle and effective way to restore balance, reduce suffering, and help preserve vitality as the years unfold.

Just as chronic inflammation accelerates decline, practices that resolve it can slow the pace of aging. By easing pain and restoring flow, the combination of acupuncture and exercise may not only improve joint health but also support the larger goal of healthy longevity.

The Slow Fire and the Path to Longevity

Aging is not only the wearing down of years but also the gradual accumulation of unresolved fire within the body. What modern science calls "inflammaging," TCM has long described as lingering Heat and stagnation. Both views recognize that when inflammation does not resolve, it shifts from being protective to corrosive, draining vitality and weakening the spirit.

The message that emerges from both traditions is clear. Healing does not come from extinguishing fire altogether but from guiding it back into rhythm. When the flames of inflammation rise, the body must be supported in resolving them. Acupuncture, nourishing foods, mindful movement, and daily practices of balance all help the immune system complete its work, clearing excess while restoring what has been consumed.

To live with longevity is to cultivate this harmony. Each time inflammation is guided to resolution, the body repairs more deeply. Each time Heat and Dampness are cleared, clarity and strength return. Over a lifetime, these moments of resolution become the foundation of resilience. The slow fire of aging does not need to consume vitality. With balance, it can be transformed into renewal, protecting both body and spirit. In this way, life is not only extended but also lived with clarity, energy, and purpose.

32

Acupuncture and Cellular Health

Ancient wisdom and modern science intersect in their view of what sustains vitality and longevity. In TCM, this foundation is called *jing*, or essence. Jing is described as the original blueprint of life, the wellspring of growth, development, reproduction, and resilience.[1] It is what makes each person unique, shaping both constitution and vitality. Part of this essence, *pre-heaven jing*, is inherited from the parents and is considered difficult to alter once adult life begins.[2] Yet it is not a static inheritance. *Pre-heaven jing* interacts continuously with *post-heaven jing*, which is generated through food, breath, and the rhythm of daily living. When nourishment is balanced and life is harmonious, the essence is supported. When it is squandered through overwork, emotional strain, or poor diet, the reserves are consumed more rapidly. Breath practices, meditation, Tai Chi, and Qigong have long been described as ways to preserve jing. They slow the pace of decline and help reconnect body and spirit.[3]

When jing is strong, growth is steady, fertility flourishes, and recovery is swift. When it is depleted, vitality fades, immunity weakens, and aging accelerates. Jing was understood not only as physical vitality but also as the "root of life," a principle linking body, mind, and spirit in continuity.[4] Jing can be envisioned as a reservoir that holds the body's deepest reserves. At birth, each of us is given a basin of water that sets the foundation for our vitality. Daily nourishment, through food, air, rest, and balanced living, acts as rain that replenishes it. When life is harmonious, the reservoir remains full, sustaining resilience. If strain, overwork, or neglect outpace its renewal, the waters diminish, and both body and spirit become vulnerable.

Modern research translates this ancient idea into cellular terms. Vitality and longevity depend on the health of our cells, influenced by mitochondrial efficiency, oxidative stress, and the signaling pathways that regulate repair.[5] Researchers speak of the "hallmarks of aging," a framework that maps how cells change over time. Among these hallmarks are genomic instability, telomere shortening, deregulated nutrient sensing, and shifts in intercellular communication.[6] Each hallmark reflects a different way in which our inherited "essence" can erode over time. Just as jing must be conserved to preserve life, these cellular systems must remain in harmony to sustain resilience.

Among the most important regulators of aging are cytokines, the body's tiny protein messengers. These molecules carry instructions between cells and coordinate immune responses. One in particular, interleukin-11 (IL-11), illustrates how biology echoes classical theory. In youth, IL-11 plays a constructive role, supporting fertility, development, and tissue growth. But when overactive in adulthood, it becomes pathogenic, driving fibrosis, cellular senescence, and chronic disease.[7] This dual role reflects the concept of jing. When essence is abundant and well-directed, life flourishes. When it is consumed or imbalanced, decline and disease follow.[8]

The convergence of these perspectives deepens the meaning of jing. It is more than a mystical concept of vitality. It also resonates with today's discoveries in genetics and epigenetics. Our inherited essence provides the foundation for life. Lifestyle choices such as diet, rest, breath, movement, and mindful living determine how steadily that foundation supports us over time. When these practices nourish jing, they also protect the very cellular systems that determine how gracefully we age. In this way, cultivating essence is not only the poetry of ancient medicine but also a practical framework for modern longevity.[9]

What ancient texts described as essence, modern science now describes as cellular integrity. Both traditions point to the same truth. Vitality depends on balance. Acupuncture becomes a meeting point in this understanding. It has been shown to modulate oxidative stress, improve mitochondrial efficiency, and calm inflammatory activity in ways that echo the conservation of jing.

From this shared perspective, TCM speaks of jing as the root of vitality, while modern biology points to cellular integrity as the measure of resilience across the years. The health of our cells, influenced by mitochondrial efficiency, oxidative stress, inflammatory activity, and cellular signaling, determines how effectively we resist disease and how gracefully we age. When these cellular systems function in harmony, the body sustains its resilience. When they become impaired, the aging process accelerates and vitality diminishes.

Resilience and the Aging Process

Current research increasingly recognizes the importance of resilience. This refers to the ability to recover, adapt, and maintain balance in the face of stressors. Resilience is as vital to longevity as the biological markers of aging.

Resilience can be seen as a unifying principle that connects many dimensions of aging research.[10] Resilience can also be seen at the cellular level. It depends on the capacity of mitochondria, DNA repair mechanisms, and signaling networks. Together they restore balance after disruption. Resilience moves through many layers of life. Systemically, it is seen in the body's capacity to regulate inflammation, resist infection, and recover from illness. Psychosocially, it reveals itself in emotional adaptability, social bonds, and a sense of purpose.

The story of aging is more than the build-up of damage over time. It is also the fading of resilience. Early in life, cells and systems bounce back quickly after stress, maintaining harmony. As we age, this recovery slows. Failures in resilience reveal themselves in chronic inflammation, impaired repair processes, and a reduced ability to return to baseline after stress. These changes accelerate the trajectory of aging and increase vulnerability to disease.

This framework echoes TCM's perspective on jing, or essence, as the foundation of vitality. Just as jing preserves the ability to restore balance and sustain life, resilience represents the biological and psychosocial capacities that buffer us against decline. Both perspectives arrive at the same truth. Longevity is not only about reducing damage. It is also about strengthening the body's natural ability to restore balance.

Mitochondria, Oxidative Stress, and Vitality

Mitochondria, often called the powerhouses of the cell, are central to how we generate and sustain energy. These tiny structures not only fuel the heart, muscles, and brain but also influence how well the body adapts to stress and repair. In producing energy, mitochondria naturally release reactive oxygen species (ROS). In healthy amounts, ROS serve as important messengers that trigger cellular defense and renewal. But when levels become excessive, they overwhelm the system, damaging DNA, proteins, and cell membranes. Over time, this imbalance contributes to inflammation, tissue decline, and the diseases of aging.

Research suggests that protecting mitochondrial health may be one of the most important strategies for preserving vitality across the years. Scientists are exploring ways to help mitochondria manage oxidative stress, keeping it at a level where it supports healing rather than causing harm. The goal is not to eliminate stress entirely, but to restore balance so that cells can continue to repair and communicate effectively.[11]

TCM offers a complementary perspective. Jing, or essence, is described as the deep reservoir of vitality that fuels growth, fertility, and resilience. When cared for, this reservoir supports the body through life's changes. When depleted, it leaves us more vulnerable to decline. Mitochondria mirror this principle on a cellular level, acting as reservoirs of energy and signaling that must be protected to maintain strength and endurance.

From both views, vitality depends less on fighting decline outright and more on nurturing the systems that sustain life. By tending to mitochondrial health, through lifestyle, balanced nourishment, and supportive practices, we echo the ancient teaching of conserving essence, allowing vitality to endure.

Acupuncture and the Energy Within the Cell

Depression is an illness that echoes through the body's deepest rhythms, disrupting energy, sleep, appetite, and clarity. Modern research points to mitochondria, the cell's powerhouses, as central players in this process. These tiny structures are responsible for producing adenosine triphosphate (ATP), the body's energy currency that fuels the processes needed to maintain cellular balance. When mitochondria lose their rhythm, energy supply falters. Oxidative stress rises. The body's ability to regulate repair diminishes. This dysfunction does more than exhaust the body. It fuels chronic inflammation and interferes with the neural pathways that support resilience and emotional balance. [12]

It has been discovered that in depression, mitochondrial structure and function are consistently altered.[13] There is a reduced efficiency of the electron transport chain, excessive production of reactive oxygen species, and impaired clearance of damaged mitochondria. Over time, this imbalance contributes to cellular aging and weakens the body's ability to respond to stress.

Research suggests that acupuncture is a potential modulator of these processes. Acupuncture has been shown to support mitophagy, the orderly recycling of worn-out mitochondria, while at the same time encouraging the growth of new ones. It improves the efficiency of the respiratory chain and reduces the burden of oxidative stress. It also helps preserve the balance between mitochondrial fusion and fission, two processes essential for maintaining healthy cellular networks. Acupuncture also appears to stabilize the mitochondrial membrane, preventing premature cell death and allowing neurons to better regulate mood-related signals.

When viewed through the lens of TCM, these findings resonate with the classical understanding of qi and jing. Depression was often described as the stagnation or depletion of vital essence. Today's science shows that this stagnation may be reflected at the cellular level, where mitochondria struggle to generate and regulate energy. Just as ancient physicians described acupuncture as a method to restore the free flow of qi, modern science suggests it may restore the harmony of the energy-producing systems within each cell. In this way, acupuncture becomes a bridge between body and mind, renewing the cellular spark that sustains vitality and emotional balance.

Acupuncture, Jing, and Mitochondrial Vitality

When the body is deprived of movement, the muscles begin to wither, not only in form but also in the deeper essence that sustains vitality. Deep in the fibers, mitochondria lose efficiency. Energy leaks away, oxidative stress accumulates, and the inner spark that fuels resilience begins to dim. In TCM, this decline is more than physical. It touches jing, the essence stored in the kidneys that sustains growth, endurance, and longevity.

Emerging clinical findings show that acupuncture may help guard this inner storehouse. By stimulating Stomach 36 and Gallbladder 34, points long associated with vitality and the nourishment of sinews, acupuncture was able to preserve muscle mass and support mitochondrial health. Instead of succumbing fully to wasting, the muscle fibers maintained their strength. Their mitochondria functioned with greater efficiency, directing energy toward repair rather than loss. In essence, acupuncture helped the body conserve its treasures, protecting both form and function. This preservation was not only structural but energetic. In states of decline, the body often shifts into driving signals that favor breakdown over renewal. Acupuncture helped to bring these signals back into balance, reducing unnecessary strain on the body's reserves. It did not force growth, but harmonized energy flow so that what was essential could be protected. This echoes the classical view that health and longevity depend on safeguarding jing. It is about using it wisely and not exhausting it recklessly.[14]

In this way, acupuncture becomes more than a therapy for pain or circulation. It acts as a guardian of vitality, ensuring that the body's inner engines burn steadily rather than erratically. By protecting mitochondrial function and slowing the drain of essence, acupuncture helps preserve the foundation of life itself. It reminds us that longevity is not simply about extending years. It is also about conserving the deep well of energy that allows us to live those years with strength, clarity, and connection.

Acupuncture, Oxidative Stress, and the Spark of Longevity

Every cell in the body is constantly balancing fire and repair. On one side is oxidative stress. This is the wear and tear caused by reactive oxygen species, often called free radicals. On the other side is the body's antioxidant defense system, a network of enzymes and pathways that quench these sparks before they burn too deeply. When the balance tips too far toward oxidative stress, the results are significant : damaged DNA, dysfunctional mitochondria, and accelerated aging of tissues. This imbalance has been strongly linked to neurodegenerative conditions like Alzheimer's and Parkinson's disease.[15]

Research has shown that acupuncture can influence this intricate dance of protection and repair. Studies reveal that it activates a master regulatory pathway in the body known as Nrf2.[16] When awakened, Nrf2 enters the nucleus of the cell and activates protective genes. This initiates the production of powerful antioxidants such as superoxide dismutase and glutathione peroxidase. These molecules sweep through the cell, neutralizing free radicals, reducing inflammation, and protecting neurons from death.

Acupuncture's effects go even deeper. It not only reduces oxidative damage, it also supports the repair of proteins, lipids, and DNA already harmed by stress. It helps mitochondria work more efficiently, producing energy without as much toxic byproduct. By guiding pathways such as PI3K/Akt and BDNF, acupuncture supports neurogenesis, the birth of new brain cells. At the same time, it quiets inflammation driven by NF-κB, creating an inner environment where repair and renewal can unfold. In practical terms, this means acupuncture may help preserve memory and protect dopamine-producing neurons. It may also slow the buildup of harmful proteins such as beta-amyloid plaques and alpha-synuclein tangles, which underlie cognitive decline and movement disorders.

From a TCM perspective, oxidative stress resembles the "smoldering heat" that consumes yin and erodes jing, the essence of life stored in the kidneys. Once this essence is depleted, vitality wanes, and the mind and body lose their ability to adapt and endure. By calming internal fires and strengthening the body's natural defenses, acupuncture nourishes jing, safeguards the spirit, and protects the brain, which is the seat of clarity and memory.

What this research highlights is something ancient practitioners long understood. Acupuncture is not just a tool for relieving symptoms, but a guardian of longevity. By enhancing the body's natural antioxidant defenses and restoring balance at the cellular level, it helps preserve the very essence of vitality, keeping the flame of life steady against the winds of time.

The Meeting Point of Essence and Science

Ancient medicine described essence, or jing, as the foundation of life. Science describes cellular integrity, mitochondria, antioxidants, repair pathways, as the foundation of resilience. Though the languages differ, both point toward the same truth: longevity depends on how well we conserve and protect the body's deepest reserves.

Acupuncture emerges as a bridge between these worlds. It strengthens mitochondrial efficiency, calms oxidative stress, and restores balance in signaling pathways that otherwise push the body toward decline. At the same time, it reflects the classical mandate to safeguard jing. By preserving this reservoir of vitality, growth, recovery, and clarity can endure.

Longevity is not merely about postponing age, but about sustaining the spark that allows life to be lived with strength, purpose, and connection. By harmonizing cellular energy with the flow of essence, acupuncture teaches that vitality does not come from the outside. It arises within, where it must be nurtured and protected so that life can unfold with strength and clarity.

In this shared vision, jing and mitochondria are two mirrors of the same reality. They reflect the body's capacity to renew itself. When these systems are tended with care through nourishment, balance, and supportive practices like acupuncture, the years become not a slow unraveling but a continuing expression of resilience. This is the art of longevity. It is the work of conserving the essence, protecting the cell, and allowing the flame of life to burn steady across time.

33

Essence Woven in Time - Telomeres and the Sentinels of Longevity

Longevity is about how well the body weathers time, preserves clarity, and sustains vitality. In recent decades, science has begun to uncover a molecular thread that helps explain this process. At the very ends of our chromosomes lie telomeres. These tiny caps act like the tips of shoelaces, keeping our genetic material from unraveling. Each time a cell divides, the telomeres shorten slightly. When they become too short, the cell can no longer replicate and either shuts down or self-destructs.[1]

This gradual fraying is not just a clock of aging but a record of how we live. Stress, poor sleep, trauma, and adversity accelerate telomere loss, while movement, rest, and resilience help preserve them. Research shows that telomeres reflect both our biology and our lived experience. They offer a bridge between science and the ways of life that either deplete or replenish us.[2]

As discussed in earlier chapters, TCM speaks of jing, the essence that underlies growth, reproduction, and vitality. Jing is inherited from our parents yet shaped continually by how we eat, breathe, rest, and live.[3] In many ways, telomere science mirrors this wisdom. Just as jing can be squandered or nourished, telomeres can be worn down by imbalance or supported through harmony.

The immune system further ties these perspectives together. Telomere research often focuses on white blood cells, guardians of repair and defense. When their telomeres shorten too quickly, the body grows more vulnerable to inflammation and disease.[4] In TCM this parallels the concept of zheng qi, the upright energy that protects us from illness. Strong zheng qi, like preserved telomere length, reflects balance, resilience, and the ability to endure.[5]

Together, these insights suggest that aging is not a fixed destiny. The pace of decline can be influenced by how well we regulate stress, how deeply we rest, and how consistently we live in rhythm with the cycles of nature. Protecting telomeres is another way of saying we are protecting essence. Cultivating harmony preserves vitality, so that life is not only long but also strong, clear, and rooted.

In the pages that follow, we will look more closely at what telomere science reveals about the quality of longevity, not just its length. Studies of centenarians show how preserved telomeres support resilience and independence in advanced age. Research on acupuncture suggests that protecting telomeres supports more than cellular health. It also extends into memory, clarity, and repair of the aging brain. New findings on electroacupuncture show that telomerase, the enzyme that maintains telomeres, defends neurons during times of stress. Together, these threads weave a picture of how vitality can be preserved across the years. Bridging molecular science with the ancient wisdom of balance and restoration.

Telomeres and the Threads of Longevity

Science has revealed that at the ends of our chromosomes lie protective caps called telomeres. With each cell division, these caps shorten slightly, like the gradual fraying of a thread. When they reach a critical point, the cell can no longer replicate and instead enters senescence or programmed death. This natural process prevents damaged cells from multiplying unchecked, but it also marks the passage of time within our tissues.[6]

Research exploring the relationship between lifestyle, stress, and cellular aging has shown that telomeres reflect not only inherited biology but also lived experience. Chronic stress, poor sleep, and early adversity are linked with accelerated shortening, while resilience, movement, and restorative rest support their preservation. In this way, telomeres act as a molecular record of how the body adapts to the conditions of life.[7]

As stated in earlier chapters, TCM describes the body's reserves of vitality through the concept of jing. We have already explored how jing represents both inheritance and the way life is nourished over time. Here, telomere science provides a parallel view. The patterns of shortening or preservation mirror the ways jing can be consumed by imbalance or supported through harmony. Rather than restating the full framework, it is enough to note that both perspectives affirm that vitality is not only given at birth but shaped by the choices and rhythms of daily life.

The immune system further connects these ideas. Much of the research on telomeres focuses on white blood cells, which are central to defense and repair. When these cells lose telomere length too quickly, the body becomes more vulnerable to inflammation, disease, and premature aging.

Both traditions point to the same truth. The speed of aging is not fixed. It is influenced by how well we regulate stress, rest, nourish ourselves, and live in rhythm with our environment. To protect telomeres is to protect essence. To cultivate harmony is to preserve vitality, allowing the years of life to carry strength as well as length.

Telomere Length and Healthy Longevity

Research on people who live beyond one hundred raises an important question. Is telomere length a measure of lifespan itself, or is it more closely tied to the quality of health in advanced age? Research by Terry and colleagues (2014) examined this question. They compared telomere length in healthy centenarians with those of the same age who were living with multiple chronic illnesses and functional decline.[8]

The researchers studied men and women between the ages of 97 and 108, dividing them into two groups. One group remained relatively independent in daily activities and free of major conditions such as heart disease, dementia, diabetes, and stroke. The other group required assistance and carried at least two significant illnesses. The results were revealing. Centenarians in good health had significantly longer telomeres than those in poor health.

This finding suggests that telomeres are not only linked to reaching extreme ages. They might be directly tied to the vitality within those years. Longer telomeres appeared to protect against frailty and chronic disease. Shorter telomeres were linked with the burden of illness. In this way, telomere length may serve as a biological marker of functional resilience rather than of longevity alone.

Acupuncture, Telomeres, and Memory

Scientists have discovered that when telomerase, the enzyme that helps maintain our telomeres, is lacking or not working well, the brain tends to age more quickly. This can show up as problems with memory, focus, and learning new things. The question asked was whether acupuncture could help slow or even reverse some of these changes.[9]

They focused on an important point often used for vitality, ST36, and compared two styles of acupuncture. Manual acupuncture is the traditional twisting and manipulation of the needle by hand. Electroacupuncture uses a gentle current through the needles to provide steady, repeatable stimulation.

The results showed that electroacupuncture gave stronger benefits. People receiving this treatment performed better in memory-related tasks. Even more interestingly, brain analysis showed an increase in certain protective chemicals. One of these is called TrkB,^1 which helps nerve cells grow, repair, and stay flexible. The other is NF-κB,^2 which acts as a master switch for cell protection, turning on pathways that defend against stress and inflammation. When these signals are active, the brain is better able to repair itself and maintain healthy function.

TCM would see this as a reminder that acupuncture is not simply about adding extra energy into the body. Its real power lies in helping restore balance when inner reserves have been strained. Electroacupuncture, with its steady and consistent rhythm, seemed especially effective in guiding the brain back into repair and protection.

What this research suggests is that acupuncture may do more than ease discomfort in the moment. It may also support the deeper processes that keep the brain clear, resilient, and capable of learning well into later life.

Electroacupuncture, Telomerase, and Protecting the Aging Brain

As people grow older, surgery can sometimes bring unexpected challenges to memory and clear thinking. This problem, often called postoperative cognitive decline, is linked to the way the aging brain responds to stress. When the body is placed under strain, harmful molecules known as free radicals rise sharply. This rise causes inflammation that spreads. These chemicals also alter the brain's ability to repair and "clean house".[10]

A recent study by Wei Wang et al. (2023), looked at whether electroacupuncture could help protect the brain under these conditions. The focuses was on a protein called telomerase reverse transcriptase (TERT).[11] TERT is best known for its role in maintaining telomeres, the protective caps at the ends of chromosomes. It also has important protective functions in the brain. Inside the mitochondria, the cell's energy factories, TERT shields neurons from oxidative stress. It also supports autophagy, the process that clears away damaged proteins.

The findings were significant. Without support, the stress of surgery was linked with lower telomerase activity This reduced TERT levels in brain tissue, causing higher inflammation, and sluggish autophagy. Memory and learning functions suffered as a result.

Electroacupuncture changed this picture. Treatment given before surgery helped preserve telomerase activity and kept TERT levels steady, especially in the mitochondria. It also calmed inflammation, improved the brain's natural ability to clear waste, and supported stronger performance in memory-related tasks. When telomerase was blocked, most of these benefits disappeared, showing that TERT is central to how electroacupuncture protects the brain.

In practical terms, this suggests that electroacupuncture may strengthen the brain's defenses during times of strain. By protecting telomerase and TERT, it helps keep the brain clear and resilient. It also supports recovery. This protection is especially valuable for memory and cognition in later life.

Summary of Telomere Studies and Longevity

Findings from these trials highlight that telomeres are not only markers of lifespan but also guardians of vitality. Longer telomeres have been linked with greater independence and resilience in advanced age. Shorter telomeres are tied to frailty, inflammation, and cognitive decline. Acupuncture research adds another layer. It shows that telomerase, the enzyme that maintains telomeres, also supports brain repair, memory, and cellular defense during times of stress.

From both scientific and traditional perspectives, protecting telomeres is another way of protecting essence. It allows the years of life to carry clarity, adaptability, and strength instead of decline.

While telomeres reveal how deeply vitality is woven into our cells, the immune system shows how this vitality is expressed in daily life. Among its many defenders, natural killer cells stand out as sentinels that patrol for threats and maintain resilience. The following section explores how these guardians of immunity connect with both longevity and the wisdom of balance.

Defenses of Longevity

Genuine rejuvenation is more than simply being free of disease. It is the body's ability to repair itself, adapt to change, and remain steady in a world of constant challenges. In TCM, this dynamic resilience is carried by wei qi. It is the protective energy that circulates just beneath the surface of the body. wei qi acts as a shield against external threats while also preserving inner balance.[12] In modern biomedical terms, this parallels the immune system, with its quick-acting first responders and longer-lasting adaptive defenses. Both systems are shaped by the ANS, which determines how the body responds to stress and maintains homeostasis.

Research confirms this bridge between ancient insight and contemporary science. By restoring balance in the ANS, acupuncture has been shown to influence immunity in powerful ways. Studies demonstrate that it can calm chronic inflammation, enhance the body's defense against pathogens, regulate the activity of white blood cells, and even support the repair of immune tissues when they are weakened.

Natural killer cells, often called NK cells, are one of the body's front-line defenders. Unlike other immune cells that need time to recognize and "remember" a threat, NK cells can act immediately. They patrol the body, searching for cells that are damaged, stressed, or infected, and respond with swift precision. In this way, they serve as guardians of balance, eliminating danger before it can spread.

What makes NK cells unique is their ability to sense when something is "off." Healthy cells display signals on their surface that tell NK cells to leave them alone. But when a cell is infected by a virus or is otherwise compromised, those signals often disappear. NK cells recognize this absence as a warning sign and move quickly to neutralize the threat.

Beyond direct defense, NK cells also act as messengers. Once activated, they release chemical signals that alert and guide other parts of the immune system. These signals shape inflammation, encourage the growth of other immune cells, and help bridge innate defenses with longer-lasting adaptive immunity.

In the bigger picture of longevity, NK cells embody the same principle described in TCM as wei qi, the protective energy at the body's surface. Just as wei qi shields against external invasion and preserves inner harmony, NK cells provide a living shield within the blood and tissues. Their efficiency in responding to threats, coordinating repair, and maintaining vigilance is essential for resilience across the years.[13]

Natural Killers and the Secret of Long Life

What allows some people to live past one hundred years while still retaining strength and clarity? Researchers Mattia E. Ligotti et al. (2023) in Sicily, home to one of the world's "blue zones" of longevity, asked this very question.[14] They studied the immune systems of semi- and supercentenarians, men and women living into their nineties, hundreds, and beyond, and found something remarkable about their Natural Killer (NK) cells.

In this study, scientists compared immune cell profiles across ages 19 to 110. They discovered that NK cell levels rise steadily with age, and in centenarians, they are significantly elevated compared to younger people. Interestingly, the increase was observed in both men and women, though it was even more pronounced in males. Far from being a sign of dysfunction, these higher NK cell levels appear to represent an *adaptation. A* refined form of immune resilience that supports healthy longevity.

Immune aging is often described as decline. Yet it may also be a different kind of adaptation. In other words, the immune system of the longest-lived individuals does not simply weaken. It reorganizes, finding new strategies to protect the body across the decades. NK cells, with their ability to clear threats quickly and orchestrate defense, may be one of the keys that allow centenarians to survive the insults of time and still flourish.

From the perspective of TCM, this echoes the strength of wei qi. Just as wei qi adjusts with the seasons and life stages, these findings suggest that NK cells evolve with age. They become a flexible line of defense that helps preserve vitality. In this way, the wisdom of the immune system mirrors the wisdom of long life itself. It is a wisdom of adaptation, balance, and the capacity to renew in the face of change.

Acupuncture and the Natural Killer Connection

Natural Killer (NK) cells are some of the immune system's most fascinating players. Unlike other defenders that need to be trained to recognize invaders, NK cells come ready to act. They patrol constantly, scanning for cells that look off, and respond with swift precision. Think of them as vigilant guardians that keep the body's internal environment in balance.[15]

What makes NK cells remarkable is their flexibility. They can directly destroy compromised cells using powerful molecular weapons. At the same time, they send out signals that rally other parts of the immune system. In this way, NK cells don't just fight threats, they coordinate defense, repair, and long-term resilience.[16]

The intriguing hypothesis explored in this review is that acupuncture may amplify NK cell activity. Evidence from studies suggests that acupuncture, especially at the immune-regulating point ST36, can increase NK cell numbers and boost their effectiveness16. For example, after acupuncture, patients have shown higher levels of IFN-γ, a chemical signal that helps NK cells activate and strengthen the body's broader defenses. In some studies, NK cell activity that was previously low returned to normal after a series of acupuncture sessions.

How does this work? Experts propose that acupuncture triggers a kind of "cross-talk" between the nervous and immune systems. Needling specific points can release natural messengers such as nitric oxide and beta-endorphins. These molecules not only calm pain and stress but also directly engage NK cells, stimulating them to multiply, activate, and release their protective arsenal.

The broader message is that acupuncture may be doing more than easing symptoms. By enhancing the vigilance and strength of NK cells, it could be helping the body sustain its balance and resilience over the long haul. In TCM, this mirrors the role of wei qi. Just as wei qi adapts and fortifies the body's boundary, NK cells serve as an inner shield, one that acupuncture may help sharpen and sustain.

How Acupuncture Tunes the Immune Symphony

Acupuncture has long been described in TCM as a way to restore balance and awaken the body's natural healing capacity. Modern science is beginning to show how this may work. It reveals that acupuncture can act like a conductor, helping different parts of the immune system stay in harmony with one another.[17]

At its core, acupuncture taps into the body's communication networks. Stimulating acupoints sends signals through nerves that reach the brain and ripple outward to influence hormones, immune cells, and inflammatory pathways. Rather than targeting a single molecule or pathway, acupuncture seems to guide entire systems back toward equilibrium.

Research demonstrates that acupuncture affects both the innate immune system, which provides rapid first-line defense, and the adaptive immune system, which offers memory and longer-term protection.[18] Mast cells, positioned near the skin and blood vessels, respond to needling by releasing chemical messengers such as histamine and serotonin. These substances promote local healing and help translate mechanical stimulation into nerve signals. Macrophages, the immune system's cleanup crew, can also be influenced. Acupuncture encourages them to shift from a destructive, pro-inflammatory mode to a repair-oriented mode, supporting recovery and easing chronic inflammation. Neutrophils, the body's fast responders, are regulated in a similar way, with acupuncture preventing them from causing excessive damage during infections or injuries. Natural Killer cells, which patrol the body for stressed or abnormal cells, have been shown to increase in both number and activity following acupuncture, enhancing the body's vigilance and defense. Even within the brain and nervous system, cells such as astrocytes and microglia can be calmed, reducing the type of runaway neuroinflammation that contributes to conditions like stroke or neurodegeneration.

Beyond individual cells, acupuncture engages broader reflex networks. Signals travel along pathways like the vagus nerve, which helps quiet inflammation through a pathway called the cholinergic anti-inflammatory pathway. Other reflex loops involve the sympathetic nervous system and the brain-gut axis, suggesting that acupuncture has the capacity to restore balance across widely separated systems of the body.

The adaptive immune system is also influenced. Acupuncture has been shown to balance the activity of T helper cells, keeping pro-inflammatory responses in check while supporting regulatory cells that prevent autoimmune flare-ups. In this way, it encourages harmony between defense and tolerance.

Taken together, these findings create a picture of acupuncture as a therapy that works on the level of systems rather than symptoms. Instead of addressing a single disease pathway, it engages the body's network of nerves, hormones, and immune cells to re-establish balance. In the language of TCM, acupuncture strengthens wei qi and restores homeostasis. In modern biomedical terms, it modulates inflammation, supports resilience, and promotes healing on multiple fronts.

This dual perspective, one rooted in ancient wisdom and the other in modern systems physiology, helps explain why acupuncture has endured for thousands of years. It does not simply mask illness but guides the body back toward its natural state of adaptability, protection, and repair.

Guardians of Vitality

The story of telomeres reminds us that longevity is not measured only in time. It is carried in the way life is lived. Each choice, each rhythm of rest and renewal, leaves its trace. Just as jing can be nurtured or depleted, telomeres reflect whether we meet the years with strength or with decline.

The immune system tells the same story. White blood cells and natural killer cells are more than defenders. They are mirrors of vitality, showing how well the body protects, repairs, and adapts. When they are strong, balance holds. When they falter, decline sets in.

Both science and Chinese medicine affirm this truth. Vitality is not fixed at birth. It is cultivated. It is shaped by balance, by resilience, by the capacity to return to harmony after stress.

To protect telomeres is to protect essence. To protect essence is to protect life itself. When body, mind, and spirit move in balance, the years do not simply accumulate. They carry clarity, adaptability, and strength. Longevity, at its heart, is not just about length of years. It is about the quality carried within them.

VII

Rhythms of Renewal

Daily Rituals for Longevity and Balance

"In the past, people practiced the Tao, the Way of Life. They understood the principle of Balance, of yin and yang, as represented by the transformation of the energies of the energies of the universe. Thus, they formulated practices such as Dao-in, an exercise combining stretching, massaging, and breathing to promote energy flow, and meditation to help maintain and harmonize themselves with the universe."

— Qi Bo

34

Living in Rhythm - Daily Tools for Autonomic Balance

Healing unfolds not just through what we learn, but through the quiet rhythms we return to. The research throughout this book has shown how effectively acupuncture regulates the ANS. We have explored how it promotes parasympathetic activity and helps reduce stress. Yet beyond its physiological effects, its deeper medicine lies in restoring rhythm to the body and mind.

In TCM, health is not considered a fixed state but a dynamic relationship between internal and external rhythms. These rhythms include the cycles of the seasons, the breath, digestion, sleep, and emotion. Health is shaped by the body's ongoing relationship with these natural patterns. They are not isolated processes, but rhythmic expressions that reflect and respond to the world around us. When these patterns fall out of sync, resilience begins to fade. But when we return to them, when we begin to restore their flow, the conditions for healing naturally arise. As the *Huang Di Nei Jing Su Wen* states, *"Hence, yin [qi], yang [qi], and the four seasons, they constitute the end and beginning of the myriad beings. They are the basis of life"*.[1]

There is an ancient rhythm within the body. It breathes, digests, heals, and restores without our conscious instruction. This rhythm is the heartbeat of the ANS. It orchestrates the quiet miracles of life. The slowing of the pulse after fear. The release of digestive enzymes. The calming of tears after a cry.

We've seen throughout this book how rhythm shapes well-being. When the nervous system can shift with ease between action and recovery, the body thrives. But modern pressures often freeze us in high alert. This lingering sympathetic charge slowly wears down our capacity for rest, resilience, and internal harmony.

While acupuncture is a powerful tool for restoring parasympathetic tone, healing cannot be outsourced to a treatment table alone. It can be lived. Moment by moment. Through conscious rhythm and embodied rituals.

Section VII invites us into this reclamation. It is a shift from science to practice. From mechanism to meaning. Just as acupuncture restores nervous system regulation through carefully placed points and timing, we too can align our lives through intentional rituals and daily awareness. These simple tools, such as breathwork, acupressure, stillness, and emotional reflection, have been shown to regulate vagal tone. They increase HRV and lower sympathetic arousal.[2]

These tools are also ancient. Rooted in traditions that recognized the power of pattern and presence. These are not elaborate wellness routines or strict regimens. They are acts of remembrance. Remembering how to breathe, how to eat, how to listen to the body. Grounded in both TCM and contemporary research, these daily rituals are designed to gently return to ourselves.

Whether you are waking in the morning, preparing a meal, or winding down before sleep, your body is listening. Every breath. Every pause. Every moment of stillness becomes a conversation with your nervous system. The goal is to return to our natural state of rhythm and balance.

Let us return to it. Together.

Note: This section is shared for educational and self-care purposes only. It does not constitute medical advice or therapeutic instruction.

35

Morning Grounding Practices - Waking the Body with Rhythm and Intention

The first moments after waking are more than just a transition from sleep to consciousness. They offer a powerful moment to orient the nervous system for the day ahead. In TCM, early morning is seen as a time of renewal, linked to lung and large intestine function in the body's meridian clock.[1] Modern research echoes this view. The cortisol awakening response, a spike in cortisol 30 to 45 minutes after waking, plays a key role in mobilizing energy and preparing the brain and body for daytime function. How you rise determines how you move through the world.[2]

According to the TCM organ clock, the hours between 5:00 a.m. and 7:00 a.m. correspond to the large intestine meridian. This time is linked to elimination, both physical and emotional, supporting clarity of mind and healthy digestive function. Energetically, it is a moment for letting go of stagnation and encouraging the movement of qi throughout the body. This is also reflected mentally in our ability to let go of the past.[3] From a biomedical perspective, this phase of the morning also coincides with the cortisol awakening response, a natural rise in the body's alertness hormone that helps prepare us for daily activity.[4] When we honor this process with gentleness rather than rushing, we lay a neurological foundation for greater resilience and emotional balance throughout the day.

A grounding morning ritual does not need to be elaborate. Its power often lies in its simplicity and intention. The key is to engage the sensory and regulatory systems gently, before the pressures of screens, decisions, and external input take over. Simple practices like mindful breathing, warm water, or quiet movement invite the nervous system into a state of presence, calm, and connection. Research shows that slow, controlled breathing enhances parasympathetic tone and suppresses stress-related sympathetic activity, helping to balance the nervous system.[5]

Whenever possible, allow your body to wake naturally or to soft, soothing sounds. Harsh alarms can immediately trigger sympathetic nervous system activation, pulling you into a stress response before your feet even touch the floor. If an alarm is needed, opt for a chime or vibration. Choose something that honors the transition between sleep and wakefulness.[6]

Begin your day with hydration and natural light. A glass of warm water with lemon rehydrates the tissues, stimulates digestion, and supports healthy elimination. Stepping into early morning sunlight, ideally within the first 30 minutes of waking, sends signals to the brain that help regulate melatonin and cortisol levels. This simple habit supports the alignment of your circadian rhythm.[7]

Before reaching for your phone or stepping into obligation, take a few minutes to reconnect with your body through movement. This might include Qigong-style shaking to stimulate circulation, light tapping to awaken the skin, or gentle neck and shoulder rolls to ease stiffness from sleep. Even three deep, intentional breaths with a hand placed on the chest or belly can signal the vagus nerve and help shift the nervous system toward a state of parasympathetic calm. Research shows that Qigong exercises support ANS balance and activate the parasympathetic response. Meditative movement practices such as Qigong have also been associated with improved blood flow, increased HRV, and reduced stress.[8]

Once your body is gently awakened, pause to orient the mind. The nervous system responds not only to posture and breath but also to the meanings we bring. Begin your day with a moment of mindfulness, a brief prayer, a sentence in a journal, or a quiet inquiry such as "What does my body need today to function at its best?" or "What does balance feel like?"

In TCM, this practice nurtures the *Shén*, or spirit, which resides in the heart and is governed by clarity, and intention. A calm *Shén* supports emotional regulation and fosters coherence between the heart and the brain. This is a state associated with greater adaptability and well-being.[9]

A morning ritual is not a task. It is an invitation to meet yourself with presence, not pressure., to step into your day aligned with rhythm, not reaction.

Morning Practice Prompt - Begin with Rhythm

Tomorrow morning, before checking your phone or stepping into the day:

1. **Hydrate**: Drink a glass of warm water. Feel the temperature awaken your digestion.
2. **Step into light**: Open a window or walk outside. Let natural light touch your eyes and skin.
3. **Breathe**: Take three slow, deep breaths with one hand on your belly. Inhale softly. Exhale longer.
4. **Move**: Gently roll your shoulders or tap down the arms and legs to awaken circulation.
5. **Reflect**: Ask yourself, *What rhythm do I want to carry into today?*

36

Breathwork for Vagal Stimulation - Returning to Calm, One Exhale at a Time

Breathing is one of the only autonomic functions we can consciously control. In doing so, we gain a direct channel into the nervous system itself. Each inhale and exhale offers a choice to upregulate or downregulate, to stimulate or to soften. Breath is not just a physiological necessity. It is a form of medicine, long recognized in TCM and Qigong, and increasingly supported by modern neurobiology as a vital tool for cultivating inner balance.[1]

The Breath - Nervous System Connection

The breath is more than a mechanical act of survival. It is a messenger, a mediator, and in many ways, a medicine. Across both ancient traditions and modern neuroscience, breath is recognized as a direct interface between the body and the nervous system. When the rhythm of breath changes, so too does our internal state.

The length and depth of the exhale, carry powerful physiological messages. Slow, extended exhalation stimulates the vagus nerve and activates the parasympathetic branch of the ANS. In contrast, shallow, rapid breathing reinforces sympathetic activation. It signals a state of stress, preparing the body for action but making it harder to access internal safety and regulation. Breath becomes both a cause and a consequence of our emotional reality.[2]

New findings continue to reveal that breathing at a rate slower than ten breaths per minute produces measurable changes across both the autonomic and central nervous systems. HRV and respiratory sinus arrhythmia increase, reflecting parasympathetic activation. Meanwhile, brainwave studies show that slow breathing enhances alpha activity and reduces theta power, creating a state of calm attentiveness. The only available fMRI data suggest that slow breathing activates not only the brainstem but also the prefrontal cortex, thalamus, and hypothalamus. These regions are associated with mood regulation, executive function, and interoceptive awareness. These shifts translate into tangible emotional outcomes: reduced anxiety, improved mood, and heightened clarity.[3]

While breathing is regulated by the brainstem for metabolic needs, it is also profoundly shaped by the limbic system, which is the emotional brain. Findings indicate that inhalation and exhalation rhythms are linked to oscillations in the piriform cortex and amygdala, areas involved in olfaction, emotional memory, and fear processing. This synchronization means that every breath influences emotional tone, and every emotional state leaves its imprint on the breath. Inhalation through the nose even activates sensory pathways that modulate emotional centers, linking breath to both smell and safety perception. When breath is disrupted by trauma, anxiety, or chronic stress, the emotional brain becomes dysregulated. Yet when breath is consciously slowed, it becomes a stabilizing force, bringing coherence to the nervous system and restoring inner balance.4

A 2023 study by Sakurai and colleagues adds clinical further clinical insight. In their trial of healthy Japanese women, participants practiced consciously slow breathing. The results showed a clear predominance of parasympathetic activity, measurable through changes in heart rate and subjective reports of relaxation. The body responded not only to the rhythm of breath but also to the intention behind it. The act of slowing down was enough to shift physiology toward repair and ease.[5]

These insights are echoed in the expanding field of embodied cognition, which explores how the body shapes perception, emotion, and self-awareness. Studies show that controlled breathing can modulate the relationship between the brain and body, helping individuals feel more grounded and present. Emerging technologies now use this principle to create digital tools that pair slow breathing with immersive feedback environments to ease respiratory distress and support calm. In this model, the breath becomes a gateway for reconnection with the self.[6]

The breath is not a passive process. It is an active agent of change. Through breath, we can calm the heart, balance the brain, regulate emotion, and reclaim access to the deeper rhythms of safety and presence. This is not metaphor. It is measurable biology. It is also timeless medicine.

The Science of Safety - Breath and the Polyvagal Lens

One of the most influential frameworks for understanding how breath influences the nervous system is the Polyvagal Theory. This perspective deepens the conversation around breath by revealing how the vagus nerve is not only a biological structure but also a mediator of emotional, physiological, and social well-being.

The theory identifies two distinct branches of the vagus nerve. The older, unmyelinated branch is shared with most vertebrates and is associated with freeze responses and shutdown under extreme threat. The newer, myelinated branch, unique to mammals, is responsible for regulating social engagement, calming the heart, and supporting feelings of safety. This "ventral vagal pathway" is crucial for prosocial behavior, emotion regulation, and healing. When it is active, the body enters a physiological state that allows for connection, reflection, and restoration.

The breath is one of the most accessible ways to activate this ventral vagal pathway. Because respiration is both automatic and voluntary, it allows humans to directly influence their internal state through conscious rhythm and pacing. Slow, controlled breathing sends signals to the brainstem that the environment is safe. This downregulates defensive systems and promotes parasympathetic dominance. The result is not only a calmer nervous system, but also an increased ability to think clearly, relate to others, and heal from stress.

This framework also reframes the very meaning of well-being. Health is not defined solely by the absence of disease or stress but by the presence of physiological safety. This state can be measured through indicators such as HRV and facial expression and is often cultivated through rhythmic sensory experiences, especially the breath.

Interventions such as breathwork, safe social interaction, vocal toning, and nasal breathing have all been shown to shift the nervous system toward regulation. In this way, breath serves as a portal through which we access the neurophysiological states necessary for balance, emotional stability, and genuine connection. Breath becomes the language of safety, spoken not only by the lungs but by the vagus nerve itself.

This theory explains why slow breathing techniques improve HRV, why exhalation calms the system, and why emotional shifts are possible simply through rhythm. Breath becomes the language of safety, spoken not only by the lungs but by the vagus nerve itself.

Breath as Medicine - Qigong, Qi, and the Rhythm of the Heart

In Qigong, breath is inseparable from qi. Practitioners are taught to breathe slowly, through the nose, and to coordinate breath with both intention and movement. With each inhale, they gather qi. With each exhale, they direct it through the channels of the body. This practice reflects what modern science now refers to as respiratory sinus arrhythmia. This is the natural increase in heart rate during inhalation and the decrease during exhalation. It is considered a key indicator of healthy vagal tone.[8]

The scientific foundation for this approach is deeply rooted in Qigong, a Chinese breathing practice that combines slow nasal breathing, mindful awareness, and gentle movement to influence both the physical body and the energetic system. Breath, in this tradition, is an active force rather than a passive act. It is a method for cultivating internal awareness and supporting physiological regulation. Its purpose is to guide qi smoothly through the meridians, maintaining harmony among breath, body, and mind.[9]

What stands out is how closely this ancient understanding aligns with modern models of autonomic balance. Early observations noted that Qigong breathing lowers the respiratory rate, slows the heart, and produces a calm, centered state. These responses are now recognized as signs of parasympathetic activation. Such physiological changes can be measured through higher HRV and more pronounced respiratory sinus arrhythmia. In essence, what was once described as the smooth flow of qi through the body now finds its parallel in the rhythmic oscillations of the cardiovascular system during conscious, steady breathing.

Regular practice has also been shown to improve emotional stability, mental clarity, and physical resilience. These benefits mirror modern findings linking breath regulation to vagal tone, baroreflex sensitivity, and coherent heart-lung rhythms. What ancient practitioners understood as the cultivation of qi, contemporary science now describes through measurable patterns of nervous system regulation.

Together, these perspectives reveal the same truth. Conscious breathing, especially when paired with mindful awareness, restores harmony to the body's internal systems. Breath is both a biological necessity and a vehicle for healing, presence, and vitality. It serves as a bridge between physiology and spirit.

Inhale, Exhale, Heal - A Scientific Comparison of Breath Techniques in Therapy

Several breathing techniques have been shown to support ANS regulation. Slowing the breath to around six breaths per minute can significantly increase HRV, which is a key marker of parasympathetic strength and resilience to stress. Techniques such as 4-6 breathing, where you inhale for a count of four and exhale for a count of six, or box breathing, which uses equal counts for inhaling, holding, exhaling, and holding again, are frequently used to bring coherence to the cardiovascular system and emotional state. Although many of these approaches are now integrated into therapy, questions remain about their relative effectiveness.

A 2021 randomized controlled study looked at the impact of two specific breathwork interventions on HRV when used in a psychotherapy setting.[10] Participants were randomly assigned to one of three groups: a guided six-breaths-per-minute pacer, a compassion-focused soothing rhythm breathing group, or a control group that watched a calming nature video. The researchers measured HRV through electrocardiogram readings and also tracked heart rate and blood pressure before, during, and after the intervention. Following the breathing session, participants completed writing exercises designed to induce self-criticism, followed by self-compassion. These exercises mimicked the emotional fluctuations often addressed in therapy.

The results showed that both breathing interventions significantly increased HRV, specifically as measured by standard deviation of NN intervals (SDNN), when compared to the nature video. The group using the six-breaths-per-minute pacer produced the highest low-frequency HRV and LF/HF ratio, suggesting a greater effect on baroreflex sensitivity and autonomic flexibility. Although participants in this group struggled to maintain the target pace and averaged closer to 12 breaths per minute, the effort itself still produced measurable benefits. This suggests that intentional engagement with slower breathing supports physiological regulation. The soothing rhythm breathing group also improved HRV, though to a slightly lesser extent. These findings support the use of breathwork in psychotherapy as a practical method to help restore balance to the nervous system and build emotional resilience.

Further exploration into the comparative effectiveness of different breathing styles was examined in 2024 analysis.[11] Researchers examined three commonly used techniques: square breathing, 4-7-8 breathing, and two variations of six breaths per minute. One used a 4:6 inhale-to-exhale ratio, and the other maintained a balanced 5:5 rhythm. With 84 college-aged participants, the team measured HRV, end-tidal CO_2 ($PETCO_2$), and mood before and after each breathing session using a 3-lead electrocardiogram and capnometry.

The results confirmed that breathing at six breaths per minute, particularly with a 4:6 ratio, produced the greatest increases in HRV. This supports existing evidence that extending the exhalation phase enhances vagal tone. Square breathing and 4-7-8 breathing, while widely used in clinical and wellness settings, were less effective in improving HRV. None of the breathing methods produced significant changes in mood over the short term, and all led to mild reductions in PETCO$_2$. This indicates a tendency toward over-breathing during slower-paced techniques, which could be a concern if not properly guided. Practitioners may need to monitor CO$_2$ levels or emphasize gentle pacing to prevent potential side effects.

This research offers growing insight that slow, conscious breathing can influence HRV and enhance autonomic regulation. Among the techniques tested, six breaths per minute appears to provide the most physiological benefit. Although more research is needed to assess long-term outcomes and individual variability, integrating structured breathwork into psychotherapy presents a promising, accessible, and non-invasive way to help individuals regulate stress and reconnect with a sense of inner safety.

Vibration as Medicine - Humming, Chanting, and the Wisdom of the Lungs

Humming, chanting, and extended sighs activate the vagus nerve through its connection to the vocal cords and inner ear, helping to regulate the ANS. In TCM, the voice is linked to the lung system, which governs both breath and the movement of qi throughout the body. Vocal expression is considered a way to release stagnation, restore harmony, and support the Shen, or spirit. These practices are not merely cultural or spiritual. They are embodied techniques for self-regulation, grounded in both ancient energetic principles and modern neurophysiology.

Recent discoveries continue to affirm the physiological relevance of these practices. Recent studies have assessed HRV during humming, sleep, physical activity, and emotional stress.[12] Humming produced the lowest stress index of all conditions measured, indicating the highest parasympathetic activation. Compared with the calming effects of sleep, gentle humming showed even greater potential to downregulate sympathetic arousal and promote nervous system stability. These results support the use of sound and vibration-based practices, such as Bhramari pranayama, as practical tools for daily stress recovery and autonomic recalibration.

Further evidence comes from a 2011 pilot fMRI study investigated the neurohemodynamic effects of OM chanting.[13] Unlike the control sound "ssss," which produced no changes in brain activity, OM chanting led to significant deactivation in several brain regions associated with emotional processing and internal regulation, including the anterior cingulate cortex, hippocampus, amygdala, and thalamus. These areas also respond to vagus nerve stimulation used in clinical settings for depression and epilepsy. The findings suggest that OM chanting may act through similar neural pathways to create calm, emotional clarity, and mental stillness.

This intersection of vocalization, respiration, and neural modulation is also reflected in Traditional Chinese practices such as Liuzijue Qigong (LQG).[14] A 2023 clinical study by Xia and colleagues examined the effects of combining conventional speech therapy with LQG in stroke patients suffering from post-stroke spastic dysarthria (PSSD), a condition marked by impaired motor speech and communication. LQG involves the coordinated use of six healing sounds, Xu, He, Hu, Si, Chui, and Xi, each synchronized with specific breath patterns and body movements. After four weeks of daily treatment, patients who practiced LQG showed significantly greater improvements in speech articulation, maximum phonation time, vocal strength, and cognitive scores compared to those receiving conventional therapy alone. The practice of vocal sound with breath not only restores speech function but also enhances mental clarity and emotional resilience.

From a TCM standpoint, each sound in LQG is believed to resonate with a particular organ system. These sounds help circulate qi, clear emotional stagnation, and restore vitality through the vibrational resonance of the voice. In modern terms, these practices activate vagal tone, regulate respiration, and modulate brain activity. Whether through humming, OM chanting, or LQG healing sounds, vocal expression becomes an accessible tool for integrating breath, intention, and nervous system regulation.

Sound is not just a metaphor for healing. It is a physiological event. These vocal practices, rooted in centuries of embodied wisdom, now find validation in HRV data, neuroimaging, and clinical trials. The voice, when aligned with breath and intention, becomes a bridge between the seen and unseen, the ancient and the measurable, the somatic and the spiritual.

Whether practiced in stillness or during movement, breathwork becomes a form of acupuncture without needles. It stimulates the internal channels, calms the mind, and restores the natural rhythm of the body.

Practice Prompt: Reclaim Calm with Your Breath

At some point today, perhaps during a moment of stress or quiet transition, pause and try this gentle practice. Begin by finding a comfortable seated or lying position. Allow your spine to lengthen slightly and your jaw to soften.

Breathe to Regulate

Place one hand over your heart and your other over your lower abdomen below your bellybutton. Focus on your breath. Breath down to your kidneys. Imagine your breath reaching all of your organs. Feel your belly expand. Gently breathe out. Relaxing tension.

Let your breath be smooth, not forced. Feel your body subtly expand on the inhale and soften on the exhale.

Repeat for two to three minutes. This pacing encourages the qi to move through all your meridians.

Anchor Your Intention

With each exhale, silently whisper to yourself:

I return to center.

Feel this phrase ripple through your body like a tuning fork, echoing through the nervous system. Let it become your breath's message, not just a thought, but a signal.

Add Gentle Sound

If you feel ready, try adding a soft humming sound on your exhale. The vibration will stimulate the vagus nerve through the vocal cords and ear pathways. This may deepen the feeling of calm and presence. Choose a tone or sound that feels comforting. OM, Mmm, or even a soft sigh are all valid.

Deepen with Visualization

Visualize your breath as a wave of light. On the inhale, draw that light into your chest and belly. On the exhale, let it wash down your arms and legs, grounding you. Let the breath carry the qi, as described in Qigong, gathering with each inhale, guiding with each exhale.

Observe with Compassion

Pause after a few rounds and check in with your body.

Has your heart rate slowed?

Has your jaw or belly softened?

Do you feel more spacious inside your chest?

This moment of awareness is a form of embodied cognition. You're not just thinking calm, you're *becoming* calm.

Integration

Carry the rhythm of this breath with you. If you notice yourself tensing or rushing later in the day, return to it. A few slow, nasal breaths can act as your internal reset button, clearing the noise, restoring coherence.

37

Nourishment as Regulation - Eating in Rhythm with the Nervous System

Food is more than fuel. It is information. Every bite you take sends signals through your nervous system. These signals influence your energy, mood, digestion, and immune response.[1] In TCM, food is seen as both nourishment and medicine. It shapes the flow of qi and blood and supports the function of the internal organs.[2] In modern physiology, we now understand that eating is a full-body event. It is orchestrated largely by the ANS, which governs digestion, absorption, and metabolic balance.[3]

A Diet for the Mind: Ancient Wisdom, Modern Science

The human brain is often described as the most complex structure in the known universe. It orchestrates thought, memory, sensation, and emotion with astonishing precision, yet it cannot do this work alone. Every spark of cognition depends on fuel, and the quality of that fuel matters. Ancient traditions of medicine have long taught that food is more than sustenance. It is medicine, energy, and information for the body and mind. Modern nutritional psychiatry now echoes this wisdom, showing that what we place on our plates directly shapes our mood, resilience, and mental clarity. Emerging research suggests that the human brain is a demanding organ.[4] It runs continuously. It processes thoughts, regulates breath and heartbeat, and manages sensory input. Even while we sleep, it remains active. To sustain this constant activity, the brain requires steady, high-quality fuel. This fuel comes directly from the food we eat. Just like a luxury car runs best on premium gasoline, the brain functions best when nourished with nutrient-rich, anti-inflammatory foods.

Science confirms a principle woven into many healing traditions. Nourishment is medicine for both brain and spirit. Food directly influences mood, mental clarity, and emotional resilience. A diet filled with vitamins, minerals, and antioxidants supports brain function and reduces oxidative stress. This stress is the cellular "rust" caused by metabolic waste. On the other hand, diets high in refined sugars and processed foods impair insulin regulation, increase inflammation, and worsen symptoms of depression and anxiety.

One key player in this relationship is serotonin. This neurotransmitter plays an important role in regulating mood, sleep, appetite, and pain. About 95% of serotonin is produced in the gut, not the brain. The gastrointestinal tract contains over 100 million neurons and trillions of microbes. These systems do far more than digest food. They help shape our emotional well-being. The gut microbiome protects the intestinal lining, reduces inflammation, improves nutrient absorption, and activates neural pathways that link directly to the brain.

Studies comparing traditional diets, such as the Mediterranean or Japanese diet, with the typical Western diet reveal significant differences in mental health. People who eat traditional diets rich in vegetables, fruits, whole grains, fish, and fermented foods have a 25 to 35 percent lower risk of depression. These traditional diets are naturally low in processed sugars and refined foods. In contrast, such processed foods are staples of the Western diet and are closely tied to chronic inflammation.

As research continues to uncover the connection between food and mental health, one message stands out. Our food choices are not just about calories or weight. They shape how we feel, think, and cope. Choosing a nutrient-dense, gut-friendly diet can help the brain function with greater clarity, creativity, and calm.

Nourishing the Nervous System Through the Gut

The connection between the gut and the brain is a well-documented system of communication that influences everything from mood to cognition. emerging studies have started to explore how nutrition and gut microbiota affect mental health through what is known as the microbiota-gut-brain axis.[5]

This axis is a biological pathway that links the digestive system to the brain. It involves immune signals, metabolic byproducts, and direct communication via the vagus nerve. The research highlights how diet plays a central role in shaping this relationship. Poor nutrition does not just impact physical health. It can disrupt the gut microbiome and lead to inflammation, mood imbalances, and cognitive decline.

The brain requires a steady supply of nutrients to meet its high energy demands. When we eat processed, inflammatory foods, the microbiome becomes less diverse and less stable. This shift can impair the production of neurotransmitters like serotonin and GABA. It can also increase systemic inflammation, which is often linked to anxiety and depression.

On the other hand, diets rich in fiber, antioxidants, omega-3 fats, and fermented foods help nourish beneficial bacteria. These microbes produce short-chain fatty acids, which help regulate inflammation and support brain health. They also improve the gut barrier and influence neural pathways that help stabilize mood and reduce stress responses.

This research reinforces the idea that food is not just fuel. It is a form of communication with the nervous system. The researchers suggest that nutritional interventions focused on gut health may be a powerful tool for supporting mental well-being. As evidence grows, food is being redefined. It is medicine for the brain and a foundation for emotional resilience.

Food as Medicine - A Core Principle of Chinese Healing

What we eat does more than sustain us. Each bite carries the potential to heal, to restore, or to disturb the body's inner balance. For centuries, Chinese medicine has described food and medicine as companions on the same path, reminding us that nourishment and treatment are not separate but reflections of the same principle of harmony. This enduring concept, known as medicine and food homology, holds that many foods also serve medicinal purposes and that certain medicinal substances can be used in daily nourishment. It reflects a holistic understanding that diet and healing are not separate but deeply intertwined.[6]

From this perspective, the boundary between food and medicine is seamless. Substances that are safe for regular consumption and offer therapeutic benefits are recognized within Chinese health traditions. The principle teaches that by eating with intention, we can prevent illness, support internal balance, and promote healing.

Countless foods illustrate this harmony in practice. Ginger supports digestion and helps dispel cold. Goji berries nourish the eyes and immune system. Ginseng promotes vitality and strengthens qi. Jujube and lotus seeds calm the mind, soothe digestion, and encourage restful sleep. These ingredients flow naturally between cuisine and medicine, embodying gentle yet powerful qualities that sustain health.

Modern research continues to validate these ancient insights. Many of these foods demonstrate antioxidant, anti-inflammatory, and immune-regulating effects. Still, researchers emphasize the need for ongoing study to clarify mechanisms and ensure safe, effective use.

As interest in functional foods and integrative nutrition continues to grow, the wisdom of medicine and food homology offers a bridge between tradition and science. Simple choices, such as adding ginger to morning tea or goji berries to soup, remind us that healing often begins in the most ordinary rituals of nourishment. The path forward lies in collaboration with honoring both the ancient roots and modern understanding of food as medicine.

The Nervous System Eats Too

Research has introduced a thoughtful framework for understanding how stress, digestion, and mindfulness are deeply interconnected. This relationship, often described as the stress–digestion–mindfulness triad, offers insight into how our mental state can either support or disrupt digestive function. It also reveals how mindful eating can help restore balance.[7]

Stress, especially when chronic, has a significant impact on the gastrointestinal system. It alters gut motility, disrupts the microbiome, reduces nutrient absorption, and increases inflammation. These changes can contribute to a range of digestive challenges, from indigestion and bloating to more complex conditions such as irritable bowel syndrome. The ANS plays a central role in this process. When the body remains in a state of sympathetic activation or "fight or flight," digestion becomes impaired and energy is diverted away from the gut.

Mindfulness offers a powerful and accessible way to reverse this pattern. When we slow down, pay attention, and engage with our meals consciously, we activate the parasympathetic nervous system. This state of rest and digest supports enzyme production, improves motility, and allows the gut to function more efficiently. By eating with awareness, we nourish not only the body but also the mind.

Unlike diet-centered approaches, mindful eating does not focus on what to eat, but on how we eat. It invites awareness of hunger and fullness cues, appreciation of flavor and texture, and presence at the table. Simple practices such as pausing before a meal, chewing slowly, minimizing distractions, and engaging the senses can transform the act of eating into a healing ritual.

Mindful eating is particularly supportive for those with stress-sensitive digestive conditions. It can ease symptoms, regulate appetite, and enhance the overall experience of nourishment. These effects occur not solely through food itself, but through the nervous system's response to the act of eating. As understanding of the gut–brain connection continues to expand, mindfulness is increasingly recognized as a tool for both emotional regulation and digestive health. Eating with intention and presence becomes more than a lifestyle choice. It becomes a form of medicine.[8]

In Chinese medicine, the spleen and stomach are considered the central organs of digestion and transformation. They do not simply digest food, they digest life. When these organs are overworked or neglected, symptoms such as bloating, fatigue, worry, and lowered immunity may appear. The spleen thrives on regularity, warmth, and mindfulness. Meals that are eaten on time, in a calm environment, and prepared with care are considered more nourishing than any supplement or superfood.

According to the Chinese organ clock, the optimal time to eat is between 7:00 and 9:00 a.m., when the stomach's energy is at its peak. From 9:00 to 11:00 a.m., the spleen takes over, transforming food into qi and blood. Eating a warm, balanced breakfast during this window is believed to enhance digestive strength, improve mental clarity, and support sustained energy throughout the day.[9]

Traditional wisdom also emphasizes the importance of warm, cooked foods, especially in the morning and during the colder months. Cold or raw foods are thought to weaken the spleen's ability to transform nutrients, leading to sluggish metabolism and diminished digestive fire. Soups, porridges, and herbal teas are more than comforting, they are gentle tools of regulation. The act of nourishment, when done with rhythm and presence, becomes a daily ritual of balance. You are not only feeding your body. You are sending a message of safety to your nervous system.

Practice Prompt - A Moment Before the First Bite

Before your next meal, pause. Let this moment become a small ceremony of presence.

Sit down without distractions. Put your phone away. Allow yourself to arrive fully at the table.

Take one full breath in. Feel your belly expand. Then exhale slowly, letting your shoulders drop. Soften your gaze.

Look at your plate. Take a moment to notice the colors, textures, and scents of your food. Ask gently:

What part of this meal is nourishing my body? What part is nourishing my mind? My spirit?

If you are eating breakfast, reflect on the wisdom of the body's rhythm. Place your hands over your belly. Silently tell your nervous system:

"I am safe to receive."

"There is time."

"This food will become my energy, my thoughts, and my strength."

Chew slowly. Taste your food fully. Set down your utensil between bites. Let eating be a full-body experience. Let it be slow enough for your parasympathetic nervous system to awaken and support digestion.

If you notice worry or restlessness arise, gently return to the breath. One inhale. One exhale. You are here. You are nourished.

This is more than eating. It is nervous system regulation. It is restoration. It is medicine.

38

The Night Gate - Calming Rituals for the Shen and Vagal Tone

With the setting sun and fading light, the body is called to soften and slow. In both TCM and circadian biology, evening is considered a sacred window. This is a time to transition from doing to being, from action to restoration. Yet in the modern world, this transition is often overlooked. Bright lights, screen time, emotional residue, and overstimulation can keep the nervous system in overdrive, long past nightfall.[1]

Light at the Wrong Time - A Circadian Risk

Modern life has introduced a quiet but persistent disruption to our biology. The glow of phones, computers, and city lights does more than brighten our nights. It alters the very rhythms that guide our mood, energy, and rest. While we may not notice these shifts immediately, the body remembers. The nervous system responds. The brain adapts. And slowly, the internal harmony we rely on begins to falter.

In a 2016 study, researchers Tomoko Ikeno and Lily Yan explored what happens when light interrupts the darkness.[2] Using a controlled model, they exposed subjects to a four-hour pulse of light in the middle of their usual dark phase. This pattern mirrored what many people now experience, a glow at midnight, a flickering screen in bed, or a porch light cutting through the silence of night. After just two weeks, the effects were clear.

The subjects exposed to this nighttime light lost the natural coherence of their daily rhythms. Unlike those in the control group, they no longer anticipated dawn or dusk. Their activity became irregular, fragmented, and out of sync. When researchers examined the brain, they found that the body's master clock, located in the suprachiasmatic nucleus, had lost its steady rhythm of clock gene expression. Proteins like PER1 and PER2, which normally rise and fall in a tight daily cycle, no longer followed predictable patterns. In other parts of the brain, the disruption varied. The amygdala shifted its rhythm. The paraventricular nucleus lost its timing completely. Some regions, like the hippocampus, remained more stable. But the overall network of timing signals lost its unity.

Emotional changes reflected this disruption. Subjects exposed to light in the middle of the night showed greater signs of anxiety. They were less likely to explore new environments and more prone to signs of stress. On a molecular level, their brains exhibited reduced levels of BDNF, a critical growth factor for emotional resilience and neural repair. This reduction occurred in key emotional centers including the amygdala, hippocampus, and medial prefrontal cortex.

The study offers a powerful insight. The circadian system is not a simple light switch. It is a delicate network of oscillators that must remain in communication. When one part loses time, others begin to drift. When artificial light arrives at the wrong hour, it does more than disturb sleep. It quietly erodes our emotional foundation.

Ikeno and Yan's research is not just a warning about technology or overexposure. It is a reminder of our biological need for darkness. Healthy sleep is not only about setting down our phones or adjusting our routines. It is about learning to trust the deep cycles of light and shadow that once governed every part of our physiology. When the world dims, the nervous system recalibrates. It slows. It rests. It restores. When light remains constant, that process is interrupted.

This research brings scientific support to what TCM has long taught. Rhythm creates health, and rhythm depends on nature's cues. Aligning with the sun, honoring the stillness of night, and protecting the boundary between day and rest are not just spiritual ideas. They are deeply physiological practices. Light is powerful. So is its absence.

When we honor the body's internal clock, we support not only sleep but also emotional strength, clarity, and calm. In a world that moves faster and glows brighter each year, that truth becomes more essential than ever.

Ancient Tools for Modern Sleep Disorders

Sleep is more than rest. It is rhythm. Like the tides, the body is guided by patterns: light and dark, activity and rest, alertness and surrender. These rhythms are orchestrated by the body's internal clock, known as the circadian system. When that clock is disrupted, everything from mood to metabolism can be thrown off course.[3]

Circadian Rhythm Sleep-Wake Disorders (CRSWDs) are becoming increasingly common in our modern world. Shift work, international travel, screen exposure, and chronic stress all pull us out of sync with the natural cues of day and night. The result is insomnia, brain fog, fatigue, and emotional imbalance. Traditional treatments, such as melatonin, stimulants, or sedatives, often fail to address the root of the issue. But there is another way.[4]

Acupuncture, long used to restore balance, offers a powerful way to support circadian health. Though it was developed in a time before clocks and cortisol tests, its effects reach deeply into the same mechanisms that modern science now recognizes as essential to rhythm and regulation. Recent clinical trials have explored how acupuncture can help correct circadian rhythm disorders, shedding light on both the clinical outcomes and the neurochemical mechanisms behind them.[5]

The circadian system is not governed by willpower. It is guided by a master clock in the brain, the suprachiasmatic nucleus, and by a network of peripheral clocks throughout the body. These internal rhythms influence sleep and wake cycles, hormone secretion, digestion, body temperature, and even cellular repair. When this network becomes disrupted, the effects ripple through every system, leading not only to poor sleep but to widespread imbalance in health and mood.

Studies have identified several forms of circadian disruption, including delayed sleep phase syndrome, jet lag, shift-work disorder, and non-24-hour rhythm disturbances. In each of these conditions, the body's internal timing is out of sync with environmental cues.

Acupuncture has been shown to influence this system on both behavioral and biological levels. Clinical and preclinical trials demonstrate that it can improve sleep quality, reduce fatigue, and restore the healthy expression of circadian genes. In human studies, stimulation of points such as PC6, HT7, and SP6 improved sleep scores, lowered cortisol, and increased parasympathetic activity as reflected by HRV. Night-shift workers who received laser stimulation at PC6 showed better autonomic balance and reduced blood pressure, while treatments using SP6 and HT7 were linked with decreased stress hormones and better overall sleep.

These effects occur through multiple pathways. Acupuncture calms the body and restores the internal timing system that regulates sleep and alertness. In the brain, it influences the suprachiasmatic nucleus, the central circadian clock, while also affecting peripheral clocks in organs such as the liver, heart, and kidneys. This regulation extends to genes associated with rhythmic function, including Clock, Bmal1, Per1, and Cry1.

Beyond gene expression, acupuncture modulates key neurotransmitters. It increases calming messengers like GABA and serotonin while balancing dopamine, norepinephrine, and cortisol. These neurochemical shifts promote equilibrium in the nervous system, reducing stress and encouraging rest. Some studies have also found higher melatonin levels following treatment, suggesting that acupuncture may strengthen the body's natural sleep–wake rhythm.

Acupuncture can even act as a non-light-based cue for the body's internal clock. This is particularly valuable for individuals who travel across time zones or work night shifts, where light cues are distorted. Rather than masking symptoms, acupuncture helps re-establish the body's natural rhythm from within.

The implications of this research extend far beyond sleep. Circadian rhythms govern immunity, metabolism, cardiovascular function, and emotional well-being. Chronic misalignment is associated with increased risk of depression, diabetes, and even cancer. By restoring harmony at both cellular and systemic levels, acupuncture may offer protective effects that resonate throughout the entire body.

Chinese medicine teaches that illness often arises from disconnection. This is a disconnection from nature, from others, and from the deeper rhythms within. Acupuncture, by restoring those connections, helps guide the body back toward harmony. The restoration of rhythm becomes more than a physiological process. It becomes a return to balance, to presence, and to rest.

When Sleep Breaks, So Does Balance

Sleep is not passive. It is a vital state of regulation that resets the body's inner rhythms and restores emotional and physiological balance. Yet in the modern world, full and uninterrupted sleep has become increasingly rare. Late nights, early alarms, and constant stimulation fragment the cycles that were once protected by darkness and silence. What seems like a mild inconvenience, a few hours lost here or there, can gradually accumulate into profound shifts in the nervous system.

Research has shown that even short periods of restricted or disrupted sleep can alter how the body processes and responds to stress. When rest is compromised, the ANS, the network that governs our baseline of calm and arousal, shifts toward sympathetic dominance. The body remains alert, the heart becomes more reactive, and recovery is harder to access.[6]

Sleep loss also activates the hypothalamic-pituitary-adrenal axis, the system responsible for releasing cortisol in response to stress. When sleep is reduced or fragmented, cortisol levels rise. This pattern not only reflects stress but also amplifies it. The body begins to anticipate threat even when none exists, creating a state of heightened vigilance. Everyday challenges feel heavier, and emotions become harder to regulate. Over time, this constant activation erodes resilience.

Changes also occur within the brain itself. Receptors involved in serotonin signaling lose sensitivity, and feedback mechanisms that normally quiet the stress response become less efficient. The brain adapts to sleep loss by becoming more reactive and less flexible. This same pattern is seen in chronic stress conditions and mood disorders, suggesting that ongoing sleep restriction may create physiological vulnerability to anxiety and depression.

The effects extend far beyond mood. Short sleep duration has been linked to higher rates of hypertension, cardiovascular disease, and metabolic dysfunction. These patterns may share a common root in the chronic overactivation of stress pathways. When sleep is disturbed, the nervous system cannot recalibrate. What should be a time of renewal becomes a time of silent strain.

This research affirms what many people sense but find difficult to describe. Disrupted sleep does not only leave us tired. It leaves us wired. It changes the tone of the nervous system, placing a hidden weight on both body and mind. Deep rest, the kind that emerges when the parasympathetic system is engaged, is not a luxury. It is a biological necessity and a form of repair. To heal, we must reclaim it.

The Heart, the Liver, and the Landscape of Sleep

As discussed in Chapter 13, the heart is said to house the *Shen*, or spirit, which governs consciousness, thought, emotion, and sleep.[7] The quality of sleep reflects the state of both the *Shen* and the *Hun*. This includes how easily one falls asleep, how deeply one stays asleep, and whether dreams are calm, vivid, or disturbing. When the heart is well-nourished by blood and yin, the *Shen* is anchored, and sleep becomes deep and restorative. But when the heart is imbalanced due to deficiency, internal heat, or emotional agitation, the *Shen* becomes restless. This can lead to difficulty falling asleep, frequent waking, dream-disturbed sleep, or a sense of mental unrest upon waking.[8]

In Chapter 17 we explored The *Hun*, or ethereal soul, which resides in the liver. While the *Shen* governs conscious awareness, the *Hun* is responsible for dreaming, vision, and the movement of the spirit during the night. At rest, both should be peacefully housed and anchored. This anchoring depends on the strength and stability of blood and yin, which provide the nourishment and stillness needed for sleep to unfold. At night, yin energy naturally dominates. This inward, cooling, and restorative force allows the mind and spirit to return to center. If the ethereal soul is not anchored, it can result in the *Hun* wandering at night. This leads to excessive dreaming or dream-disturbed sleep. The person may feel mentally exhausted in the morning, as though they were active all night.[9]

When blood is deficient, the *Shen* may struggle to settle at the beginning of the night, leading to difficulty falling asleep. If yin is deficient, sleep may come easily but become disrupted, with frequent waking and difficulty returning to sleep. This distinction helps guide diagnosis. Difficulty initiating sleep points to blood deficiency. Frequent waking suggests yin deficiency. In both cases, the spirit lacks proper containment, and rest becomes elusive.[10]

The heart and liver work together to support emotional balance and healthy sleep. The heart provides containment. The liver ensures smooth circulation of qi and blood. When both are in harmony, the spirit is calm, the *Hun* is integrated, and the body enters restorative rest. When either is disturbed, sleep becomes a space where unprocessed emotions linger. The mind cannot settle. The spirit cannot return. And the body is left reaching for rest it cannot find.[11]

Twilight Medicine: Regulating the Nervous System through Evening Rituals

New insights confirm that intentional evening rituals can enhance vagal tone and HRV, supporting deep, restorative rest. Simple practices like dimming lights an hour before bed, avoiding stimulating content or conversations, and allowing quiet moments before sleep help cue the body that it's time to downshift.[12]

Herbal teas such as chamomile or lavender, soft ambient music, warm baths, and gentle breathwork can support this transition. Sipping a warm beverage in silence is seen as a way to anchor the spirit and create space for reflection.

Perhaps most importantly, consistency matters. Going to bed and waking at the same time each day, even on weekends, helps regulate the circadian clock and train the body to move smoothly between daytime activity and nighttime restoration.

Evening is more than a time of sleep; it is an invitation to surrender, to let go of the day, reconnect with the breath, and allow the deeper rhythms of healing to take root.

Reflection Prompt - A Ritual of Rest

As you prepare for sleep tonight, give yourself the gift of an intentional transition. Create a space between your day and your rest, a sacred pause where your body is invited to soften and your spirit is welcomed back home.

Try this simple ritual to signal safety, calm, and closure to your nervous system:

- Dim the lights. Let the room begin to quiet visually. Reduce stimulation to support the natural rise of melatonin. Use warm, amber light, to gently mimic dusk.
- Prepare a warm herbal tea. Choose calming herbs like chamomile, lavender, and sleep-inducing tea mixtures. As you sip, hold the mug with both hands. Let the warmth move through you and invite your mind to slow.
- Close your eyes. Take three deep, intentional breaths. Inhale gently through your nose. Exhale even slower, also through the nose, feeling the breath leave the body like a tide drawing out.
- Place your hands over your heart or belly. Feel the rhythm beneath your palms. Soften your shoulders. Drop your awareness inward. With a quiet voice or inner whisper, repeat:
- "It is safe to rest. I release this day. My body remembers how to restore."

Let these words be more than a mantra. Each time you practice this, you are teaching your nervous system a new rhythm, one of ease, safety, and return.

Sleep is not just the absence of wakefulness. It is an active process of repair. Your body knows the way back.

39

Restoring Rhythm - Touch as Medicine for Emotion and Longevity

Emotions do not live only in the mind. They echo through the breath, the muscles, the heartbeat, and the subtle energy beneath the skin. When we feel anxious, overwhelmed, or heartbroken, the body responds instantly. The posture shifts, the breath shortens, and the heart races or withdraws. Over time, these physiological responses become patterned, shaping how we engage with the world.[1]

Touch offers a direct and immediate way to shift the body's internal state. It activates sensory pathways that speak to the nervous system in a language older than words. In moments of tension, even a gentle hand placed with intention can slow the heart, deepen the breath, and restore a sense of inner safety. Within TCM, specific zones on the body are known to influence the flow of qi and the stability of the spirit. Areas such as the chest, forehead, and wrists are not random, they are entry points into the deeper rhythms of regulation. When touch is paired with breath and presence, it becomes a form of medicine, grounding us back into the body and gently guiding the system toward calm.[2]

This chapter begins with that understanding, that emotions are real, tangible, and traceable within the body. And if emotions are carried in the tissues, then healing must also happen through the body. Touch becomes one of our most powerful tools. It sends signals of safety to the brain. It calms the heart. It soothes the breath. specific areas of the body are seen as gateways to regulating the spirit and restoring balance to the organ systems. When combined with mindful breath and presence, even the simplest touch becomes a method of returning home to ourselves.

Here, we explore how practices like acupressure and gua sha can be used to support emotional regulation, calm the ANS, and foster longevity. These ancient therapies work by releasing stagnation, promoting qi flow, and helping the body shift out of survival mode and into restoration. They are more than cosmetic rituals or temporary fixes. They are accessible, embodied practices for cultivating emotional balance, nervous system resilience, and a deeper sense of safety within.

This chapter invites you to reconnect with your emotional body, to learn where your feelings live, and to gently guide them into movement, release, and peace.

Where Feelings Live - Mapping Emotions in the Body

Emotions do not arise only in thought. They move through the body, leaving traces in breath, posture, and sensation. Long before words are formed, the body carries the imprint of joy, fear, anger, or grief. Modern science is beginning to map what ancient wisdom has always known. Feeling is as much a bodily experience as it is a state of mind. A study published by Lauri Nummenmaa and colleagues (2014) explored how emotions are experienced in the body, not just in the mind.[3] Using a method called "body mapping," the team asked over 700 participants from Finland, Sweden, and Taiwan to color areas of a human silhouette where they felt increased or decreased activity in response to specific emotions.

What emerged was a remarkably consistent set of "bodily maps" that revealed where people most commonly feel emotions. Happiness was felt as warmth in the face and chest. Anger surged through the arms and upper body. Sadness caused heaviness in the limbs. Fear showed up in the chest and abdomen. Even more nuanced emotions like love and pride had distinct physical signatures.

These patterns were not random. They appeared consistently across cultures, which suggests that the way we physically experience emotion may be a universal human trait. The body speaks the language of emotion clearly and consistently, often before the mind has a chance to label what is happening.

This research affirms what many healing traditions have long taught. Emotions live in the tissues. They ripple through the skin, influence the breath, and affect the internal organs. When emotions go unprocessed, they can leave imprints like tight shoulders, clenched jaws, or a sunken chest. When given space to move, they also have the power to soften, open, and restore.

From Skin to Spirit - The Neuroscience of Touch

Touch is far more than a sensory experience. It is a foundational form of communication that shapes development, emotional regulation, and physical health. Touch has long been recognized in research as playing a critical role in early life.[4] It supports brain development, secure attachment, and nervous system maturation. The absence of nurturing touch, on the other hand, has been linked to emotional distress, dysregulation, and behavioral difficulties.

Touch continues to influence well-being throughout life. Friendly touch can increase social bonding, improve compliance, and convey nuanced emotional messages such as empathy, gratitude, or reassurance. On a neurological level, affective touch activates the orbitofrontal cortex and caudate, regions associated with pleasure, emotional processing, and decision-making.

The physiological effects of touch are just as powerful. Moderate pressure stimulation, like that used in massage or intentional self-touch, can lower heart rate, reduce blood pressure, and decrease cortisol levels. At the same time, it increases oxytocin, the "bonding hormone," and activates the vagus nerve, supporting parasympathetic activity. These shifts promote relaxation, connection, and immune resilience.

Touch also appears to influence brain chemistry. Moderate pressure touch has been shown to increase serotonin, reduce substance P (a neuropeptide associated with pain), and shift frontal brain activity in ways that support mood, attention, and emotional balance. In studies, these changes correspond with improvements in depression, anxiety, immune function, and cognitive performance.

Together, these findings confirm what many healing traditions already teach. Intentional touch regulates the body, nourishes the spirit, and offers one of the most accessible tools for calming the nervous system and supporting long-term resilience.

The Science of Slow Touch

One of the most primal ways the body communicates safety is through tough. In recent years, research has focused on a specific type of touch known as affective touch. This form of touch is a gentle, slow stroke across the skin that activates specialized nerve fibers called C-tactile afferents. These fibers are most densely located in areas with fine body hair, such as the forearms, and they respond not to pressure or heat, but to the quality of gentle contact.

Research by Köteles and colleagues (2024) examined how this kind of slow, soothing touch affects both sensation and nervous system regulation.[5] In the study, eighty-five participants received slow stroking at a pace of 5 centimeters per second for three minutes. This was compared to rhythmic touching and to a control condition involving skin focused attention.

The results showed that slow stroking felt the most pleasant to participants. It produced a deep sense of comfort and calm, independent of personality traits or levels of body awareness. Interestingly, even though slow stroking and rhythmic touching felt different in terms of intensity and pleasantness, both produced similar effects on the ANS.

Both forms of touch led to a shift toward parasympathetic dominance, which is the body's natural state of rest and recovery. Heart rate decreased. HRV increased. Breathing slowed. Skin conductance patterns also changed, signaling a relaxed but alert state. These shifts mirror what happens during deep exhalation or when we feel truly safe in the presence of another.

One of the most remarkable findings was that the calming physiological effects were not directly tied to how pleasant the touch felt. In other words, even if a person did not find the touch especially enjoyable, their body still moved into a more relaxed and regulated state. This suggests that gentle touch works independently of preference or mood. The body listens and responds, even if the mind is uncertain.

These clinical findings support the ancient understanding that intentional touch is medicine. Whether applied through gua sha, acupressure, or simple human connection, it offers a powerful gateway into the parasympathetic state. Slow, mindful touch helps regulate the nervous system, reduce stress, and bring the body into balance. It is one of the most accessible tools we have to support emotional healing, physiological restoration, and longevity.

Unwinding the Mind - Head Meridian Massage for Stress Relief

In moments of stress, the body often tightens around the head. The jaw clenches, the scalp contracts, and the mind races. These patterns reflect what TCM has understood for centuries. The head is a powerful convergence point of meridians. This is where energy pathways meet and influence both spirit and physiology.

A study conducted by Ya-Ting Lee (2016) explored how head meridian acupoint massage can relieve stress.[6] In this study analysts used a method called grey data model analysis to track subtle yet measurable shifts in the body. Participants in the study received a targeted massage focused on key acupoints along the head, including areas connected to the gallbladder, bladder, and governing vessel meridians.

The results demonstrated that after a brief period of massage, participants experienced a significant reduction in stress indicators. The results showed lowered blood pressure, heart rate, and subjective reports of mental tension. The grey datamodel, designed to analyze small-sample and uncertain systems, revealed a consistent trend. Even simple head-based acupoint massage created a measurable shift toward parasympathetic regulation.

What makes this research particularly relevant is how it affirms both modern and ancient wisdom. The head, often viewed as the domain of thought, is also deeply connected to the body's stress-response system. Acupoints like Baihui (DU20), Yintang, and the points around the temples and occiput are more than energetic landmarks. They are gateways to calming the nervous system, especially when activated through rhythmic, mindful touch.

For readers seeking practical ways to regulate their emotions and support longevity, this study suggests that relief may be just above the neck. A few minutes of acupoint massage, focused on the scalp, temples, or forehead, can provide immediate nervous system support. It is a gentle way to release tension, restore mental clarity, and reconnect the spirit with the body.

Self-Massage for Skin, Spirit, and Longevity

As modern life becomes more demanding, stress often leaves its imprint not just on the mind but also on the skin. The face, in particular, reflects our internal state. Tension settles in the jaw, forehead, and around the eyes. Over time, these patterns become etched into the tissue, contributing to fine lines, dullness, and a sense of fatigue in both appearance and mood.

In a clinical trial conducted by, Frédéric Flament and fellow researchers (2023) investigated how a daily facial self-massage practice could influence visible signs of stress on the skin.[7] They also examined its impact on subjective emotional well-being. Fifty women between the ages of 40 and 60 participated in a two-week protocol, performing a guided three-minute self-massage routine each day. The routine included 14 specific movements. These movements included stretching, flicking, tapping, friction, and smoothing. They also applied botanical oils designed to support both glide and nourishment.

The results showed participants experienced measurable improvements in skin vitality. Fine lines were reduced by nearly 24 percent. Skin plumpness increased, radiance improved by over 16 percent, and signs of drooping (ptosis) diminished. Subjectively, the response was even more profound. More than 85 percent of participants reported that their skin felt smoother, more supple, and visibly rejuvenated. Most importantly, 100 percent of the women said the massage improved their sense of emotional well-being.

While this trial focused on aesthetics, its deeper implications point toward longevity. Touch-based rituals like self-massage activate the parasympathetic nervous system, reduce stress hormone levels, and increase oxytocin. These shifts support emotional regulation and help the body move from chronic tension into a state of repair. Over time, this contributes to healthier aging not just on the surface, but within the deeper networks of the nervous system.

Daily self-massage offers more than cosmetic benefit. It is a gentle, embodied way to reconnect with the self, soften the effects of stress, and promote long-term resilience. In TCM, regular touch rituals are understood to harmonize qi, nourish the spirit, and maintain the vitality of the face as a reflection of internal balance. As the skin softens, the nervous system also shifts, and the entire system begins to remember what it means to feel safe, present, and well.

Gua Sha Through Time - Ancient Origins, Timeless Wisdom

Long before it entered today's beauty routines or clinical studies, gua sha was practiced in courtyards, and villages across East Asia. Its origins reach deep into the folk traditions of China, where it was known not as a cosmetic indulgence, but as a form of emergency medicine and preventive care. The term "gua" means to scrape, while "sha" refers to the reddish marks or petechiae that often appear after the treatment, a sign that stagnant qi and blood were being released from the surface of the body.[8]

The origins of gua sha are difficult to define, but historical evidence places its roots in the earliest writings of Chinese medicine. References in the *Huang Di Nei Jing Su Wen* describe the use of stone tools for external treatments, which many scholars view as early forms of scraping therapy. This practice is often linked to bian stone therapy, considered a precursor to modern gua sha. By the sixth century, commentators such as Quan Yuanqi expanded on these methods, classifying different types of stone instruments according to their therapeutic use.[9]

The sister text of the *Su Wen*, the *Ling Shu* (Spiritual Pivot), expands on these tools through the description of the Nine Needles. The first three of these were non-insertive instruments used to rub, press, and scrape the body surface. The second needle, known as the enshin, had a rounded, egg-shaped tip and was intended for massaging between the flesh without piercing, to regulate the qi. The third, the *teishin*, featured a spoon-shaped tip and was used to stimulate the channels and move stagnant qi without penetration. These tools and their functions bear a clear resemblance to the principles underlying gua sha therapy today.[10]

Additional historical references appear in later dynastic texts. In *Effective Formulas Handed Down for Generations* (1337 CE), physician Wei Yi Lin describes a scraping technique applied to the neck, elbows, knees, and wrists to induce light bleeding and sweating, followed by herbal decoctions to facilitate recovery. This method not only highlights the therapeutic use of scraping but also refers to sha, the reddish petechiae that rise to the surface and signify the release of pathogenic heat.[11]

Although scraping therapies like gua sha became less visible in official medical literature for centuries, likely overshadowed by the rise of acupuncture and herbal pharmacology, they endured as folk remedies throughout East Asia. In many households, especially in rural areas, spoons were the tool of choice to perform gua sha. This improvisational tradition laid the groundwork for modern gua sha practice, where simple tools evolved into professionally designed instruments now used by licensed practitioners and integrative health professionals around the world.[12]

Today, gua sha is experiencing a global resurgence, not only as a beauty ritual, but as a tool for nervous system regulation, pain relief, immune support, and healthy aging. Recent observations suggest that gua sha increases microcirculation, promotes anti-inflammatory effects, and boosts immune responsiveness.[13] These findings echo the ancient belief that when the body is gently stimulated through the skin, it remembers how to heal.

When viewed through the lens of longevity, gua sha is more than an aesthetic practice. It is a ritual of reconnection, to circulation, to breath, to the intelligence of the immune system, and to the emotional patterns stored in the tissues of the face and body. The same simple scraping strokes used centuries ago now stand alongside cutting-edge research, bridging the past and future of integrative wellness.

Circulation and Longevity - Gua Sha's Microvascular Magic

Research is now catching up to this ancient wisdom. In a pilot study led by Arya Nielsen (2007) examined how gua sha affects microcirculation, the blood flow within the smallest vessels of the skin.[14] Using laser Doppler imaging, the study measured changes in surface circulation before and after a single gua sha treatment in healthy volunteers.

The results showed a significant increase in microcirculation at the treatment site, and that this enhanced blood flow persisted for more than 25 minutes after the session ended. This suggests that gua sha does more than just move blood to the surface temporarily. It may support deeper tissue oxygenation, cellular nourishment, and detoxification.

Healthy microcirculation is essential for longevity. As we age, blood flow to the skin and superficial tissues tends to decline. This reduces nutrient delivery, impairs temperature regulation, and slows wound healing. By restoring circulation to areas where it has become sluggish or stagnant, gua sha may help slow visible and biological aging processes. It invigorates not just the skin, but the internal terrain beneath it.

In addition to its circulatory effects, gua sha has been shown in other studies to reduce inflammation, activate the immune system, and relieve pain. When practiced regularly and gently, especially as part of a calming ritual paired with breathwork, it offers a way to care for both the nervous system and the vascular system, two key players in aging and resilience.

This research gives scientific grounding to what TCM has always taught. When the surface flows freely, the internal systems can heal. Gua sha is more than a beauty tool. It is a longevity practice, a way to keep the rivers of the body open, flowing, and full of life.

Skin as Messenger - Gua Sha and the Immune System

In TCM, the skin is more than a boundary. It is a bridge between the internal and external world, a surface where defensive qi circulates and immunity is expressed. When stimulated correctly, the skin becomes a powerful communicator, signaling the body to awaken its healing capacities.

Modern medicine now supports this ancient idea. In 2016 researchers, Tingting Chen et al., explored how gua sha treatment could influence immune function, particularly in response to vaccination.[15] In this controlled experiment, gua sha was applied to the skin of subjects prior to administering an intradermal vaccine. The goal was to determine whether this stimulation could enhance the immune system's ability to recognize and respond to the antigen.

The results were significant. Subjects that received gua sha prior to vaccination showed a significantly stronger immune response, including higher levels of activated immune cells and greater production of antibodies. These effects were not simply mechanical. The clinicians found that gua sha enhanced immune cell recruitment in the skin and activated local inflammation pathways that prime the body to defend and repair. The skin, when gently stimulated, became more responsive and engaged.

What this study reveals is that gua sha may act as a natural immune modulator. It creates a momentary controlled stress signal on the skin that the body interprets as a call to strengthen its defenses. This insight carries profound implications for health and longevity. As the immune system ages, its responsiveness tends to decline. The ability to recognize threats, produce antibodies, and mount efficient repair slows down. Practices that gently stimulate immune vigilance, without overstimulating the system, may support immune resilience well into older age.

Gua sha, especially when used as a ritual of rest and renewal, offers more than circulatory or muscular relief. It supports the skin's natural immune intelligence. It reminds the body how to respond, recover, and regulate. When integrated regularly, this gentle practice may help maintain one of the most essential pillars of longevity, a strong, adaptable, and intelligent immune response.

Gua Sha vs. Facial Rolling - A Scientific Look at Beauty and Balance

In the world of self-care and skin rituals, both facial rollers and gua sha tools have gained popularity. But do they truly create changes in the face? Beyond surface-level beauty, can these tools influence the muscle tone, circulation, and vitality of the tissues they touch? A 2024 randomized controlled trial led by Sun-Hee Ahn and colleagues set out to explore these questions.[16] The trial compared the effects of gua sha massage and facial rolling on several physical parameters, including facial contour, skin elasticity, and muscle tone. Participants were divided into two groups, each receiving either a gua sha treatment or a facial roller massage over a period of several weeks.

The results showed that both treatments improved facial appearance, but gua sha had a significantly greater effect on enhancing facial contour and muscle tone. Participants in the gua sha group showed visible lifting and sculpting along the jawline and cheeks. They also reported more noticeable improvements in tension release, circulation, and overall skin vitality.

One of the reasons for this difference may lie in the nature of gua sha itself. The technique involves slow, intentional strokes with slight pressure, which stimulate lymphatic flow, release fascial adhesions, and engage deeper layers of the tissue. Facial rolling, while gentle and soothing, does not reach the same depth or activate the muscle and connective tissue in the same way.

Although the trial focused on external results, it also hints at something deeper. Gua sha, when practiced with breath and presence, can help quiet the mind, soften stored emotional tension in the face, and shift the body into a parasympathetic state. As muscles release and circulation improves, the nervous system also receives the message that it is safe to relax.

This internal shift is not only restorative in the moment. Over time, it may support longevity. A youthful face is more than a cosmetic goal, it is a visible marker of internal balance, vitality, and health. Signs like skin elasticity, muscle tone, and healthy circulation reflect how well the nervous, lymphatic, and immune systems are functioning beneath the surface. By integrating gua sha as a daily or weekly ritual, individuals are not just lifting the face. They are tending to the very systems that preserve resilience, slow cellular aging, and support graceful longevity from within.

For those seeking to integrate beauty rituals with emotional well-being and nervous system balance, gua sha offers more than a lifted face. It becomes a tool for regulation, presence, and connection, supporting both external glow and internal harmony.

Your Nervous System Knows

You do not need elaborate tools to restore balance. You need breath. You need presence. You need your own hands. A palm placed gently over the heart, the belly, or the forehead can become a powerful act of self-regulation. These gestures are not trivial. They are ancient. The skin, rich with sensory receptors, translates touch into safety, and safety into healing. When the body feels safe, the nervous system remembers how to return to stillness.

Practices like gua sha and acupressure extend this wisdom. With slow, intentional strokes or focused pressure along specific points, you can awaken circulation, support lymphatic movement, ease muscular holding, and soften stored emotional tension. These techniques, passed down through generations and now supported by research, speak the body's original language: connection, rhythm, and flow.

Touch activates the rivers beneath the skin. It enhances microcirculation, delivering oxygen and nutrients to the tissues. It supports the immune system by recruiting the body's defenses to the surface. It lifts and tones facial muscles not just for beauty, but as a reflection of inner vitality. When practiced regularly, these rituals regulate the nervous system, calm the mind, and invite the body into a state of rest and repair. This is the terrain where longevity is cultivated.

True resilience is not about avoiding challenges. It is about meeting life with presence. It is the ability to return to rhythm after disruption. To soften. To breathe. To reconnect with the steady intelligence that lives inside your body. Longevity does not live in a single supplement or treatment. It lives in moments of care. In how we tend to ourselves day by day. In rituals that restore rhythm to the breath, clarity to the mind, and vitality to the tissues. Gua sha becomes a map. Meridian massage becomes a rhythm. Acupressure becomes a dialogue. And breath becomes a bridge. Together, they bring us home.

Longevity Ritual - A Daily Practice for Regulation and Renewal

This is a self-care ritual for nervous system balance, immune support, and long-term vitality. Let it be simple. Let it be intuitive. You do not need to do it all. You just need to begin.

Meridian Massage (12 Channels of Life Flow)

With your fingertips or palms, gently tap or rub along each accessible meridian channel for 15 to 30 seconds. Begin with the arms, move to the torso, and finish with the legs.

- **Lung**: Inner upper arm
- **Large Intestine**: Lateral arm
- **Pericardium**: Center of inner arm
- **Triple Burner**: Outer arm
- **Heart:** Inner arm, pinky side
- **Small Intestine**: Back of arm, ulnar side
- **Stomach**: Front of thighs and outer shins
- **Spleen**: Inner thigh to side of ribs
- **Liver**: Top of foot and Inner leg
- **Gallbladder**: Side of leg and body
- **Kidney**: Sole of foot up inner leg
- **Bladder**: Back of legs, spine (you can use a foam roller), and neck. Follow the flow.

Let your breath lead. You are awakening the body's internal rivers.

Facial Gua Sha for Vital Glow

Apply a small amount of oil or balm. Using a gua sha tool or your fingertips:

- Gently and slowly sweep from chin to ear along the jawline
- Glidesofly from the nose to the cheekbones
- Lift gently along the brow and forehead
- Gently move down the sides of the neck Move slowly. Let the warmth rise. Feel tension melt from the face and jaw.

Acupressure Points for Restoration

Gently add light pressure to each point.

- **ST36**: On the front of the lower leg, about four finger-widths below the bottom of the kneecap, just to the outside of the shin bone. Massaging this point supports immunity, boosts energy, and strengthens vitality.
- **PC6**: On the inner forearm, about three finger-widths up from the wrist crease, in the middle between the two tendons. Pressing here calms

the heart, eases the stomach, and soothes anxiety.

- **HT7:** On the inside of the wrist crease, in line with the pinky finger. You will feel a small hollow at the wrist joint. Pressing here helps calm the mind, anchor the spirit, and ease anxiety.

Hold each point gently for 30 to 60 seconds. Inhale through the nose. Exhale through the mouth. Imagine light or warmth moving into each point.

Auricular Massage

Gently massage the outer ear using your thumbs and fingers:
- Roll from the earlobe upward
- Trace the outer rim and inner ridge
- Gently press the center and tragus
- Focus briefly on the Shen Men point in the upper inner ear

This stimulates the vagus nerve and supports emotional grounding.

Breath and Mantra

Place one hand on your heart or lower abdomen below belly button. Settle into stillness.
- Inhale gently
- Exhale softly. Silently say: "I return to center. I nourish the surface. I protect what lies within." Repeat for three to five rounds. Let your system soften. Let the wisdom of your body guide you home.

When to Refrain from Practicing Gua Sha/Acupressure

For your safety, refrain from practicing gua sha, massage, acupressure if any of the following apply. Always consult your physician before use, especially if you have underlying health conditions.
- Active infections
- Tumors or suspicious growths
- Bleeding or clotting disorders
- Bruises, open wounds, or lesions
- Chronic or acute skin conditions
- Use of anticoagulant medications
- Facial implants (consult your physician prior to facial gua sha)

If a minor skin concern is present, such as a pimple, mole, or wart, simply avoid that specific area.

40

The Rhythm of Return - Acupuncture, Autonomic Healing, and the Way Back to Balance

The path to balance is not a straight line. It moves like breath. Rising, falling, and returning. Healing is not a single event or fixed destination. It is a rhythm. A remembering. A slow reawakening of the body's ability to restore and recalibrate itself in response to life.

This journey has invited you to walk between two worlds. On one side, the science of the ANS. On the other, the ancient wisdom of TCM. Each chapter has traced the threads that connect these worlds, not as competing paradigms, but as complementary lenses for understanding the human body, spirit, and capacity for renewal.

We have explored how the nervous system shapes every aspect of our health. It regulates heart rate, breath, digestion, immunity, and sleep. It influences emotion, memory, and our sense of safety. When the nervous system becomes dysregulated, so do the rhythms of life. Chronic stress, trauma, environmental strain, and emotional overload can push us into survival mode. In this state, the body forgets how to rest. The spirit forgets how to trust.

Healing is possible. Not by overriding the body, but by listening to it.

Not through control, but through relationship.

Acupuncture/acupressure, breathwork, gua sha, ritual, food, and rest, these practices are not simply therapeutic tools. They are invitations. Each one activates the body's innate intelligence and opens the door to balance.

Restoring the Internal Landscape

This book has shown that the body is more than tissue and chemistry. It is a landscape that is alive, responsive, and shaped by the unseen. The Five Spirits, Shen, Hun, Po, Yi, and Zhi, reflect how emotion, memory, and will, live within that landscape. They are not abstract ideals. They are maps of human experience.

When the Shen is scattered, the mind loses clarity.

When the Hun is unanchored, sleep becomes restless and dreams disturbed.

When the Po is weighed down, grief becomes heavy and somatic.

When the Yi is taxed, worry and overthinking disrupt digestion.

When the Zhi is weak, the will to move forward dissolves.

To restore the nervous system is also to restore these spirits. It is to nourish the organs that house them. It is to reconnect the body's functions with the emotional, psychological, and energetic levels of being.

This book has not separated the mechanical from the mystical. It has brought them into dialogue. It has shown that fascia and meridians, vagus tone, qi flow, cytokines and dampness are all part of the same web. They speak different languages but point to the same truth, healing is relational. It happens through reconnection.

The Future of Acupuncture in Nervous System Medicine

As we stand at the intersection of ancient practice and modern research, acupuncture emerges not only as a treatment, but as a paradigm. It shows us what it means to heal through rhythm, not resistance.

Thousands of years ago, Chinese physicians observed the body with deep reverence. They studied the cycles of nature and applied them to human physiology. They saw how wind, cold, damp, and heat affected both climate and constitution. They named channels of flow. They described the interdependence of organ systems. They charted a medicine of movement and stillness.

Today, researchers measure what those physicians sensed through observation thousands of years ago. Acupuncture has been shown to affect the ANS, reduce sympathetic overactivation, enhance vagal tone, and modulate inflammation. Studies confirm its effects on HRV, neurotransmitter release, sleep quality, and mood regulation. The language has changed, but the principles remain.

Acupuncture is particularly supportive in its ability to *rewire the stress response*. Chronic stress alters the baseline of the nervous system. What was once a temporary defense state becomes a constant undercurrent. The body begins to organize itself around threat, even in the absence of danger. This reshapes hormonal patterns, immune function, digestion, and emotional resilience.

Acupuncture does not push the body to change. It invites it. With precision and gentleness, the needle engages the sensory system in a way that initiates regulation. Points are chosen not randomly, but intentionally. Many lie along fascial planes, over major nerve junctions, or near vascular bundles. These access points allow communication with deep regulatory mechanisms. These mechanisms governing not just pain and movement, but breath, circulation, digestion, and calm.

In a world saturated by stimulation, this subtlety is radical. Acupuncture slows the pace. It interrupts the loop of urgency. It offers a felt sense of safety that the body can internalize.

Reweaving a New Model of Care

This book has asked us to reconsider what it means to offer care. Not just as intervention, but as presence. The healing relationship is central. Whether through the hand on the shoulder, the needle placed with intention, or the ritual of breath, healing is a co-regulated experience.

The nervous system responds to touch, tone, and attention. It does not only respond to pharmaceuticals or procedures. It responds to presence, rhythm, and trust.

Acupuncture models this kind of care. It asks both practitioner and patient to slow down and listen to what is subtle. In doing so, it becomes not only medicine for the body, but medicine for the times we live in.

Our current culture prizes speed, productivity, and disconnection from nature. It leaves little space for slowness, digestion, or repair. The nervous system suffers under this weight. We see the consequences in rising rates of burnout, anxiety, digestive disorders, and autoimmune conditions. The body cannot sustain unending acceleration. Healing begins when we remember how to stop, feel, and breathe again.

Riding the Wave of Regulation

This book began with a question. What does it mean to be wired for balance?

The answer is not simple. It is not a single formula. It is a process. To be wired for balance is to honor your capacity to shift between states. To move between sympathetic activation and parasympathetic restoration. Between doing and being. Between effort and ease.

It is the ability to respond, without becoming reactive. To feel, without becoming overwhelmed. To rest, without guilt. To know the difference between urgency and importance. To trust that your body has the wisdom to heal when given the chance.

Science and spirit are not in opposition. They are two rivers feeding the same ocean.

The meridian is no longer just a poetic metaphor. It is a communication channel embedded in fascia, nerves, and fluid.

The vagus nerve is no longer just a medical term. It is a bridge between emotion and physiology, between safety and connection.

The needle is no longer just a clinical tool. It is a compass that helps the body find its way home.

The role of the practitioner is not to fix, but to listen. To offer ritual, rhythm, and touch. To help the patient feel their body as a place of wisdom, not dysfunction.

The role of the reader, the patient, the seeker, is to begin that dialogue within themselves. To learn the patterns. To feel the shifts. To respond with kindness.

Continuing the Rhythm Through Self Care Rituals

Healing is not a single moment. It is a practice. It lives in the daily choices we make to return to center. Breath by breath. Meal by meal. Touch by touch.

To support this integration, Ancient Vitality Tools was created as a companion to this book and as a living extension of its wisdom. The Wired for Balance Companion Journal invites you to reflect on your inner state, your sleep, your emotions, and your nervous system patterns day by day. The Self-Care Ritual Deck offers practices from each chapter, rooted in both Chinese medicine and modern neuroscience, to help regulate your system through breath, movement, intention, and sensory presence.

This collection is continuing to grow. In the months ahead, new offerings will be introduced, including the Five Spirit Journals, each attuned to the emotional and physiological landscape of the Shen, Hun, Po, Zhi, and Yi. These guided spaces will help you work gently with the inner movements of grief, vision, will, worry, and the heart-mind.

Over time, Ancient Vitality Tools will expand into seasonal kits, ritual tools, oils, and practices aligned with the rhythms of nature and the wisdom of the meridians. Each creation is being designed with care to support longevity, resilience, and harmony with life.

This is more than a book. It is a doorway. You are invited to continue the journey.

Final Reflections

As we move forward, perhaps we will see that healing is not something we force through effort or analysis, but something that unfolds as we return to rhythm and let the body remember its own pace.

Acupuncture reminds us of that rhythm. So does breath. So does sleep. So does stillness.

To practitioners. May your presence be your medicine. May your hands carry both precision and compassion. May you continue to walk between ancient knowledge and emerging science.

To readers and patients. May you feel empowered to rest. To reflect. To reclaim the pace that nourishes your nervous system. May you return to the wisdom that lives within you.

Balance is not a fixed point.
It is a rhythm.
A wave we learn to ride.
A pattern we learn to recognize.
A memory we learn to trust.
"The part can never be well unless the whole is well."
— Plato, *Charmides*

Notes

Introduction Endnotes

1. Wei Huang et al., "Autonomic Activation in Insomnia: The Case for Acupuncture," *Journal of Clinical Sleep Medicine* 7, no. 1 (February 15, 2011): 95-102, PMCID: PMC3041619, https://doi.org/10.5664/jcsm.28048; Yun-tao Ma, Mila Ma, and Zang-Hee Cho, *Biomedical Acupuncture for Pain Management: An Integrative Approach* (St. Louis, MO: Elsevier Health Sciences, 2005), xiii.
2. Ben Kavoussi and Brian E. Ross, "The Neuroimmune Basis of Anti-Inflammatory Acupuncture," *Integrative Cancer Therapies* 6, no. 3 (September 2007). https://doi.org/10.1177/1534735407305892.
3. Ma, Ma, and Cho, *Biomedical Acupuncture*, xvi.
4. Tzu-Hsin Wei and Ching-Liang Hsieh, "Effect of Acupuncture on the p38 Signaling Pathway in Several Nervous System Diseases: A Systematic Review." *International Journal of Molecular Sciences* 21, no. 13 (2020): 4693. https://doi.org/10.3390/ijms21134693.
5. Hyeonho Kim, Hye Rim Jung, Jae Beom Kim, and Dae Jung Kim, "Autonomic Dysfunction in Sleep Disorders: From Neurobiological Basis to Potential Therapeutic Approaches," *Journal of Clinical Neurology* 18, no. 2 (March 2022): 140–151, https://doi.org/10.3988/jcn.2022.18.2.140; Kevin J. Tracey, "The Inflammatory Reflex." *Nature* 420, no. 6917 (2002): 853–859. https://doi.org/10.1038/nature01321; Valentin A. Pavlov and Kevin J. Tracey, "The Vagus Nerve and the Inflammatory Reflex—Linking Immunity and Metabolism," *Nature Reviews Endocrinology* 8, no. 12 (2012): 743–754, https://doi.org/10.1038/nrendo.2012.189.

6. Shih-Tsung Huang et al., "Increase in the Vagal Modulation by Acupuncture at Neiguan Point in the Healthy Subjects," *American Journal of Chinese Medicine* 33, no. 1 (2005): 157–64, https://doi.org/10.1142/S0192415X0500276X; Dieu-Thuong Thi Trinh et al., "Heart Rate Variability during Auricular Acupressure at the Left Sympathetic Point on Healthy Volunteers: A Pilot Study," *Frontiers in Neuroscience* 17 (June 1, 2023), doi.org/10.3389/fnins.2023.1116154.

7. Ted J. Kaptchuk, *The Web That Has No Weaver: Understanding Chinese Medicine*, 2nd ed. (New York: McGraw-Hill, 2000), 215-238; Paul U. Unschuld and Hermann Tessenow, *Huang Di Nei Jing Su Wen: An Annotated Translation of Huang Di's Inner Classic – Basic Questions*, vol. 1 (Berkeley: University of California Press, 2011), 95-135.

8. Leon I. Hammer, *Dragon Rises, Red Bird Flies: Psychology and Chinese Medicine*, rev. ed. (Seattle: Eastland Press, 2005), 302-303, 310-314; Ma, Ma, and Cho, *Biomedical Acupuncture for Pain Management*, 1-9.

9. Ma, Ma, and Cho, *Biomedical Acupuncture for Pain Management*, 1-9, 25, 52-56.

10. Ted J. Kaptchuk, *The Web That Has No Weaver*, 132-141; Ding Li, *Acupuncture, Meridian Theory, and Acupuncture Points* (San Francisco: China Books & Periodicals, 1992), 3-14; Helene M. Langevin and Jason A. Yandow, "Relationship of acupuncture points and meridians to connective tissue planes" *The Anatomical Record* 269, no. 6 (2002): 257–265. https://doi.org/10.1002/ar.10185.

11. Langevin and Yandow, "Relationship of Acupuncture Points and Meridians," 257-265.

12. Alicia C. Ahn et al., "Electrical Impedance of Acupuncture Meridians: The Relevance of Subcutaneous Collagenous Bands," *PLoS ONE* 5, no. 7 (2010): e11907, https://doi.org/10.1371/journal.pone.0011907.

13. Ma, Ma, Cho, *Biomedical Acupuncture*, 17-35; Langevin and Yandow, "Relationship of Acupuncture Points and Meridians", 257-265.

Chapter 1 Endnotes

1. Elaine N. Marieb, *Human Anatomy & Physiology*, 2nd ed. (San Francisco: Pearson Benjamin Cummings, 2005), 9.
2. David Shier, Jackie Butler, and Ricki Lewis, *Hole's Human Anatomy & Physiology*, 9th ed. (Boston: McGraw-Hill, 2006), 5.
3. Sandy Fritz, *Mosby's Essential Sciences for Therapeutic Massage*, 4th ed. (St. Louis, MO: Mosby, 2012), 4.
4. Yun-tao Ma, Mila Ma, and Zang-Hee Cho, *Biomedical Acupuncture for Pain Management: An Integrative Approach* (St. Louis, MO: Elsevier Churchill Livingstone, 2005), 6-7; Marieb, *Human Anatomy & Physiology*, 9.
5. Fritz, *Mosby's Essential Sciences for Therapeutic Massage*, 4th ed., 25.
6. Leon Hammer, *Dragon Rises, Red Bird Flies: Psychology & Chinese Medicine*, 2nd ed. (New York: Ballantine Books, 2010), 60.
7. Giovanni Maciocia, *The Foundations of Chinese Medicine: A Comprehensive Text for Acupuncturists and Herbalists*, 2nd ed. (London: Churchill Livingstone, 2005), 116–122.
8. Robert S. Feldman, *Psychology 105*, 11th ed. (New York: Pearson, 2013), custom edition for University of New Mexico, 25.
9. Marieb, *Human Anatomy & Physiology*, 10.
10. Fritz, *Mosby's Essential Sciences*, 4th ed., 27.
11. Marieb, *Human Anatomy & Physiology*, 12.
12. Fritz, *Mosby's Essential Sciences*, 4th ed., 27.
13. Shier, Butler, and Lewis, *Hole's Human Anatomy & Physiology*, 13.
14. Peng Gao, Xi Gao, Tairan Fu, and Dan Xu, "Acupuncture: Emerging Evidence for Its Use as an Analgesic (Review)." *Experimental and Therapeutic Medicine 9*, no. 5 (2015): 1577–1581. https://doi.org/10.3892/etm.2015.2348; Ning-cen Li, Ming-yue Li, Bo Chen, and Yi Guo, "A New Perspective of Acupuncture: The Interaction among Three Networks Leads to Neutralization," *Evidence-Based Complementary and Alternative Medicine*, (2019): Article ID 2326867, https://doi.org/10.1155/2019/2326867.
15. Kathleen K.S. Hui et al., "Acupuncture Modulates the Limbic System and Subcortical Gray Structures of the Human Brain: Evidence from

fMRI Studies in Normal Subjects," *Human Brain Mapping* 9, no.1 (2000): 13–25, DOI: 10.1002/(sici)1097-0193(2000)9:1<13::aid-hbm2>3.0.co;2-f, PMCID: PMC6871878; Vitaly Napadow et al,. "The Status and Future of Acupuncture Mechanism Research." *The Journal of Alternative and Complementary Medicine* 14, no. 7 (2012): 861–869. doi: 10.1089/acm.2008.SAR-3,https://pmc.ncbi.nlm.nih.gov/articles/PMC3155097/.

16. Adrián Hernández-Vicente et al., "Heart Rate Variability and Exceptional Longevity," *Frontiers in Physiology* 11 (September 17, 2020): 566399, doi: 10.3389/fphys.2020.566399; Sz. Hamvas et al., "Acupuncture Increases Parasympathetic Tone, Modulating HRV: Systematic Review and Meta-Analysis," *Complementary Therapies in Medicine* 72 (March 2023): 102905, https://doi.org/10.1016/j.ctim.2022.102905; Stefanie Hillebrand et al., "Heart Rate Variability and First Cardiovascular Event in Populations without Known Cardiovascular Disease: Meta-Analysis and Dose–Response Meta-Regression," *EP Europace* 15, no. 5 (May 2013): 742–49, https://doi.org/10.1093/europace/eus341.

Chapter 2 Endnotes

1. Elaine N. Marieb, *Human Anatomy & Physiology*, 2nd ed. (San Francisco: Pearson Benjamin Cummings, 2005), 9.
2. Robert S. Feldman, *Psychology 105*, 11th ed. (New York: Pearson, 2013), custom edition for University of New Mexico, 70; Sandy Fritz, *Mosby's Essential Sciences for Therapeutic Massage*, 4th ed. (St. Louis, MO: Mosby, 2012), 27.
3. Marieb, *Human Anatomy & Physiology*, 9-10; David Shier, Jackie Butler, and Ricki Lewis, *Hole's Human Anatomy & Physiology*, 9th ed. (Boston: McGraw-Hill, 2006), 27.
4. Marieb, *Human Anatomy & Physiology*, 9-12.
5. Fritz, *Mosby's Essential Sciences*, 4th ed., 27; Marieb, *Human Anatomy & Physiology*, 9-12.

6. Fritz, *Mosby's Essential Sciences*, 4th ed., 27
7. Shier, Butler, and Lewis, *Hole's Human Anatomy & Physiology*, 204; Marieb, *Human Anatomy & Physiology*, 9-12; Qian-Qian Li et al., "Acupuncture Effect and Central Autonomic Regulation," *Evidence-Based Complementary and Alternative Medicine* 2013 (May 26, 2013): 267959, doi: 10.1155/2013/267959.
8. Shier, Butler, and Lewis, *Hole's Human Anatomy & Physiology*, 204; Marieb, *Human Anatomy & Physiology*, 9-12.
9. Kevin J. Tracey, "The Inflammatory Reflex." *Nature* 420, no. 6917 (2002): 853–859. https://doi.org/10.1038/nature01321; Kathleen K. S. Hui et al., "Acupuncture Modulates the Limbic System and Subcortical Gray Structures of the Human Brain: Evidence from fMRI Studies in Normal Subjects," *Human Brain Mapping* 9, no. 1 (February 16, 2000): 13–25, PMID: 10643726; https://doi.org/10.1002/(SICI)1097-0193(2000)9:1<13::AID-HBM2>3.0.CO;2-F; Vitaly Napadow et al, "Effects of electroacupuncture versus manual acupuncture on the human brain as measured by fMRI." *Human Brain Mapping* 24, no. 3 (2005): 193–205. **https://doi.org/10.1002/hbm.20081.**
10. Giovanni Maciocia, *The Foundations of Chinese Medicine: A Comprehensive Text for Acupuncturists and Herbalists*, 2nd ed. (Edinburgh: Elsevier Churchill Livingstone, 2005), 25; Leon Hammer, *Dragon Rises, Red Bird Flies: Psychology and Chinese Medicine* (Eastland Press, 2005), 60.
11. Stephen W. Porges, "Polyvagal Theory: A Science of Safety," *Frontiers in Integrative Neuroscience* 16 (May 10, 2022): 871227, PMC9131189, DOI: 10.3389/fnint.2022.871227; Julian F. Thayer and Richard D. Lane, "A Model of Neurovisceral Integration in Emotion Regulation and Dysregulation," *Journal of Affective Disorders* 61, no. 3 (2000): 201–216, DOI: 10.1016/s0165-0327(00)00338-4; Wei Zhou and Peyman Benharash, "Effects and Mechanisms of Acupuncture Based on the Principle of Meridians," *Journal of Acupuncture and Meridian Studies* 7, no. 4 (August 2014): 190–93, https://doi.org/10.1016/j.jams.2014.02.007; Andrei Efremov, "Psychosomatics: Communication of the Central Nervous System through Connection to Tissues,

Organs, and Cells," *Clinical Psychopharmacology and Neuroscience* 22, no. 4 (September 6, 2024): 565–77, PMID: 39420604, doi: 10.9758/cpn.24.1197.

12. Shier, Butler, and Lewis, *Hole's Human Anatomy & Physiology*, 203.
13. Marieb, *Human Anatomy & Physiology*, 342.
14. Fritz, *Mosby's Essential Sciences*, 4th ed., 134.
15. Tom Tam, *Healing Cancer with the Nervous System* (Oriental Culture Institute, 2012), 14.
16. Yun-tao Ma, Mila Ma, and Zang-Hee Cho, *Biomedical Acupuncture for Pain Management: An Integrative Approach* (St. Louis, MO: Elsevier Churchill Livingstone, 2005), 3.
17. Tam, *Healing Cancer with the Nervous System*, 14.
18. Ma, Ma, and Cho, *Biomedical Acupuncture for Pain Management*, 3.
19. Yan-Wei Li et al., "The Autonomic Nervous System: A Potential Link to the Efficacy of Acupuncture," *Frontiers in Neuroscience* 16 (December 8, 2022): 1038945, doi: 10.3389/fnins.2022.1038945; Ji-Sheng Han, "Acupuncture and Endorphins." *Neuroscience Letters* 361, no. 1–3 (2004): 258–261. https://doi.org/10.1016/j.neulet.2003.12.019; Zezhi Fan et al, "Effects and mechanisms of acupuncture analgesia mediated by afferent nerves in acupoint microenvironments." *Frontiers in Neuroscience* 17 (2024): 1239839. https://doi.org/10.3389/fnins.2023.1239839.
20. Hui et al., "Acupuncture Modulates the Limbic System and Subcortical Gray Structures of the Human Brain: Evidence from fMRI Studies in Normal Subjects," *Human Brain Mapping* 9, no.1 (2000): 13–25, DOI: 10.1002/(sici)1097-0193(2000)9:1<13::aid-hbm2>3.0.co;2-f, PMCID: PMC6871878; Hammer, *Dragon Rises, Red Bird Flies: Psychology & Chinese Medicine*, 60; Bo Sun et al., "Treatment of Depression with Acupuncture Based on Pathophysiological Mechanism," *International Journal of General Medicine* 17 (January 31, 2024): 347–57, PMID: 38314195; Jingwen Cui et al., "Research Progress on the Mechanism of the Acupuncture Regulating Neuro-Endocrine-Immune Network System," *Veterinary Sciences* 8, no. 8 (July 30, 2021): 149, PMID:

34437474.

21. Hui et al., "Acupuncture Modulates the Limbic System," 13–25; Alcedo, Joy, Thomas Flatt, and Elena Pasyukova. "The Role of the Nervous System in Aging and Longevity." *Frontiers in Genetics* 4 (2013): 124. https://doi.org/10.3389/fgene.2013.00124; Zheng, Jinyan, Jun Zhu, Yan Wang, and Zhenzhen Tian. "Effects of acupuncture on hypothalamic-pituitary-adrenal axis: Current status and future perspectives." *Journal of Integrative Medicine* 22, no. 4 (2024): 446–459. PMID: 38955651, DOI: 10.1016/j.joim.2024.06.004, https://pubmed.ncbi.nlm.nih.gov/38955651/; Morningside Acupuncture NYC. "Acupuncture's Effect on the Autonomic Nervous System." *Morningside Acupuncture NYC Blog*. Accessed July 7, 2025. https://www.morningsideacupuncturenyc.com/blog/acupuncture-effect-on-nervous-system.

22. Han, "Acupuncture and Endorphins," 258–261; Zhi-Qi Zhao, "Neural Mechanism Underlying Acupuncture Analgesia," *Progress in Neurobiology* 85, no. 4 (August 2008): 355–375, https://doi.org/10.1016/j.pneurobio.2008.05.004.

23. Macicoa, *The Foundations of Chinese Medicine*, 89-91

24. Joyce Shaffer, "Neuroplasticity and Clinical Practice: Building Brain Power for Health," *Frontiers in Psychology* 7 (July 26, 2016): 1118, PMID: 27507957; Patrícia Marzola et al., "Exploring the Role of Neuroplasticity in Development, Aging, and Neurodegeneration," *Brain Sciences* 13, no. 12 (November 21, 2023): 1610, doi: 10.3390/brainsci13121610; Wei Zhou and Peyman Benharash, "Effects and Mechanisms of Acupuncture Based on the Principle of Meridians," *Journal of Acupuncture and Meridian Studies* 7, no. 4 (August 2014): 190–193, 10.1016/j.jams.2014.02.007; Hui et al., "Acupuncture Modulates the Limbic System," 13–25.

25. Monica Bucci, Sara S. Marques, David Oh, and Nadine Burke Harris. "Toxic Stress in Children and Adolescents." *Advances in Pediatrics* 63, no. 1 (2016): 403–428. https://doi.org/10.1016/j.yapd.2016.04.002; Joseph M. Zullo, Bruce A. Drake, Michael J. Aron, et al., "Regulation

of lifespan by neural excitation and REST," *Nature* 574, no. 7778 (October 2019): 359–364, DOI:10.1038/s41586-019-1647-8

26. Claudio Franceschi et al., "Inflammaging and Anti-Inflammaging: A Systemic Perspective on Aging and Longevity Emerged from Studies in Humans," *Mechanisms of Ageing and Development* 128, no. 1 (2007): 92–105, https://doi.org/10.1016/j.mad.2006.11.016; Hui et al., "Acupuncture Modulates the Limbic System," 13–25; Jing, Cao et al., "Analgesic Effects Evoked by Real and Imagined Acupuncture: A Neuroimaging Study." *Cerebral Cortex* 29, no. 8 (2019): 3220–3231. https://doi.org/10.1093/cercor/bhy190; Chueh-Yi Tsai et al., "Acupuncture Improves Neurological Function and Anti-Inflammatory Effect in Patients with Acute Ischemic Stroke: A Double-Blinded Randomized Controlled Trial," *Complementary Therapies in Medicine* 82 (June 2024): 103049, PMID: 38729273, DOI: 10.1016/j.ctim.2024.103049; Zhou and Benharash, "Effects and Mechanisms of Acupuncture."

27. Maciocia, *The Foundations of Chinese Medicine*, 41-71

28. Thayer and Lane, "A Model of Neurovisceral Integration," 201–216; Porges, *The Polyvagal Theory*; Hui et al., "Acupuncture Modulates the Limbic System," 13–25; Fred Shaffer and J. P. Ginsberg. "An Overview of Heart Rate Variability Metrics and Norms." *Frontiers in Public Health* 5 (2017): 258. https://doi.org/10.3389/fpubh.2017.00258.

Chapter 3 Endnotes

1. Yun-tao Ma, Mila Ma, and Zang-Hee Cho, *Biomedical Acupuncture for Pain Management: An Integrative Approach* (St. Louis, MO: Elsevier Churchill Livingstone, 2005), 2.

2. Tom Tam, *Healing Cancer with the Nervous System* (Oriental Culture Institute, 2012), 14; Ma, Ma, and Cho, *Biomedical Acupuncture for Pain Management*, 3.

3. Yuwei Li et al., "The Autonomic Nervous System: A Potential Link to the Efficacy of Acupuncture," *Frontiers in Neuroscience* 16 (December

8, 2022): 1038945, https://doi.org/10.3389/fnins.2022.1038945.
4. Elaine N. Marieb, *Human Anatomy & Physiology*, 2nd ed. (San Francisco: Pearson Education Inc., 2005), 502.
5. Tam, *Healing Cancer with the Nervous System*, 21.
6. Ma, Ma, and Cho, *Biomedical Acupuncture for Pain Management*, 5; Christopher H. Gibbons, "Basics of Autonomic Nervous System Function," in *Handbook of Clinical Neurology*, vol. 160 (2019): 407–18, DOI: 10.1016/B978-0-444-64032-1.00027-8.
7. Tam, *Healing Cancer with the Nervous System*, 15; Robert S. Feldman, *Psychology 105*, 11th ed. (New York: McGraw-Hill Education, 2013), 70.
8. Marieb, *Human Anatomy & Physiology*, 2nd ed, 343; Sandy Fritz, *Mosby's Fundamentals of Therapeutic Massage*, 4th ed. (St. Louis: Mosby/Elsevier, 2012), 150.
9. Qian-Qian Li et al., "Acupuncture Effect and Central Autonomic Regulation," *Evidence-Based Complementary and Alternative Medicine* 2013, Article ID 267959, https://doi.org/10.1155/2013/267959; Ma, Ma, and Cho, *Biomedical Acupuncture for Pain Management*, 3; Fritz, *Mosby's Fundamentals of Therapeutic Massage*, 4th ed. (2012), 150.
10. Bruno Bonaz et al., "The Vagus Nerve in the Neuro-Immune Axis: Implications in the Pathology of the Gastrointestinal Tract," *Frontiers in Immunology* 8 (2017): Article 1452, https://doi.org/10.3389/fimmu.2017.01452; Julian F. Thayer and Richard D. Lane, "The Role of Vagal Function in the Risk for Cardiovascular Disease and Mortality," *Biological Psychology* 74, no. 2 (2007): 224–242, https://doi.org/10.1016/j.biopsycho.2005.11.013; Toku Takahashi, "Acupuncture for Functional Gastrointestinal Disorders," *Journal of Gastroenterology* 41, no. 5 (May 2006): 408–417, https://doi.org/10.1007/s00535-006-1773-6.
11. Li et al., "Acupuncture Effect and Central Autonomic Regulation."
12. Thayer and Lane, "Role of Vagal Function"; Claudio Franceschi et al., "Inflammaging: A New Immune–Metabolic Viewpoint for Age-Related Diseases," *Nature Reviews Endocrinology* 14, no. 10 (2018):

576–590. https://doi.org/10.1038/s41574-018-0059-4
13. Donald Shaffer and J. P. Ginsberg, "An Overview of Heart Rate Variability Metrics and Norms," *Frontiers in Public Health* 5 (2017): 258. https://doi.org/10.3389/fpubh.2017.00258
14. Klaus Streitberger et al., "Effects of Verum Acupuncture Compared to Placebo Acupuncture on Quantitative EEG and Heart Rate Variability in Healthy Volunteers." *Journal of Alternative and Complementary Medicine* 14, no. 5 (June 2008): 505–513, PMID: 18537467, DOI: 10.1089/acm.2007.0552; Joanne W. Y. Chung, V. C. Yan, and H. Zhang., "Effect of Acupuncture on Heart Rate Variability: A Systematic Review." *Evidence-Based Complementary and Alternative Medicine* 2014 (2014): Article ID 819871. https://doi.org/10.1155/2014/819871; Zheng, J. Y., J. Zhu, Y. Wang, and Z. Z. Tian. "Effects of Acupuncture on Hypothalamic–Pituitary–Adrenal Axis: Current Status and Future Perspectives." *Journal of Integrative Medicine* 22, no. 4 (July 2024): 445–458. https://doi.org/10.1016/j.joim.2024.06.004.
15. Hyungjun Kim et al., "Reduced Tactile Acuity in Chronic Low Back Pain Is Linked with Structural Neuroplasticity in Primary Somatosensory Cortex and Is Modulated by Acupuncture Therapy." *NeuroImage* 217 (2020): 116899. https://doi.org/10.1016/j.neuroimage.2020.116899; Kenneth K.S. Hui et al., "Acupuncture Modulates the Limbic System and Subcortical Gray Structures of the Human Brain: Evidence from fMRI Studies in Normal Subjects," *Human Brain Mapping* 9, no.1 (2000): 13–25, DOI: 10.1002/(sici)1097-0193(2000)9:1<13::aid-hbm2>3.0.co;2-f, PMCID: PMC6871878.
16. Hui et al., "Acupuncture Modulates the Limbic System," *Human Brain Mapping* 9, no. 1 (2000): 13–25; Nick Errington-Evans., "Randomised Controlled Trial on the Use of Acupuncture in Adults with Chronic, Non-Responsive Anxiety." *Acupuncture in Medicine* 30, no. 1 (2012): 21–26. DOI: 10.1136/acupmed-2014-010524; Dae-Sung Hwang et al., "Sympathomodulatory effects of Saam acupuncture on Heart Rate Variability in night-shift-working nurses." *Complementary Therapies in Medicine* 19, Suppl. 1 (2011): S33–S40. https://doi.org/10.1016/

j.ctim.2010.11.001.
17. Ning Li et al., "The Anti-Inflammatory Actions and Mechanisms of Acupuncture from Acupoint to Target Organs via Neuro-Immune Regulation," *Journal of Inflammation Research* 14 (2021): 7191–7224, https://doi.org/10.2147/JIR.S341581; Streitberger et al., "Effects of Verum Acupuncture Compared to Placebo Acupuncture; Chung, Yan, and Zhang, "Effect of Acupuncture on Heart Rate Variability," *Journal of Alternative and Complementary Medicine* 14, no. 5 (June 2008): 505–513, https://doi.org/10.1089/acm.2007.055.
18. Toku Takahashi, "Acupuncture for Functional Gastrointestinal Disorders," *Journal of Gastroenterology* 41, no. 5 (2006): 408–417, PMID: 16799881, DOI: 10.1007/s00535-006-1773-6.

Chapter 4 Endnotes

1. Elaine N. Marieb, *Human Anatomy & Physiology*, 6th ed. (San Francisco: Pearson Benjamin Cummings, 2005), 480; David Shier, Jackie Butler, and Ricki Lewis, *Hole's Human Anatomy & Physiology*, 11th ed. (Boston: McGraw-Hill, 2006), 233-235.
2. Bruno Bonaz, Valérie Sinniger, and Séverine Pellissier, "The Vagus Nerve in the Neuro-Immune Axis: Implications in the Pathology of the Gastrointestinal Tract," *Frontiers in Immunology* 8 (November 2, 2017): 1452, https://doi.org/10.3389/fimmu.2017.01452.
3. Christopher H. Gibbons, "Basics of Autonomic Nervous System Function," in *Handbook of Clinical Neurology*, vol. 160 (2019): 407–418, https://doi.org/10.1016/B978-0-444-64032-1.00027-8; Robert S. Feldman, *Psychology 105*, custom ed. for University of New Mexico (New York: McGraw-Hill Education, 2013), 70; Fritz, *Mosby's Essential Sciences for Therapeutic Massage*, 4th ed., 70.
4. Yun-tao Ma, Mila Ma, and Zang-Hee Cho, *Biomedical Acupuncture for Pain Management: An Integrative Approach* (St. Louis, MO: Elsevier Churchill Livingstone, 2005), 7.
5. Marieb, *Human Anatomy & Physiology*, 480.

6. Bonaz, "The Vagus Nerve in the Neuro-Immune Axis," 1452.
7. Kathleen S. Hui et al., "Acupuncture Modulates the Limbic System and Subcortical Gray Structures of the Human Brain: Evidence from fMRI Studies in Normal Subjects," *Human Brain Mapping* 9, no.1 (2000): 13–25, DOI: 10.1002/(sici)1097-0193(2000)9:1<13::aid-hbm2>3.0.co;2-f, PMCID: PMC6871878; Qian-Qian Li et al., "Acupuncture Effect and Central Autonomic Regulation," Evidence-Based *Complementary and Alternative Medicine* 2013 (2013): Article ID 267959. https://doi.org/10.1155/2013/267959; Xiao-Yu Wang, et al., "Effects of Electroacupuncture at PC6 and ST36 on Heart Rate Variability in Anesthetized Mice." *World Journal of TCM* 1, no. 3 (July–September 2015): 67–70. https://doi.org/10.15806/J.ISSN.23118571.2014.0015.https://journals.lww.com/wtcm/fulltext/2015/01030/effects_of_electroacupuncture_at_pc6_and_st36_on.7.aspx.
8. Hui et al., "Acupuncture Modulates the Limbic System." ; Wang et al., "Effects of Electroacupuncture at PC6 and ST36," Li et al., "Acupuncture Effect and Central Autonomic Regulation."; Stephanie C. Tjen-A-Looi, Liang-Wu Fu, Zhi-Ling Guo, and John C. Longhurst, "Modulation of Neurally Mediated Vasodepression and Bradycardia by Electroacupuncture through Opioids in Nucleus Tractus Solitarius," *Scientific Reports* 8 (2018): 1900. https://doi.org/10.1038/s41598-018-19672-9; Ma, Ma, and Cho, *Biomedical Acupuncture for Pain Management*, 3.
9. Giovanni Maciocia, *The Foundations of Chinese Medicine: A Comprehensive Text for Acupuncturists and Herbalists*, 2nd ed. (Edinburgh: Elsevier Churchill Livingstone, 2005), 48-64.
10. Bonaz, "The Vagus Nerve in the Neuro-Immune Axis"; Wei He et al., "Auricular Acupuncture and Vagal Regulation." *Evidence-Based Complementary and Alternative Medicine* 2012 (2012): Article ID 786839. https://doi.org/10.1155/2012/786839.
11. Bonaz, "The Vagus Nerve in the Neuro-Immune Axis"; Li, "Acupuncture Effect and Central Autonomic Regulation."; Wang, "Effects of Electroacupuncture at PC6 and ST36."; He, "Auricular Acupuncture

and Vagal Regulation.";Tjen-A-Looi, "Modulation of Neurally Mediated Vasodepression."
12. Julian F. Thayer, and Richard D. Lane. "A model of neurovisceral integration in emotion regulation and dysregulation." *Journal of Affective Disorders* 61, no. 3 (2000): 201–216.https://doi.org/10.1016/S0165-0327(00)00338-4; Fred Shaffer and J. P. Ginsberg, "An Overview of Heart Rate Variability Metrics and Norms," *Frontiers in Public Health* 5 (2017): article 258, https://doi.org/10.3389/fpubh.2017.00258; M. N. Jarczok et al., "First Evaluation of an Index of Low Vagally-Mediated Heart Rate Variability as a Marker of Health Risks in Human Adults: Proof of Concept," *Journal of Clinical Medicine* 8, no. 11 (2019): 1940, https://doi.org/10.3390/jcm8111940.
13. Thayer and Lane, "A Model of Neurovisceral Integration."; Shaffer and Ginsberg, "Overview of Heart Rate Variability."; Jarczok et al., "Index of Low Vagal Heart Rate Variability as Health Marker."
14. John A. Chalmers, Daniel S. Quintana, Maree J.-Anne Abbott, and Andrew H. Kemp, "Anxiety Disorders Are Associated with Reduced Heart Rate Variability: A Meta-Analysis," *Frontiers in Psychiatry* 5 (July 11, 2014): 80, https://doi.org/10.3389/fpsyt.2014.00080.; Jarczok et al., "Index of Low Vagal Heart Rate Variability as Health Marker."
15. Thayer and Lane, "A Model of Neurovisceral Integration."
16. Konrad Streitberger et al., "Effects of Verum Acupuncture Compared to Placebo Acupuncture on Quantitative EEG and Heart Rate Variability in Healthy Volunteers," *Journal of Alternative and Complementary Medicine* 14, no. 5 (June 2008): 505–513, PMID: 18537467, DOI: 10.1089/acm.2007.0552; Eugenijus Kaniusas et al., "Current Directions in the Auricular Vagus Nerve Stimulation I – A Physiological Perspective," *Frontiers in Neuroscience* 13 (2019): Article 854, https://doi.org/10.3389/fnins.2019.00854; Duyan Geng, Xuanyu Liu, Yan Wang, and Jiaxing Wang, "The Effect of Transcutaneous Auricular Vagus Nerve Stimulation on Heart Rate Variability in Healthy Young People," *PLOS ONE* 17, no. 2 (February 10, 2022): e0263833, https://doi.org/10.1371/journal.pone.0263833.

17. Dieu-Thuong T. T. Trinh et al., "Heart Rate Variability during Auricular Acupressure at the Left Sympathetic Point on Healthy Volunteers," *Frontiers in Neuroscience* 17 (2023): Article 1116154, https://doi.org/10.3389/fnins.2023.1116154; Gerhard Litscher et al., "Transcontinental and Translational High-Tech Acupuncture Research Using Computer-Based Heart Rate and 'Fire of Life' Heart Rate Variability Analysis," *Chinese Journal of Integrative Medicine* 16, no. 2 (2010): 102–7, DOI: 10.1016/S2005-2901(10)60031-3; "iPhone & iPad App Measures Acupuncture Stress Reduction." *Acupuncture Today 14,* no. 7 *(July 2013). Accessed July 9, 2025. https://www.healthcmi.com/Acupuncture-Continuing-Education-News/547-iphoneipadappacupuncturehrvstress.*
18. Esther Cherland, review of *The Polyvagal Theory: Neurophysiological Foundations of Emotions, Attachment, Communication, Self-Regulation,* by Stephen W. Porges, *Canadian Journal of Psychiatry* 57, no. 5 (2012): 322–323. https://pmc.ncbi.nlm.nih.gov/articles/PMC3490536/.
19. Bonaz, "The Vagus Nerve in the Neuro-Immune Axis."; Cherland, review of *The Polyvagal Theory,* 322.
20. Li et al., "Acupuncture Effect and Central Autonomic Regulation."

Chapter 5 Endnotes

1. Tzu-Hsuan Wei and Ching-Liang Hsieh, "Effect of Acupuncture on the p38 Signaling Pathway in Several Nervous System Diseases: A Systematic Review," *International Journal of Molecular Sciences* 21, no. 13 (June 30, 2020): 4693, https://doi.org/10.3390/ijms21134693; Paul U. Unschuld, Hermann Tessenow, and Zheng Jinsheng, *Huang Di Nei Jing Su Wen,* vol. 1 (Berkeley and Los Angeles, CA: University of California Press, 2011), 2.
2. Wei Zhou and Peyman Benharash, "Effects and Mechanisms of Acupuncture Based on the Principle of Meridians," *Journal of Acupuncture and Meridian Studies* 7, no. 4 (August 2014): 190–193, https://doi.org/10.1016/j.jams.2014.02.007; Unschuld, *Huang Di Nei Jing Su*

Wen, 59.
3. Unschuld, *Huang Di Nei Jing Su Wen*, 59.
4. Paul U. Unschuld, *Huang Di Nei Jing Ling Shu: The Ancient Classic on Needle Therapy* (Oakland, CA: University of California Press, 2016), 11.
5. Sandy Fritz, *Mosby's Essential Sciences for Therapeutic Massage*, 4th ed. (Maryland Heights, MO: Elsevier Inc., 2012), 5.
6. Qi-Quan Li, Guang-Xia Shi, Qi Xu, Jie Wang, Cun-Zhi Liu, and Lin-Peng Wang, "Acupuncture Effect and Central Autonomic Regulation," *Evidence-Based Complementary and Alternative Medicine* (May 26, 2013): Article ID 267959, https://doi.org/10.1155/2013/267959.
7. Unschuld, *Huang Di Nei Jing Ling Shu*, 35.
8. Yan-Wei Li et al., "The The Autonomic Nervous System: A Potential Link to the Efficacy of Acupuncture," *Frontiers in Neuroscience* 16 (December 8, 2022): Article 1038945, https://doi.org/10.3389/fnins.2022.1038945.
9. Vitaly Napadow et al., "Brain Encoding of Acupuncture Sensation—Coupling On-line Rating with fMRI," *NeuroImage* 47, no. 3 (2009): 1055–1065, https://doi.org/10.1016/j.neuroimage.2009.05.079.
10. Li et al., "The The Autonomic Nervous System,"
11. Kevin Tracey, "The Inflammatory Reflex," *Nature* 420, no. 6917 (2002): 853–859, https://doi.org/10.1038/nature01321.
12. R. Ader, N. Cohen, D. Felton, "Psychoneuroimmunology: Interactions Between the Nervous System and the Immune System," *The Lancet* 345, no. 8942 (January 14, 1995): 99–103, https://doi.org/10.1016/s0140-6736(95)90066-7.

Chapter 6: Trauma and the ANS

1. Yun-tao Ma, Mila Ma, and Zang-Hee Cho, *Biomedical Acupuncture for Pain Management: An Integrative Approach* (St. Louis, MO: Elsevier Churchill Livingstone, 2005), 7.
2. Sandy Fritz, *Mosby's Essential Sciences for Therapeutic Massage*, 4th ed.

(Maryland Heights, MO: Elsevier, 2012), 46.

3. Fritz, *Mosby's Essential Sciences*, 4th ed., 46; Ma, Ma, and Cho, *Biomedical Acupuncture for Pain Management*, 7.

4. Luca Rossi, "Understanding the Neurobiology of Traumatic Shock and Pain." *Journal of Trauma and Rehabilitation* 2023. https://doi.org/10.4172/Jtr.1000129, https://www.scitechnol.com/peer-review/understanding-the-neurobiology-of-traumatic-shock-and-pain-oR38.php?article_id=23256; Erin Berenz, "5 Ways Trauma Changes Your Brain and Body (And How You Can Start Taking Back Control)." *Anxiety and Depression Association of America* (ADAA), March 11, 2025. https://adaa.org/learn-from-us/from-the-experts/blog-posts/consumer/ways-trauma-changes-your-brain-and-body; Hailey Shafir, "Trauma & the Brain: Understanding the Effects." *Choosing Therapy*, June 24, 2025. https://www.choosingtherapy.com/trauma-brain/; Yan-Wei Li et al., "The Autonomic Nervous System: A Potential Link to the Efficacy of Acupuncture," *Frontiers in Neuroscience* 16 (2022): 1038945, DOI: 10.3389/fnins.2022.1038945.

5. B. D. Perry and R. Pollard, "Homeostasis, Stress, Trauma, and Adaptation: A Neurodevelopmental View of Childhood Trauma," *Child and Adolescent Psychiatric Clinics of North America* 7, no. 1 (January 1998): 33–51, viii, https://doi.org/10.1016/S1056-4993(18)30258-X.

6. Leon Hammer, *Dragon Rises, Red Bird Flies: Psychology and Chinese Medicine*, rev. ed. (Seattle: Eastland Press, 2010), 273.

7. Ibid

8. Laurie Kelly McCorry, "Physiology of the Autonomic Nervous System," *American Journal of Pharmaceutical Education* 71, no. 4 (August 15, 2007): 78, doi: 10.5688/aj710478; Fritz, *Mosby's Essential Sciences*, 4th ed., 46;

9. Thayer, Julian F., and Richard D. Lane. "A Model of Neurovisceral Integration in Emotion Regulation and Dysregulation." *Journal of Affective Disorders* 61, no. 3 (2000): 201–216, https://doi.org/10.1016/S0165-0327(00)00338-4.

10. Hammer, *Dragon Rises, Red Bird Flies*, 60.
11. Satsangi, Anurag Kumar, and Maria Paola Brugnoli. "Anxiety and Psychosomatic Symptoms in Palliative Care: From Neuro-Psychobiological Response to Stress, to Symptoms' Management with Clinical Hypnosis and Meditative States." *Annals of Palliative Medicine* 7, no. 1 (2018): 75–111. https://doi.org/10.21037/apm.2017.07.01; Robert S. Feldman, *Psychology 105*, custom ed. for University of New Mexico (New York: McGraw-Hill Education, 2013), 489-491.
12. Feldman, *Psychology*, 489-491.
13. Hammer, *Dragon Rises, Red Bird Flies*, 60-66
14. Stephen W. Porges, "Polyvagal Theory: A Science of Safety." *Frontiers in Integrative Neuroscience* 16 (2022): 871227. DOI:10.3389/fnint.2 022.871227; Maria Paola Brugnoli, "Clinical Hypnosis for Palliative Care in Severe Chronic Diseases: A Review and the Procedures for Relieving Physical, Psychological and Spiritual Symptoms," *Annals of Palliative Medicine* 5, no. 4 (October 2016): 280–297,DOI: 10.21037/apm.2016.09.04
15. Hammer, *Dragon Rises, Red Bird Flies*, 273.
16. A. D. Craig, "How Do You Feel? Interoception: The Sense of the Physiological Condition of the Body." *Nature Reviews Neuroscience* 3, no. 8 (2002): 655–666. https://doi.org/10.1038/nrn894. Feldman, *Psychology*, 489-491.
17. Maggie Schauer and Thomas Elbert. "Dissociation Following Traumatic Stress: Etiology and Treatment." *Zeitschrift für Psychologie/Journal of Psychology* 218, no. 2 (2010): 109–127.https://doi.org/10.1027/0044-3409/a000018.
18. Giovanni Maciocia, *Foundations of Chinese Medicine: A Comprehensive Text for Acupuncturists and Herbalists* (Philadelphia: Churchill Livingstone, 2005), 153-163
19. Hammer, *Dragon Rises, Red Bird Flies*, 273
20. Bessel A. van der Kolk, "The Body Keeps the Score: Memory and the Evolving Psychobiology of Posttraumatic Stress," *Harvard Review of Psychiatry* 1, no. 5 (1994): 253–65, https://doi.org/10.3109/1067322

9409017088.
21. Feldman, *Psychology*, 490-491.
22. Brugnoli, "Clinical Hypnosis for Palliative Care," 280-297.
23. Ibid.
24. Feldman, *Psychology*, 490-491.
25. Maciocia, *Foundations of Chinese Medicine*, 99-101.

Chapter 7 end notes

1. Leon Hammer, *Dragon Rises, Red Bird Flies: Psychology and Chinese Medicine*, rev. ed. (Seattle, WA: Eastland Press, 2010), 60.
2. Ibid.
3. John P. Plummer, "Acupuncture and Homeostasis: Physiological, Physical (Postural) and Psychological," *American Journal of Chinese Medicine* 9, no. 1 (1981): 1–14, https://doi.org/10.1142/S0192415X81000020.
4. Hammer, *Dragon Rises, Red Bird Flies*, 273.
5. Yan-Wei Li et al., "The The Autonomic Nervous System: A Potential Link to the Efficacy of Acupuncture," *Frontiers in Neuroscience* 16 (December 8, 2022): Article 1038945, https://doi.org/10.3389/fnins.2022.1038945.
6. Hammer, *Dragon Rises, Red Bird Flies*, 60-66.
7. Ibid
8. Li et al., "The Autonomic Nervous System."
9. Robert S. Feldman, *Psychology 105*, 11th ed. (New York: McGraw-Hill Education, 2013).
10. Li et al., "The Autonomic Nervous System:."
11. Hammer, *Dragon Rises, Red Bird Flies*, 60-66.
12. Hammer, *Dragon Rises, Red Bird Flies*, 49.
13. Allen Chen, "An Introduction to Sequential Electric Acupuncture (SEA) in the Treatment of Stress Related Physical and Mental Disorders," *Acupuncture & Electro-Therapeutics Research* 17, no. 4 (October-December 1992): 273-83, doi: 10.3727/036012992816357675; Li et

al., "The Autonomic Nervous System."

Chapter 8: Channels and Nerves

1. David Shier, Jackie Butler, and Ricki Lewis, *Hole's Essentials of Human Anatomy and Physiology*, 9th ed. (New York: McGraw-Hill, 2006), 238; Yun-tao Ma, Mila Ma, and Zang-Hee Cho, *Biomedical Acupuncture for Pain Management: An Integrative Approach* (St. Louis, MO: Elsevier Churchill Livingstone, 2005), 6.
2. Paul U. Unschuld, *Huang Di Nei Jing Ling Shu: The Ancient Classic on Needle Therapy* (Oakland, CA: University of California Press, 2016), 179.
3. Wei Zhou and Peyman Benharash, "Effects and Mechanisms of Acupuncture Based on the Principle of Meridians," *Journal of Acupuncture and Meridian Studies* 7, no. 4 (August 2014): 190–93, https://doi.org/10.1016/j.jams.2014.02.007.
4. Unschuld, *Huang Di Nei Jing Ling Shu*, 179.
5. Zhou and Benharash, "Effects and Mechanisms of Acupuncture."
6. Ibid.
7. Kathleen K. Hui et al., "Acupuncture Modulates the Limbic System and Subcortical Gray Structures of the Human Brain: Evidence from fMRI Studies in Normal Subjects," *Human Brain Mapping* 9, no. 1 (2000): 13–25, PMCID: PMC6871878, DOI: 10.1002/(sici)1097-0193(2000)9:1<13::aid-hbm2>3.0.co;2-f
8. Zhou and Benharash, "Effects and Mechanisms of Acupuncture."
9. Unschuld, *Huang Di Nei Jing Ling Shu*, 190-191.
10. Zhou and Benharash, "Effects and Mechanisms of Acupuncture."
11. Unschuld, *Huang Di Nei Jing Ling Shu*, 180-181.
12. Zhou and Benharash, "Effects and Mechanisms of Acupuncture."
13. Rebecca P. R. Tompkins et al., "Arrangement of Sympathetic Fibers within the Human Common Peroneal Nerve: Implications for Microneurography," *Journal of Applied Physiology* 115, no. 10 (2013): 384–91, https://doi.org/10.1152/japplphysiol.00273.2013; Kanae

Umemoto et al.,"A Part of the Medial Branch of the Deep Peroneal Nerve Distributes the Dorsal Pedis Artery and Its Distribution Area Is Close to the Acupuncture Point LR3 (Taichong)," *Evidence-Based Complementary and Alternative Medicine* (April 14, 2020), https://doi.org/10.1155/2020/6760958.

14. Junichi Sugenoya et al., "Vasodilator Component in Sympathetic Nerve Activity Destined for the Skin of the Dorsal Foot of Mildly Heated Humans," *The Journal of Physiology* 507, no. 2 (March 1, 1998): 603–10, PMCID: PMC2230797, DOI: 10.1111/j.1469-7793.1998.603bt.x; B. G. Wallin, G. Sundlöf, and W. Delius, "The Effect of Carotid Sinus Nerve Stimulation on Muscle and Skin Nerve Sympathetic Activity in Man," *Pflügers Archiv* 358, no. 2 (July 21, 1975): 101–110, DOI: 10.1007/BF00583921.

15. Umemoto et al., "Deep Peroneal Nerve and LR3."

16. Rafael Torres-Rosas et al.,"Dopamine Mediates the Vagal Modulation of the Immune System by Electroacupuncture," *Nature Medicine* 20, no. 3 (2014): 291–95, https://doi.org/10.1038/nm.3479; Qian-Qian Li et al., "Acupuncture Effect and Central Autonomic Regulation," *Evidence-Based Complementary and Alternative Medicine* 2013 (2013): 1–9, https://doi.org/10.1155/2013/267959; Shenbin Liu et al.,"Somatotopic Organization and Intensity Dependence in Driving Distinct NPY-Expressing Sympathetic Pathways by Electroacupuncture," *Neuron* 108, no. 6 (2020): Article 107086, DOI: 10.1016/j.neuron.2020.07.015.

17. Torres-Rosas et al., "Dopamine Mediates the Vagal Modulation."

18. Liu et al., "NPY-Expressing Sympathetic Pathways."

19. Unschuld, *Huang Di Nei Jing Ling Shu*, 179.

20. Zhou and Benharash, "Effects and Mechanisms of Acupuncture."

21. Tom Tam, *Healing Cancer with the Nervous System* (Quincy, MA: Oriental Culture Institute, 2012), 41.

Chapter 9: Spinal Pathways and the energetics of Organ Regulation

1. Giovanni Maciocia, *Diagnosis in Chinese Medicine: A Comprehensive Guide* (Edinburgh: Churchill Livingstone, 2004), 791-802.
2. Lonny S. Jarrett, *The Clinical Practice of Chinese Medicine* (Stockbridge, MA: Spirit Path Press, 2003), 17.
3. Jarrett, *The Clinical Practice of Chinese Medicine*, 20.
4. Ibid
5. Sandy Fritz, *Mosby's Essential Sciences for Therapeutic Massage*, 4th ed. (Maryland Heights, MO: Elsevier Inc., 2012), 150-151.
6. Yun-tao Ma, Mila Ma, and Zang-Hee Cho, *Biomedical Acupuncture for Pain Management: An Integrative Approach* (St. Louis, MO: Elsevier Churchill Livingstone, 2005), 60.
7. Fritz, *Mosby's Essential Sciences*, 150-152.
8. Tom Tam, *Healing Cancer with the Nervous System* (Quincy, MA: Oriental Culture Institute, 2012), 35-39.
9. Ibid.
10. Ibid.
11. Ibid.

Chapter 10 Endontes

1. Wei Zhou and Peyman Benharash, "Effects and Mechanisms of Acupuncture Based on the Principle of Meridians," *Journal of Acupuncture and Meridian Studies* 7, no. 4 (August 2014): 190–93, https://doi.org/10.1016/j.jams.2014.02.007; Sandy Fritz, *Mosby's Essential Sciences for Therapeutic Massage*, 4th ed. (Maryland Heights, MO: Elsevier, 2012), 150-151; Tom Tam, *Healing Cancer with the Nervous System* (Quincy, MA: Oriental Culture Institute, 2012), 33.
2. Paul U. Unschuld, *Huang Di Nei Jing Ling Shu: The Ancient Classic on Needle Therapy* (Oakland, CA: University of California Press, 2016), 498.
3. Zhou and Benharash, "Effects and Mechanisms"; Tam, *Healing Cancer*, 33.
4. Fritz, *Essential Sciences*, 150-151; Tam, *Healing Cancer*, 33.

5. Zhou and Benharash, "Effects and Mechanisms."
6. Yan-Wei Li et al., "The Autonomic Nervous System: A Potential Link to the Efficacy of Acupuncture," *Frontiers in Neuroscience* 16 (December 8, 2022): 1038945, https://doi.org/10.3389/fnins.2022.1038945.
7. Lonny S. Jarrett, *The Clinical Practice of Chinese Medicine*. Stockbridge, MA: Spirit Path Press, 2015, 20.
8. Yun-tao Ma, Mila Ma, and Zang-Hee Cho, *Biomedical Acupuncture for Pain Management: An Integrative Approach* (St. Louis, MO: Elsevier Churchill Livingstone, 2005), 17-18, 67.
9. Ma, Ma, and Cho, *Biomedical Acupuncture*, 53.
10. Unschuld, *Ling Shu*, 498.
11. Mark N. Alshak and Joe M. Das, "Neuroanatomy, Sympathetic Nervous System," *StatPearls* [Internet], last updated May 8, 2023, https://www.ncbi.nlm.nih.gov/books/NBK542195/; Marieb, *Human Anatomy & Physiology*, 505; Ma, Ma, and Cho, *Biomedical Acupuncture*, 17; Emily Scott-Solomon, Erica Boehm, and Rejji Kuruvilla, "The Sympathetic Nervous System in Development and Disease," *Nature Reviews Neuroscience* 22, no. 11 (2021): 685–702, https://doi.org/10.1038/s41583-021-00523-y.
12. Alshak and Das, "Neuroanatomy, Sympathetic Nervous System,"; Marieb, *Human Anatomy & Physiology*, 505.
13. Splanchnic Nerves, "*ScienceDirect Topics*", Elsevier, https://www.sciencedirect.com/topics/neuroscience/splanchnic-nerve; Sympathetic Nervous System," Encyclopaedia Britannica, https://www.britannica.com/science/autonomic-nervous-system; Marieb, *Human Anatomy & Physiology*, 50-508.
14. Ibid
15. Alshak and Das, "Neuroanatomy, Sympathetic Nervous System."
16. Ma, Ma, and Cho, *Biomedical Acupuncture*, 53

Chapter 11 Endnotes

1. Leon Hammer, *Dragon Rises, Red Bird Flies: Psychology and Chinese*

Medicine, rev. ed. (Seattle, WA: Eastland Press, 2010), 49.
2. Yan-Wei Li et al., "The Autonomic Nervous System: A Potential Link to the Efficacy of Acupuncture," *Frontiers in Neuroscience* 16 (December 8, 2022): 1038945, https://doi.org/10.3389/fnins.2022.1038945.
3. Hammer, *Dragon Rises, Red Bird Flies*, 28.
4. Hammer, *Dragon Rises, Red Bird Flies*, 59.
5. Paul U. Unschuld, Hermann Tessenow, and Zheng Jinsheng, *Huang Di Nei Jing Su Wen*, vol. 1 (Berkeley and Los Angeles, CA: University of California Press, 2011), 68.
6. Paul U. Unschuld, *Huang Di Nei Jing Ling Shu: The Ancient Classic on Needle Therapy* (Oakland, CA: University of California Press, 2016), 129-159.
7. Yujin Choi et al., "Acupuncture for Psychosomatic Symptoms of Hwabyung, an Anger Syndrome: A Feasibility Randomized Controlled Trial," *Frontiers in Psychology* 12 (September 24, 2021): 651649, https://doi.org/10.3389/fpsyg.2021.651649.
8. Li et al., "The Autonomic Nervous System."
9. Li et al., "The Autonomic Nervous System"; Choi et al., "Acupuncture for Psychosomatic Symptoms."
10. Bessel A. van der Kolk et al., "Dissociation, Somatization, and Affect Dysregulation: The Complexity of Adaptation to Trauma," *American Journal of Psychiatry* 153, no. 7 Suppl (1996): 83–93, https://doi.org/10.1176/ajp.153.7.83.
11. Unschuld, *Huang Di Nei Jing Ling Shu*, 129.
12. Julian F. Thayer and Richard D. Lane, "The Role of Vagal Function in the Risk for Cardiovascular Disease and Mortality," *Biological Psychology* 74, no. 2 (2007): 224–242, DOI: 10.1016/j.biopsycho.2005.11.013

Chapter 12 Endnotes

1. David S. Goldstein, "Stress and the 'Extended' Autonomic System," *Autonomic Neuroscience* 236 (December 2021): 102889, https://doi.or

g/10.1016/j.autneu.2021.102889.
2. Wei Cen, Ralph Hoppe, and Ning Gu, "Mental Activity and Organ: Specific Emotions to Specific Organs?" *Journal of Complementary and Alternative Healthcare* 3, no. 1 (2017): 1–4, https://doi.org/10.19080/JCMAH.2017.03.555605.
3. Paul U. Unschuld, Hermann Tessenow, and Zheng Jinsheng, *Huang Di Nei Jing Su Wen*, vol. 1 (Berkeley and Los Angeles, CA: University of California Press, 2011), 129.
4. Unschuld, Tessenow, and Zheng, *Huang Di Nei Jing Su Wen*, vol. 1, 88.
5. Julian F. Thayer, S. S. Yamamoto, and Jos F. Brosschot, "The Relationship of Autonomic Imbalance, Heart Rate Variability and Cardiovascular Disease Risk Factors," *International Journal of Cardiology* 141, no. 2 (May 28, 2010): 122–131, https://doi.org/10.1016/j.ijcard.2009.09.543.
6. Unschuld, Tessenow, and Zheng, *Huang Di Nei Jing Su Wen*, vol. 1, 62.
7. Jih-Huah Wu, Hsueh-Yu Chen, Yu-Jung Chang, Hsiao-Ching Wu, Wen-Dien Chang, Yu-Jen Chu, and Jia-Ann Jiang, "Study of Autonomic Nervous Activity of Night Shift Workers Treated with Laser Acupuncture," *Photomedicine and Laser Surgery* 27, no. 2 (April 2009): 273–79, https://doi.org/10.1089/pho.2007.2235.
8. Giovanni Maciocia, *Diagnosis in Chinese Medicine: A Comprehensive Guide* (Edinburgh: Churchill Livingstone, 2004), 64.
9. Maciocia, *Diagnosis in Chinese Medicine*, 164-170.
10. Unschuld, Tessenow, and Zheng, *Huang Di Nei Jing Su Wen*, vol. 1, 107, 595.
11. Bruce S. McEwen, "Physiology and Neurobiology of Stress and Adaptation: Central Role of the Brain," *Physiological Reviews* 87 (2007): 873–904, https://doi.org/10.1152/physrev.00041.2006; Julian F. Thayer and Esther M. Sternberg, "Beyond Heart Rate Variability: Vagal Regulation of Allostatic Systems," *Annals of the New York Academy of Sciences* 1088 (2006): 361–372, https://doi.org/10.1196/annals.1366.014.
12. Allen Chen, "An Introduction to Sequential Electrical Acupuncture

(SEA) in the Treatment of Stress Related Physical and Mental Disorders," *Acupuncture & Electro-Therapeutics Research* 17, no. 4 (1992): 273–83, https://doi.org/10.3727/036012992816357675.
13. Peter Deadman, Mazin Al-Khafaji, and Kevin Baker, *A Manual of Acupuncture* (East Sussex, UK: Journal of Chinese Medicine Publications, 2007), 158, 436.
14. Hong Xu, Ya-Min Zhang, Hua Sun, Su-Hui Chen, and Ying-Kui Si, "Electroacupuncture at GV20 and ST36 Exerts Neuroprotective Effects via the EPO-Mediated JAK2/STAT3 Pathway in Cerebral Ischemic Rats," *Evidence-Based Complementary and Alternative Medicine* 2017 (2017): Article ID 6027421, https://doi.org/10.1155/2017/6027421; Yang Yang et al., "Acupuncture at GV20 and ST36 Improves the Recovery of Behavioral Activity in Rats Subjected to Cerebral Ischemia/Reperfusion Injury," *Frontiers in Behavioral Neuroscience* 16 (2022): Article 909512, https://doi.org/10.3389/fnbeh.2022.909512; Sang-Ho Hyun et al., "Effect of ST36 Acupuncture on Hyperventilation-Induced CO_2 Reactivity of the Basilar and Middle Cerebral Arteries and Heart Rate Variability in Normal Subjects," *Evidence-Based Complementary and Alternative Medicine* 2014 (2014): Article ID 574986, https://doi.org/10.1155/2014/574986.
15. Yujin Choi et al., "Acupuncture for Psychosomatic Symptoms of Hwabyung, an Anger Syndrome: A Feasibility Randomized Controlled Trial," *Frontiers in Psychology* 12 (2021): Article 651649, https://doi.org/10.3389/fpsyg.2021.651649.
16. Maciocia, *Diagnosis in Chinese Medicine*, 342-343; Unschuld, Tessenow, and Zheng, *Huang Di Nei Jing Su Wen*, 595.
17. Shenbin Liu et al., "A Neuroanatomical Basis for Electroacupuncture to Drive the Vagal–Adrenal Axis," *Nature* 598, no. 7882 (2021): 641–645, https://doi.org/10.1038/s41586-021-04001-4; Jian Kong et al., "Treating Depression with Transcutaneous Auricular Vagus Nerve Stimulation: State of the Art and Future Perspectives," *Frontiers in Psychiatry* 9 (2018): 20, https://doi.org/10.3389/fpsyt.2018.00020.
18. Kong et al., "Treating Depression with Vagus Nerve Stimulation,".

19. Yoshihiro Noda et al., "Acupuncture-Induced Changes of Vagal Function in Patients with Depression: A Preliminary Sham-Controlled Study with Press Needles," *Complementary Therapies in Clinical Practice* 21, no. 3 (August 2015): 193–200, https://doi.org/10.1016/j.ctcp.2015.07.002.

Chapter 13 Endnotes

1. Giovanni Maciocia, *Diagnosis in Chinese Medicine: A Comprehensive Guide* (Edinburgh: Churchill Livingstone, 2004), 100.
2. Paul U. Unschuld, Hermann Tessenow, and Zheng Jinsheng, *Huang Di Nei Jing Su Wen*, vol. 1 (Berkeley and Los Angeles, CA: University of California Press, 2011), 178.
3. Maciocia, *Diagnosis in Chinese Medicine*, 110.
4. Unschuld, *Huang Di Nei Jing Su Wen*, vol. 1, 155.
5. Maciocia, *Diagnosis in Chinese Medicine*, 292.
6. Unschuld, *Huang Di Nei Jing Su Wen*, vol. 1, 409, 583-597; Maciocia, *Diagnosis in Chinese Medicine*, 292.
7. Julian F. Thayer and Richard D. Lane, "The Role of Vagal Function in the Risk for Cardiovascular Disease and Mortality," *Biological Psychology* 74, no. 2 (2007): 224–242, https://doi.org/10.1016/j.biopsycho.2005.11.013; Maciocia, *Diagnosis in Chinese Medicine*, 292; Leon Hammer, *Dragon Rises, Red Bird Flies: Psychology and Chinese Medicine*, rev. ed. (Seattle, WA: Eastland Press, 2010), 273.
8. Ibid.
9. Soledade Soleil Meira do Valle and Harry Hong, "Acupuncture Treatment for Generalized Anxiety Disorder by Activating the Vagus Nerve and Improving Heart-Rate Variability and Heart-Rhythm Coherence: A Case-Series Study," *Medical Acupuncture* 36, no. 1 (2024), https://doi.org/10.1089/acu.2023.0036.
10. Tong Zheng Hong, "Treating Insomnia with Shen-Related Acupoints," *Biomedical Journal of Scientific & Technical Research* 24, no. 1 (2020), https://doi.org/10.26717/BJSTR.2020.24.004037.

11. Maciocia, *Diagnosis in Chinese Medicine*, 343.
12. Hammer, *Dragon Rises, Red Bird Flies*, 53.
13. Maciocia, *Diagnosis in Chinese Medicine*, 46-71.
14. Xiang-yun Yang et al., "Effectiveness of Acupuncture on Anxiety Disorder: A Systematic Review and Meta-Analysis of Randomised Controlled Trials," *Annals of General Psychiatry* 20 (2021): Article 9, https://doi.org/10.1186/s12991-021-00327-5.
15. Maciocia, *Diagnosis in Chinese Medicine*, 46-71, 243-249.
16. Elissa S. Epel et al., "Accelerated Telomere Shortening in Response to Life Stress," *Proceedings of the National Academy of Sciences of the United States of America* 101, no. 49 (2004): 17312–17315, https://doi.org/10.1073/pnas.0407162101.
17. Thayer and Lane, "Role of Vagal Function," 224.
18. Maciocia, *Diagnosis in Chinese Medicine*, 463-485.
19. Ibid.
20. Stephen W. Porges, "Polyvagal Theory: A Science of Safety," *Frontiers in Integrative Neuroscience* 16 (2022), https://doi.org/10.3389/fnint.2022.871227.
21. Maciocia, *Diagnosis in Chinese Medicine*, 463-485.

Chapter 14 Endnotes

1. Paul U. Unschuld, Hermann Tessenow, and Zheng Jinsheng, *Huang Di Nei Jing Su Wen*, vol. 1 (Berkeley and Los Angeles, CA: University of California Press, 2011), 599.
2. Paul U. Unschuld, *Huang Di Nei Jing Ling Shu: The Ancient Classic on Needle Therapy* (Oakland, CA: University of California Press, 2016), 178.
3. Giovanni Maciocia, *Diagnosis in Chinese Medicine: A Comprehensive Guide* (Edinburgh: Churchill Livingstone, 2004), 139, 159.
4. Unschuld, *Huang Di Nei Jing Ling Shu*, 148, 153.
5. Maciocia, *Diagnosis in Chinese Medicine*, 101, 139, 118.
6. Ted J. Kaptchuk, *The Web That Has No Weaver: Understanding Chinese*

Medicine (New York: McGraw-Hill, 2000), 64-5, 91.
7. Unschuld, *Huang Di Nei Jing Ling Shu*, 148.
8. Maciocia, *Diagnosis in Chinese Medicine*, 138-139.
9. Unschuld, Tessenow, and Zheng, *Huang Di Nei Jing*, vol. 1, 118.
10. Kaptchuk, *The Web That Has No Weaver*, 65,91.
11. Maciocia, *Diagnosis in Chinese Medicine*, 101.
12. Maciocia, *Diagnosis in Chinese Medicine*, 139.
13. Unschuld, Tessenow, and Zheng, *Huang Di Nei Jing*, vol. 1, 595.
14. Celine M. Li et al., "Somatic Symptom Burden, PTSD, and Dissociation: Cross-Sectional Findings from 995 International Female Mental Health Service Users," *Journal of Psychosomatic Research* 195 (August 2025): 112181, DOI: 10.1016/j.jpsychores.2025.112181
15. Sidney Zisook and Katherine Shear, "Grief and Bereavement: What Psychiatrists Need to Know," *World Psychiatry* 8, no. 2 (June 2009): 67–74, DOI: 10.1002/j.2051-5545.2009.tb00217.x
16. Holly G. Prigerson et al., "Traumatic Grief as a Risk Factor for Mental and Physical Morbidity." *American Journal of Psychiatry* 154, no. 5 (May 1997): 616–23, DOI: 10.1176/ajp.154.5.616
17. Tali Sahara, Arieh Y. Shalev, and Stephen W. Porges, "Vagal Modulation of Responses to Mental Challenge in Posttraumatic Stress Disorder," *Biological Psychiatry* 49, no. 7 (April 1, 2001): 637–643, https://doi.org/10.1016/S0006-3223(00)01045-3.
18. Mary Frances O'Connor, Harald Gündel, Kateri McRae, and Richard D. Lane, "Baseline Vagal Tone Predicts BOLD Response during Elicitation of Grief," *Neuropsychopharmacology* 32, no. 10 (October 2007): 2184–2189, https://doi.org/10.1038/sj.npp.1301342.
19. Maciocia, *Diagnosis in Chinese Medicine*, 101,139,145.
20. Unschuld, Tessenow, and Zheng, *Huang Di Nei Jing*, vol. 1,153.
21. Maciocia, *Diagnosis in Chinese Medicine*, 138-140.
22. TAPS (Tragedy Assistance Program for Survivors), "How the Body Reacts to the Loss of a Loved One," *TAPS.org*, accessed July 21, 2025, https://www.taps.org/articles/16-1/physicalreactionstoloss.
23. Zixuan Zhang et al., "Efficacy and Safety of Acupuncture in the

Treatment of Depression: A Systematic Review of Clinical Research," *The Anatomical Record* 304, no. 11 (2021): 2436–2453, https://doi.org/10.1002/ar.24783.

24. Maciocia, *Diagnosis in Chinese Medicine*,118,139.
25. O'Connor et al., "Baseline Vagal Tone Predicts BOLD Response"; Sahar, Shalev, and Porges, "Vagal Modulation of Responses."; Prigerson et al., "Traumatic Grief as a Risk Factor."
26. Institute of Medicine (US) Committee for the Study of Health Consequences of the Stress of Bereavement, *Bereavement: Reactions, Consequences, and Care*, ed. M. Osterweis, F. Solomon, and M. Green (Washington, DC: National Academies Press, 1984), https://www.ncbi.nlm.nih.gov/books/NBK217841/.
27. Julia St. Clair, "Supporting Your Nervous System During the Grieving Process," *Simply Refined Health*, accessed July 21, 2025, https://www.simplyrefinedhealth.com/supporting-your-nervous-system-during-the-grieving-process.
28. Sylvain Laborde, Emma Mosley, and Julian F. Thayer, "Heart Rate Variability and Cardiac Vagal Tone in Psychophysiological Research – Recommendations for Experiment Planning, Data Analysis, and Data Reporting," *Frontiers in Psychology* 8 (February 20, 2017): 213, https://doi.org/10.3389/fpsyg.2017.00213.
29. Zhang et al., "Efficacy and Safety of Acupuncture in the Treatment of Depression."
30. Holly R. Middlekauff et al., "Acupuncture Inhibits Sympathetic Activation During Mental Stress in Advanced Heart Failure Patients," *Journal of Cardiac Failure* 8, no. 6 (December 2002): 399–406, https://doi.org/10.1054/jcaf.2002.129656; Jun Matsumoto-Miyazaki, "Efficacy of Acupuncture Treatment for Improving the Respiratory Status in Patients Receiving Prolonged Mechanical Ventilation in Intensive Care Units: A Retrospective Observational Study," *Journal of Alternative and Complementary Medicine* 24, no. 11 (November 2018): 1076–1084, https://doi.org/10.1089/acm.2017.0365.
31. Mike Armour et al., "Acupuncture for Depression: A Systematic

Review and Meta-Analysis," *Journal of Clinical Medicine* 8, no. 8 (July 31, 2019): 1140, https://doi.org/10.3390/jcm8081140.

32. Melis YilmazBalban etal., "Daily Five-Minute Cyclic Sighing Improves Mood and Respiratory Rate More Than Mindfulness Meditation: A Remote Randomized Controlled Trial," *Cell Reports Medicine* 3, no. 9 (2022): 100895, https://doi.org/10.1016/j.xcrm.2022.100895.
33. ValentinMagnon, FrédéricDutheil, and GuillaumeT.Vallet, "Benefits from One Session of Deep and Slow Breathing on Vagal Tone and Anxiety in Young and Older Adults," *Scientific Reports* 11 (September29, 2021): Article19267, https://doi.org/10.1038/s41598-021-98736-9
34. RoderikJ.S. Gerritsen and GuidoP.H. Band, "Breath of Life: The Respiratory Vagal Stimulation Model of Contemplative Activity," *Frontiers in Human Neuroscience* 12 (October9,2018): 397, https://doi.org/10.3389/fnhum.2018.00397
35. Ting-Ting Yeh and Yi-Chieh Ho, "Immediate Effects of Structured and Natural Deep Breathing on Heart Rate Variability and Blood Pressure in Community-Dwelling Older Adults," *Experimental Gerontology* 198 (December2024): Article112644, https://doi.org/10.1016/j.exger.2024.112644.

Chapter 15 Endnotes

1. Paul U. Unschuld, Hermann Tessenow, and Zheng Jinsheng, *Huang Di Nei Jing Su Wen*, vol. 1 (Berkeley and Los Angeles, CA: University of California Press, 2011), 409.
2. Giovanni Maciocia, *Diagnosis in Chinese Medicine: A Comprehensive Guide* (Edinburgh: Churchill Livingstone, 2005), 100, 149.
3. Unschuld, Tessenow, and Jinsheng, *Huang Di Nei Jing Su Wen*, 146.
4. Maciocia, *Diagnosis in Chinese Medicine*, 147.
5. Ibid.
6. Maciocia, *Diagnosis in Chinese Medicine*, 100.
7. Unschuld, Tessenow, and Jinsheng, *Huang Di Nei Jing Su Wen*, 413.
8. Maciocia, *Diagnosis in Chinese Medicine*, 100.

9. Maciocia, *Diagnosis in Chinese Medicine*, 149.
10. Ted J. Kaptchuk, *The Web That Has No Weaver: Understanding Chinese Medicine* (New York: McGraw-Hill, 2000), 149, 159.
11. Maciocia, *Diagnosis in Chinese Medicine*, 100–101, 149; Kaptchuk, *The Web That Has No Weaver*, 79–80.
12. Paul U. Unschuld, *Huang Di Nei Jing Ling Shu: The Ancient Classic on Needle Therapy* (Oakland, CA: University of California Press, 2016), 24.
13. Maciocia, *Diagnosis in Chinese Medicine*, 144, 149, 251.
14. Ibid.
15. Ibid.
16. John B. Furness, "The Enteric Nervous System and Neurogastroenterology," *Nature Reviews Gastroenterology & Hepatology* 9, no. 5 (2012): 286–94, https://doi.org/10.1038/nrgastro.2012.32.
17. Allison E. Diamond and Aaron J. Fisher, "Comparative Autonomic Responses to Diagnostic Interviewing between Individuals with GAD, MDD, SAD, and Healthy Controls," *Frontiers in Human Neuroscience* 10 (2017): Article 677, https://doi.org/10.3389/fnhum.2016.00677.
18. Hongyun Zhang et al., "Understanding the Connection between Gut Homeostasis and Psychological Stress," *The Journal of Nutrition* 153, no. 4 (2023): 924–39, https://doi.org/10.1016/j.jnut.2023.01.026.
19. Xiang-Yun Yang et al., "Effectiveness of Acupuncture on Anxiety Disorder: A Systematic Review and Meta-Analysis of Randomised Controlled Trials," *Annals of General Psychiatry* 20, no. 1 (2021): 9, https://doi.org/10.1186/s12991-021-00327-5.
20. Soledade Soleil Meirado Valle and Harry Hong, "Acupuncture Treatment for Generalized Anxiety Disorder by Activating the Vagus Nerve and Improving Heart-Rate Variability and Heart-Rhythm Coherence: A Case-Series Study," *Medical Acupuncture* 36, no. 1 (2024): 21–26, https://doi.org/10.1089/acu.2023.0036.
21. Na-Na Yang et al., ""The Autonomic Nervous System in Acupuncture for Gastrointestinal Dysmotility: From Anatomical Insights to Clinical Medicine," *International Journal of Medical Sciences* 22, no. 11

(2025): 2620–36, https://doi.org/10.7150/ijms.107643.
22. Jacek Kolacz and Stephen W. Porges, "Chronic Diffuse Pain and Functional Gastrointestinal Disorders after Traumatic Stress: Pathophysiology through a Polyvagal Perspective," *Frontiers in Medicine* 5 (2018): Article 145, https://doi.org/10.3389/fmed.2018.00145.
23. Ibid.
24. Maciocia, *Diagnosis in Chinese Medicine*, 250, 450.
25. Maciocia, *Diagnosis in Chinese Medicine*, 150, 252.
26. Leon Hammer, *Dragon Rises, Red Bird Flies: Psychology and Chinese Medicine*, rev. ed. (Seattle, WA: Eastland Press, 2010), 347.
27. Unschuld, Tessenow, and Jinsheng, *Huang Di Nei Jing Su Wen*, 594.
28. Shu-Guang Cao et al., "Effects of Psychological Stress on Small Intestinal Motility and Expression of Cholecystokinin and Vasoactive Intestinal Polypeptide in Plasma and Small Intestine in Mice," *World Journal of Gastroenterology* 11, no. 5 (2005): 737–40, https://doi.org/10.3748/wjg.v11.i5.737.
29. Yu-Ming Chang, Mohamad El-Zaatari, and John Y. Kao, "Does Stress Induce Bowel Dysfunction?" *Expert Review of Gastroenterology & Hepatology* 8, no. 6 (2014): 583–85, https://doi.org/10.1586/17474124.2014.911659.
30. Chunying Tian et al., "The Efficacy and Safety of Acupuncture and Moxibustion Combined with Western Medicine for Obsessive Compulsive Disorder: A Protocol for Systematic Review and Meta-Analysis," *Medicine (Baltimore)* 99, no. 35 (2020): e21395, https://doi.org/10.1097/MD.0000000000021395.
31. Bin Feng et al., "Transcutaneous Electrical Acupoint Stimulation as an Adjunct Therapy for Obsessive-Compulsive Disorder: A Randomized Controlled Study," *Journal of Psychiatric Research* 80 (2016): 30–37, https://doi.org/10.1016/j.jpsychires.2016.05.015.
32. Federica Di Vincenzo et al., "Gut Microbiota, Intestinal Permeability, and Systemic Inflammation: A Narrative Review," *International Journal of Molecular Sciences* 24, no. 13 (2023): 10570, https://doi.org/10.1007/s11739-023-03374-w.

33. Susan Scutti, "Stress Makes Life's Clock Tick Faster, 'Chilling Out' Slows It Down," *Yale News*, December 6, 2021, https://news.yale.edu/2021/12/06/stress-makes-lifes-clock-tick-faster-chilling-out-slows-it-down.
34. Lewina O. Lee et al., "Optimism Is Associated with Exceptional Longevity in 2 Epidemiologic Cohorts of Men and Women," *Proceedings of the National Academy of Sciences* 116, no. 37 (August 26, 2019): 18357–62, https://doi.org/10.1073/pnas.1900712116.
35. Tarini Shankar Ghosh, Fergus Shanahan, and Paul W. O'Toole, "The Gut Microbiome as a Modulator of Healthy Ageing," *Nature Reviews Gastroenterology & Hepatology* 19, no. 9 (2022): 565–84, https://doi.org/10.1038/s41575-022-00605-x.
36. Unschuld, Tessenow, and Jinsheng, *Huang Di Nei Jing Su Wen*, 594.

Chapter 16 Endnotes

1. Giovanni Maciocia, *Diagnosis in Chinese Medicine: A Comprehensive Guide*. Edinburgh: Churchill Livingstone, 2005, 44, 155-160.
2. Leon Hammer, *Dragon Rises, Red Bird Flies: Psychology and Chinese Medicine*. Revised edition. Seattle, WA: Eastland Press, 2010, 41, 99.
3. Maciocia, *Diagnosis in Chinese Medicine*, 156.
4. Hammer, *Dragon Rises, Red Bird Flies*, 99-100.
5. Paul U. Unschuld, Hermann Tessenow, and Zheng Jinsheng, *Huang Di Nei Jing Su Wen*, vol. 1 (Berkeley and Los Angeles, CA: University of California Press, 2011), 93.
6. Unschuld, Tessenow, and Zheng, *Su wen*, vol. 1, 409.
7. Maciocia, *Diagnosis in Chinese Medicine*, 159.
8. Hammer, *Dragon Rises, Red Bird Flies*, 103; Ted J. Kaptchuk, *The Web That Has No Weaver: Understanding Chinese Medicine* (New York: McGraw-Hill, 2000), 86.
9. Unschuld, Tessenow, and Zheng, *Su wen*, vol. 1, 110.

10. Hammer, *Dragon Rises, Red Bird Flies,* 65, 109.
11. Unschuld, *Ling Shu,* 149.
12. Hammer, *Dragon Rises, Red Bird Flies,* 65, 109.
13. Kaptchuk, *The Web That Has No Weaver,* 86-87.
14. Earl K. Miller and Jonathan D. Cohen, "An Integrative Theory of Prefrontal Cortex Function," *Annual Review of Neuroscience* 24 (2001): 167–202, https://doi.org/10.1146/annurev.neuro.24.1.167.
15. Ibid.
16. Maciocia, *Diagnosis in Chinese Medicine,* 153-163.
17. Unschuld, Tessenow, and Zheng, *Suwen,* vol. 1, 157.
18. Bruce S. McEwen and John H. Morrison, "Brain on Stress: Vulnerability and Plasticity of the Prefrontal Cortex Over the Life Course," *Neuron* 79, no. 1 (July 10, 2013): 16–29, https://doi.org/10.1016/j.neuron.2013.06.028.
19. Unschuld, Tessenow, and Zheng, *Suwen,* vol. 1, 404.
20. Shinji Tanaka and Mark D. Okusa, "Cross-talk between the Nervous System and the Kidney," *Kidney International* 97, no. 3 (March 2020): 466–476, https://doi.org/10.1016/j.kint.2019.10.032.
21. Ibid.
22. Unschuld, Tessenow, and Zheng, *Suwen,* vol. 1, 595.
23. Tanaka and Okusa, "Cross-talk between the Nervous System and the Kidney," 466–476.
24. Mijna A. Kooijman et. al., "Fetal Blood Flow and Kidney Volume in Children: The Generation R Study." *Journal of the American Society of Nephrology* 26, no. 7 (2014): 1689–1696. doi: 10.1681/ASN.2013070746
25. Unschuld, Tessenow, and Zheng, *Suwen,* vol. 1, 178.
26. Kooijman et al., "Fetal Blood Flow and Kidney Volume," 1689–1696.
27. Unschuld, Tessenow, and Zheng, *Suwen,* vol. 1, 404.
28. Unschuld, Tessenow, and Zheng, *Suwen,* vol. 1, 78.
29. Elysia Poggi Davis and Curt A. Sandman, "Prenatal Psychobiological Predictors of Anxiety Risk in Preadolescent Children," *Psychoneuroendocrinology* 37, no. 8 (2012): 1224–1233, https://doi.org/10.1016/

j.psyneuen.2011.12.016.
30. Gavino Faa et al., "The Fascinating Theory of Fetal Programming of Adult Diseases: A Review of the Fundamentals of the Barker Hypothesis," *Journal of Public Health Research* 13, no. 1 (2024): 1–14, DOI: 10.1177/22799036241226817
31. Ibid.
32. Ibid.
33. Unschuld, Tessenow, and Zheng, *Suwen*, vol. 1, 404.
34. Unschuld, Tessenow, and Zheng, *Suwen*, vol. 1, 78.
35. Jesus Alejandro Estevez-Garcia, Marcela Tamayo-Ortiz, and Alison P. Sanders, "A Scoping Review of Life-Course Psychosocial Stress and Kidney Function," *Children* 8, no. 9 (2021): 810, https://doi.org/10.3390/children8090810.
36. Unschuld, Tessenow, and Zheng, *Suwen*, vol. 1, 595.
37. Thierry Steimer, "The Biology of Fear- and Anxiety-Related Behaviors," *Dialogues in Clinical Neuroscience* 4, no. 3 (2002): 231–249, https://doi.org/10.31887/DCNS.2002.4.3/tsteimer.
38. Unschuld, Tessenow, and Zheng, *Suwen*, vol. 1, 595.
39. Steimer, "The Biology of Fear- and Anxiety-Related Behaviors."
40. Sarina M. Rodrigues, Joseph E. LeDoux, and Robert M. Sapolsky, "The Influence of Stress Hormones on Fear Circuitry," *Annual Review of Neuroscience* 32 (2009): 289–313, https://doi.org/10.1146/annurev.neuro.051508.135620.
41. Unschuld, Tessenow, and Zheng, *Suwen*, vol. 1, 110.
42. Unschuld, Tessenow, and Zheng, *Suwen*, vol. 1, 595.
43. Shao-Jun Wang, Jiao-Jiao Zhang, and Li-Li Qie. "Acupuncture Relieves the Excessive Excitation of Hypothalamic-Pituitary-Adrenal Cortex Axis Function and Correlates with the Regulatory Mechanism of GR, CRH, and ACTHR." *Evidence-Based Complementary and Alternative Medicine* 2014 (March 11, 2014): Article ID 495379. https://doi.org/10.1155/2014/495379.
44. Ibid.
45. Greti Aguilera, "HPA Axis Responsiveness to Stress: Implications

for Healthy Aging," *Experimental Gerontology* 46, no. 2–3 (February–March 2011): 90–95, https://doi.org/10.1016/j.exger.2010.08.023.

46. Ladan Eshkevari, Eva Permaul, and Susan E. Mulroney, "Acupuncture Blocks Cold Stress-Induced Increases in the Hypothalamus–Pituitary–Adrenal Axis in the Rat," *Journal of Endocrinology* 217, no. 1 (April 2013): 95–104, DOI: 10.1530/JOE-12-0404

47. Dong Lin et al., "The Neuroprotective Role of Acupuncture and Activation of the BDNF Signaling Pathway," *International Journal of Molecular Sciences* 15, no. 2 (2014): 3234–3252, https://doi.org/10.3390/ijms15023234; Chenxin Miao et al., "Effect of Acupuncture on BDNF Signaling Pathways in Several Nervous System Diseases," *Frontiers in Neurology* 14 (September 13, 2023), https://doi.org/10.3389/fneur.2023.1248348.

48. Huili Jiang et al., "Antidepressant-Like Effects of Acupuncture: Insights from DNA Methylation and Histone Modifications of Brain-Derived Neurotrophic Factor," *Frontiers in Psychiatry* 9 (2018): Article 102, https://doi.org/10.3389/fpsyt.2018.00102.

49. Lin et al., "Neuroprotective Role of Acupuncture," 3234–3252.

50. Ibid.

51. Miao et al., "Effect of Acupuncture on BDNF Pathways," 2023.

52. Jiang et al., "Antidepressant-Like Effects of Acupuncture," 2018.

53. Liye Zou et al., "Effects of Mind–Body Exercises (Tai Chi/Yoga) on Heart Rate Variability Parameters and Perceived Stress: A Systematic Review with Meta-Analysis of Randomized Controlled Trials," *Journal of Clinical Medicine* 7, no. 11 (2018): Article 404, https://doi.org/10.3390/jcm7110404.

54. Zou et al., "Mind–Body Exercises and Heart Rate Variability," 2018.

Chapter 17 Endnotes

1. Paul U. Unschuld, Hermann Tessenow, and Zheng Jinsheng, *Huang Di Nei Jing Su Wen*, vol. 1 (Berkeley and Los Angeles, CA: University

of California Press, 2011), 180.
2. Giovanni Maciocia, *Diagnosis in Chinese Medicine: A Comprehensive Guide* (Edinburgh: Churchill Livingstone, 2005), 117-127.
3. Maciocia, *Diagnosis in Chinese Medicine*, 123.
4. Unschuld, Tessenow, and Zheng, *Huang Di Nei Jing Su Wen*, 156.
5. Paul U. Unschuld, *Huang Di Nei Jing Ling Shu: The Ancient Classic on Needle Therapy* (Oakland, CA: University of California Press, 2016), 152.
6. Maciocia, *Diagnosis in Chinese Medicine*, 117-127.
7. Unschuld, Tessenow, and Zheng, *Huang Di Nei Jing Su Wen*, 409.
8. Maciocia, *Diagnosis in Chinese Medicine*, 100.
9. Maciocia, *Diagnosis in Chinese Medicine*, 117-127.
10. Ibid.
11. Shu-Zhi Wang, Yi-Jing Yu, and Khosrow Adeli, "Role of Gut Microbiota in Neuroendocrine Regulation of Carbohydrate and Lipid Metabolism via the Microbiota-Gut-Brain-Liver Axis," *Microorganisms* 8, no. 4 (2020): Article 527, https://doi.org/10.3390/microorganisms8040527.
12. Maciocia, *Diagnosis in Chinese Medicine*, 143-152.
13. Maciocia, *Diagnosis in Chinese Medicine*, 117-127.
14. Miaomiao Ma, Bo Li, Zhi Qu, Shejuan Liu, and Sisi Li, "Efficacy of Probiotics in Patients with Cognitive Impairment: A Systematic Review and Meta-analysis," *PLOS ONE*, published (May 2, 2025), https://doi.org/10.1371/journal.pone.0321567.
15. Maciocia, *Diagnosis in Chinese Medicine,* 123-124; Leon Hammer, *Dragon Rises, Red Bird Flies: Psychology and Chinese Medicine*, Rev. ed. (Seattle, WA: Eastland Press, 2010), 140-142.
16. Stephen W. Porges, "Polyvagal Theory: A Science of Safety," *Frontiers in Integrative Neuroscience* 16 (May 10, 2022): 871227, https://doi.org/10.3389/fnint.2022.871227.
17. Ibid.
18. Maciocia, *Diagnosis in Chinese Medicine,* 123-124; Hammer, *Dragon Rises, Red Bird Flies*, 140-142.

19. Maciocia, *Diagnosis in Chinese Medicine,* 123-124; Hammer, *Dragon Rises, Red Bird Flies,* 60; Lonny S. Jarrett, *The Clinical Practice of Chinese Medicine* (Stockbridge, MA: Spirit Path Press, 2015), 164-165; Porges, "Polyvagal Theory."
20. Muhammad Amir, Michael Yu, Peijian He, and Shanthi Srinivasan, "Hepatic Autonomic Nervous System and Neurotrophic Factors Regulate the Pathogenesis and Progression of Non-alcoholic Fatty Liver Disease," *Frontiers in Medicine* 7 (February 26, 2020). https://doi.org/10.3389/fmed.2020.00062.
21. Bess M. Miller, Isaac M. Oderberg, and Wolfram Goessling, "The Hepatic Nervous System in Development, Regeneration, and Disease," *Hepatology* 74, no. 6 (August 15, 2021): 3513–3522. https://doi.org/10.1002/hep.32055.
22. Anisia Silva and Alexandre Caron, "Pathophysiological Mechanisms That Alter the Autonomic Brain–Liver Communication in Metabolic Diseases," *Endocrinology* 162, no. 11 (November 2021): bqab164. https://doi.org/10.1210/endocr/bqab164.
23. Donghee Kang, Dong Wook Zhao, So Yeon Ryu, et al., "Perceived Stress and Non-alcoholic Fatty Liver Disease in Apparently Healthy Men and Women," *Scientific Reports* 10 (2020): 38, https://doi.org/10.1038/s41598-019-57036-z.
24. Ibid.
25. Sarah Khan, Vinay Jahagirdar, and Elliot B. Tapper, "Tides of Emotion: Hepatologists' Role in Navigating Depression and Anxiety in Liver Disease," *Hepatology Communications* 9, no. 8 (July 14, 2025): e0741, https://doi.org/10.1097/HC9.0000000000000741.
26. Ibid.
27. Hammer, *Dragon Rises, Red Bird Flies,* 140.
28. Unschuld, Tessenow, and Zheng, *Huang Di Nei Jing Su Wen,* 107.
29. Maciocia, *Diagnosis in Chinese Medicine,* 247.
30. Unschuld, *Huang Di Nei Jing Ling Shu,* 594.
31. Unschuld, Tessenow, and Zheng, *Huang Di Nei Jing Su Wen,* 490.
32. Hammer, *Dragon Rises, Red Bird Flies,* 142, 147.

33. Hammer, *Dragon Rises, Red Bird Flies,* 141.
34. Adriana Henney et al., "Ultra-Processed Food Consumption and Non-Alcoholic Fatty Liver Disease: A Systematic Review and Meta-Analysis," *Nutrients* 15, no. 10 (2023): 2266, https://doi.org/10.3390/nu15102266.
35. Ibid.
36. Jadwiga Konieczna et al., "Does Consumption of Ultra-Processed Foods Matter for Liver Health? Prospective Analysis among Older Adults with Metabolic Syndrome," *Nutrients* 14, no. 19 (October 5, 2022): 4142, https://doi.org/10.3390/nu14194142.
37. Yi-Chuan Chen et al., "Long-Term Exposure to Ambient Air Pollution and the Incidence of Nonalcoholic Fatty Liver Disease: A Cohort Study," *International Journal of Epidemiology* 54, no. 4 (June 11, 2025): dyaf101, https://doi.org/10.1093/ije/dyaf101.
38. Yingxin Li et al., "Long-Term Exposure to Ambient Air Pollution and Serum Liver Enzymes in Older Adults: A Population-Based Longitudinal Study," *Annals of Epidemiology* 74 (October 2022): 1–7, https://doi.org/10.1016/j.annepidem.2022.05.011.
39. Lu Qi et al.,, "Acupuncture for the Treatment of Liver Cirrhosis: A Meta-analysis," *Gastroenterology Research and Practice,* 2020 (November 27, 2020): 4054781, doi: 10.1155/2020/4054781
40. Zang Xiaoming et al., "Effects of Acupuncture for Nonalcoholic Fatty Liver Disease: A Protocol for Systematic Review and Meta-Analysis," *Medicine (Baltimore)* 99, no. 47 (November 20, 2020): e23219, https://doi.org/10.1097/MD.0000000000023219.
41. Ibid.
42. Sung-A Kim, Yujin Choi, and Seung-Hun Cho, "Acupuncture for Attenuating Frontal Lobe α Band Asymmetry Induced by Anger: A Pilot Study," *Journal of Pharmacopuncture* 26, no. 3 (September 30, 2023): 276–84, https://doi.org/10.3831/KPI.2023.26.3.276

Chapter 18 Endnote

1. Paul U. Unschuld, *Huang Di Nei Jing Ling Shu: The Ancient Classic on Needle Therapy* (Oakland, CA: University of California Press, 2016), 756.

Chapter 21 Endnote

1. Qian-Qian Li et al., "Acupuncture Effect and Central Autonomic Regulation," *Evidence-Based Complementary and Alternative Medicine* 2013 (May 26, 2013): 267959, https://doi.org/10.1155/2013/267959.
2. Yan-Wei Li et al., "The Autonomic Nervous System: A Potential Link to the Efficacy of Acupuncture," *Frontiers in Neuroscience* 16 (December 8, 2022): 1038945, https://doi.org/10.3389/fnins.2022.1038945.
3. Qian-Qian Li et al., "Acupuncture Effect and Central Autonomic Regulation."
4. Qian-Qian Li et al., "Acupuncture Effect and Central Autonomic Regulation"; Yan-Wei Li et al., " The Autonomic Nervous System."
5. Yan-Wei Li et al., "Autonomic Nervous System and Acupuncture."
6. Ke Liu, Jian-Feng Jiang, and Shu-Fang Lu, "Effect Characteristics and Mechanism of Acupuncture in Autonomic Nerve Regulation," *Zhen Ci Yan Jiu* 46, no. 4 (April 25, 2021): 335–341 PMID: 33932001, DOI: 10.13702/j.1000-0607.20066, https://pubmed.ncbi.nlm.nih.gov/33932001/.
7. Yan-Wei Li et al., "The Autonomic Nervous System and Acupuncture."
8. Kouich Takamoto et al., "Effects of Acupuncture Needling with Specific Sensation on Cerebral Hemodynamics and Autonomic Nervous Activity in Humans," *International Review of Neurobiology* 111 (2013): 25–48, https://doi.org/10.1016/B978-0-12-411545-3.00002-X.
9. Krista Lynne Paulson and Barbara L. Shay, "Sympathetic Nervous System Responses to Acupuncture and Non-Penetrating Sham Acupuncture in Experimental Forearm Pain: A Single-Blind Randomised Descriptive Study," *Acupuncture in Medicine* 31, no. 2 (June 2013):

178–184, https://doi.org/10.1136/acupmed-2012-010223.
10. Yan-Wei Li et al., "The Autonomic Nervous System and Acupuncture."
11. Paulson and Shay, "Sympathetic Responses to Acupuncture," 178.
12. Holly R. Middlekauff et al., "Acupuncture Inhibits Sympathetic Activation During Mental Stress in Advanced Heart Failure Patients," *Journal of Cardiac Failure* 8, no. 6 (December 2002): 399–406, https://doi.org/10.1054/jcaf.2002.129656.

Chapter 22 Endnotes

1. David Shier, Jackie Butler, and Ricki Lewis, *Hole's Essentials of Human Anatomy and Physiology*, 9th ed. (New York: McGraw-Hill, 2006), 234.
2. Chun-Hong Liu et al., "Neural Networks and the Anti-Inflammatory Effect of Transcutaneous Auricular Vagus Nerve Stimulation in Depression," *Journal of Neuroinflammation* 17, no. 1 (2020): Article 54, https://doi.org/10.1186/s12974-020-01732-5.
3. Ben Kavoussi and B. E. Ross, "The Neuroimmune Basis of Anti-Inflammatory Acupuncture," *Integrative Cancer Therapies* 6, no. 3 (2007): 251–57, https://doi.org/10.1177/1534735407305892.
4. Wei He et al., "Auricular Acupuncture and Vagal Regulation," *Evidence-Based Complementary and Alternative Medicine* 2012 (2012): Article ID 786839, https://doi.org/10.1155/2012/786839.
5. He et al., "Auricular Acupuncture and Vagal Regulation."
6. Ibid.
7. Ibid
8. Elmar T. Peuker and Helmut J. Filler, "The Nerve Supply of the Human Auricle," *Clinical Anatomy* 15, no. 1 (2002): 35–37, DOI: 10.1002/ca.1089He et al., "Auricular Acupuncture and Vagal Regulation."; He et al., "Auricular Acupuncture and Vagal Regulation."
9. He et al., "Auricular Acupuncture and Vagal Regulation."
10. Roberto La Marca et al., "Effects of Auricular Electrical Stimulation on Vagal Activity in Healthy Men: Evidence from a Three-Armed Randomized Trial," *Clinical Science* 118, no. 8 (2010): 537–46,

https://doi.org/10.1042/CS20090264.
11. Juei-De Wang, Terry B. J. Kuo, and Cheryl C. H. Yang, "An Alternative Method to Enhance Vagal Activities and Suppress Sympathetic Activities in Humans," *Autonomic Neuroscience* 100, no. 1–2 (2002): 90–95, https://doi.org/10.1016/s1566-0702(02)00150-9.

Chapter 23 Endnotes

1. Yan-Wei Li et al., "The Autonomic Nervous System: A Potential Link to the Efficacy of Acupuncture," *Frontiers in Neuroscience* 16 (December 8, 2022): 1038945, https://doi.org/10.3389/fnins.2022.1038945.
2. S. Andersson and T. Lundeberg, "Acupuncture—From Empiricism to Science: Functional Background to Acupuncture Effects in Pain and Disease," *Medical Hypotheses* 45, no. 3 (September 1995): 271–81, DOI: 10.1016/0306-9877(95)90117-5
3. Ji-Sheng Han, "Acupuncture and Endorphins," *Neuroscience Letters* 361, no. 1–3 (May 6, 2004): 258–61, https://doi.org/10.1016/j.neulet.2003.12.019.
4. Li et al., "The Autonomic Nervous System" 1038945.
5. Nilima Shankar et al., "Autonomic Status and Pain Profile in Patients of Chronic Low Back Pain and Following Electroacupuncture Therapy: A Randomized Control Trial," *Indian Journal of Physiology and Pharmacology* 55, no. 1 (January–March 2011): 25–36, PMID: 22315807, https://pubmed.ncbi.nlm.nih.gov/22315807/.
6. Andersson and Lundeberg, "Acupuncture—From Empiricism to Science," 271.
7. Ruixin Zhang et al., "Mechanisms of Acupuncture–Electroacupuncture on Persistent Pain," *Anesthesiology* 120, no. 2 (2014): 482–503, https://doi.org/10.1097/ALN.0000000000000101.
8. Han, "Acupuncture and Endorphins," 258.
9. Michael Hauck et al., "Acupuncture Analgesia Involves Modulation of Pain-Induced Gamma Oscillations and Cortical Network Connectivity," *Scientific Reports* 7 (2017): 16307, https://doi.org/10.1038/

s41598-017-13633-4.
10. Zilei Tian et al., "Acupuncture Modulation Effect on Pain Processing Patterns in Patients With Migraine Without Aura," *Frontiers in Neuroscience* 15 (2021): 729218, https://doi.org/10.3389/fnins.2021.729218.

Chapter 24 Endnotes

1. Ling-Hui Ma et. Al, "Effect of Transcutaneous Electrical Acupoint Stimulation at Different Frequencies on Mild Hypertension: A Randomized Controlled Trial," *Complementary Therapies in Medicine* 87 (2024): 103103, https://doi.org/10.1016/j.ctim.2024.103103.
2. Yanbin Peng et al., "Electroacupuncture for Slow Flow/No-Reflow Phenomenon in Patients with Acute Myocardial Infarction Undergoing Percutaneous Coronary Intervention: Protocol for a Pilot Randomized Controlled Trial," *Frontiers in Cardiovascular Medicine* 11 (2024): 1401269, https://doi.org/10.3389/fcvm.2024.1401269.
3. Lei Lan et al., "Acupuncture Modulates the Spontaneous Activity and Functional Connectivity of Calcarine in Patients With Chronic Stable Angina Pectoris," *Frontiers in Molecular Neuroscience* 15 (2022): 842674, https://doi.org/10.3389/fnmol.2022.842674.
4. Ole Bernt Fasmer et al., "A Naturalistic Study of the Effect of Acupuncture on Heart-Rate Variability," *Journal of Acupuncture and Meridian Studies* 5, no. 1 (2012): 15–20, https://doi.org/10.1016/j.jams.2011.11.002.
5. Peng Li et al., "Long-Lasting Reduction of Blood Pressure by Electroacupuncture in Patients with Hypertension: Randomized Controlled Trial," *Medical Acupuncture* 27, no. 4 (2015): 253–261, https://doi.org/10.1089/acu.2015.1106.

Chapter 25 Endnotes

1. Toku Takahashi, "Mechanism of Acupuncture on Neuromodulation

in the Gut—A Review," *Neuromodulation: Technology at the Neural Interface* 14, no. 1 (February 2011): 8–12, https://doi.org/10.1111/j.1525-1403.2010.00295.x

2. Yu-Wei Li et al., "The Autonomic Nervous System: : A Potential Link to the Efficacy of Acupuncture," *Frontiers in Neuroscience* 16 (December 8, 2022): Article 1038945, https://doi.org/10.3389/fnins.2022.1038945.

3. Zhi Yu, "Neuromechanism of Acupuncture Regulating Gastrointestinal Motility," *World Journal of Gastroenterology* 26, no. 23 (2020): 3182–3200, https://doi.org/10.3748/wjg.v26.i23.3182.

4. Han Li and Yin-Ping Wang, "Effect of Auricular Acupuncture on Gastrointestinal Motility and Its Relationship with Vagal Activity," *Acupuncture in Medicine* 31, no. 1 (2013): 57–64, https://doi.org/10.1136/acupmed-2012-010173.

5. Zhaoxiu Liu et al., "Preventive Effects of Transcutaneous Electrical Acustimulation on Ischemic Stroke-Induced Constipation Mediated via the Autonomic Pathway," *American Journal of Physiology – Gastrointestinal and Liver Physiology* 315, no. 2 (2018): G293–G301, https://doi.org/10.1152/ajpgi.00049.2018

6. Luyao Zhang et al., "Electroacupuncture Ameliorates Acute Pancreatitis: A Role for the Vagus Nerve-Mediated Cholinergic Anti-Inflammatory Pathway," *Frontiers in Molecular Biosciences* 8 (2021): Article 647647, https://doi.org/10.3389/fmolb.2021.647647.

7. Dong Kee Jang et al., "Electroacupuncture for Abdominal Pain Relief in Patients with Acute Pancreatitis: Study Protocol for a Randomized Controlled Trial," *Trials* 19, no. 1 (2018): Article 646, https://doi.org/10.1186/s13063-018-2644-1.

8. Ying Zhu et al., "Transcutaneous Auricular Vagal Nerve Stimulation Improves Functional Dyspepsia by Enhancing Vagal Efferent Activity," *American Journal of Physiology – Gastrointestinal and Liver Physiology* 320, no. 5 (2021): G700–G711, https://doi.org/10.1152/ajpgi.00426.2020.

Chapter 26 Endnotes

1. Giovanni Maciocia, *Diagnosis in Chinese Medicine: A Comprehensive Guide* (Edinburgh: Churchill Livingstone, 2004), 129-131.
2. Ibid.
3. Wei He et al., "Auricular Acupuncture and Vagal Regulation," *Evidence-Based Complementary and Alternative Medicine* 2012 (2012): Article ID 786839, https://doi.org/10.1155/2012/786839.
4. Osamu Tanaka and Yoshito Mukaino, "The Effect of Auricular Acupuncture on Olfactory Acuity," *American Journal of Chinese Medicine* 27, no. 1 (1999): 19–24, https://doi.org/10.1142/S0192415X99000045.
5. J.P. Desborough, "The Stress Response to Trauma and Surgery," *British Journal of Anaesthesia* 85, no. 1 (2000): 109–117, https://doi.org/10.1093/bja/85.1.109; George P. Chrousos, "Stress and Disorders of the Stress System," *Nature Reviews Endocrinology* 5, no. 7 (2009): 374–381, https://doi.org/10.1038/nrendo.2009.106.
6. E. Facco et al., "Comparison Study Between Acupuncture and Pentazocine Analgesic and Respiratory Post-Operative Effects," *American Journal of Chinese Medicine* 9, no. 3 (1981): 225–235, https://doi.org/10.1142/S0192415X81000305.
7. Kazufumi Takahashi, "Effect of 2-Hz Electroacupuncture Stimulation on Respiratory Function: A Randomized Controlled Trial," *Medical Acupuncture* 33, no. 1 (2021): 49–57, https://doi.org/10.1089/acu.2020.1418.
8. He et al., "Auricular Acupuncture and Vagal Regulation."
9. Jun Matsumoto-Miyazaki et al., "Efficacy of Acupuncture Treatment for Improving the Respiratory Status in Patients Receiving Prolonged Mechanical Ventilation in Intensive Care Units: A Retrospective Observational Study," *Journal of Alternative and Complementary Medicine* 24, no. 11 (2018): 1076–1084, https://doi.org/10.1089/acm.2017.0365.

Chapter 28 Endnotes

1. Giovanni Maciocia, *The Foundations of Chinese Medicine: A Comprehensive Text for Acupuncturists and Herbalists*, 2nd ed. (Edinburgh: Churchill Livingstone Elsevier, 2005), 69, 242.
2. Paul U. Unschuld, Hermann Tessenow, and Zheng Jinsheng, *Huang Di Nei Jing Su Wen*, vol. 1 (Berkeley and Los Angeles, CA: University of California Press, 2011), 32.
3. Unschuld, Tessenow, and Zheng, *Huang Di Nei Jing Su Wen*, vol. 1, 30.

Chapter 29 Endnotes

1. Jean-Claude Barthelemy et al., "Targeting the Autonomic Nervous System as a Biomarker of Well-Ageing in the Prevention of Stroke," *Frontiers in Aging Neuroscience* 14 (2022), https://doi.org/10.3389/fnagi.2022.969352.
2. Yan-Wei Li et al., "The Autonomic Nervous System: A Potential Link to the Efficacy of Acupuncture," *Frontiers in Neuroscience* 16 (2022), https://doi.org/10.3389/fnins.2022.1038945.
3. Yuwei Chen, Mingzhu Li, and Kaixin Guo, "Exploring the Mechanisms and Current Status of Acupuncture in Alleviating Tumor Metabolism and Associated Diseases: Insights from the Central Nervous System and Immune Microenvironment," *Signal Transduction and Targeted Therapy* (2024), https://doi.org/10.1016/j.slast.2024.100208.
4. Adrián Hernández-Vicente et al., " Heart Rate Variability and Exceptional Longevity," *Frontiers in Physiology* 11 (September 2020): 566399, https://doi.org/10.3389/fphys.2020.566399.
5. Usman Zulfiqar and Donald A. Jurivich, "Relation of High Heart Rate Variability to Healthy Longevity," *The American Journal of Cardiology* 105, no. 9 (May 2010): 1181–85, https://doi.org/10.1016/j.amjcard.2009.12.022.
6. Ken Umetani et al., "Twenty-Four Hour Time Domain Heart Rate

Variability and Heart Rate: Relations to Age and Gender over Nine Decades," *Journal of the American College of Cardiology* 31, no. 3 (1998): 593–601, https://doi.org/10.1016/S0735-1097(97)00554-8.
7. Toshinori Akita et al., "Effects of Acupuncture on Autonomic Nervous Functions During Sleep: Comparison with Nonacupuncture Site Stimulation Using a Crossover Design," *Journal of Integrative and Complementary Medicine* (2022), https://doi.org/10.1089/jicm.2022.0526.
8. Hyungsun Jun et al., "Impact of Acupuncture on Mortality in Patients with Disabilities and Newly Diagnosed Heart Failure: A Nationwide Cohort Study," *Frontiers in Medicine* 12 (2025): Article 1519588, https://doi.org/10.3389/fmed.2025.1519588.

Chapter 30 Endnotes

1. Huang Di, *Huang Di Nei Jing Su Wen*, trans. Paul U. Unschuld (Berkeley: University of California Press, 2011), 175.
2. Huang Di, *Huang Di Nei Jing Su Wen*, 191–192.
3. Huang Di, *Huang Di Nei Jing Su Wen*, 653.
4. Athanase Benetos, Stéphane Laurent, Pierre Safar, and Michael E. O'Rourke, "Arterial Stiffness and Hypertension: A New Risk Factor for Cardiovascular Disease," *American Journal of Hypertension* 15, no. 8 *(2002)*: 688–697, https://doi.org/10.1016/S0895-7061(02)03029-7
5. Philip E. Gates and Douglas R. Seals, "Decline in Large Elastic Artery Compliance with Age: A Therapeutic Target for Habitual Exercise," *British Journal of Sports Medicine* 40, no. 11 (September 5, 2006): 897–899, https://doi.org/10.1136/bjsm.2004.016782.
6. Benetos et al., "Arterial Stiffness and Hypertension," *American Journal of Hypertension*, 2002.
7. Ibid.
8. Nina Terenteva, Oksana Chernykh, Marcos A. Sanchez-Gonzalez, and Alexei Wong, "Acupuncture Therapy Improves Vascular Hemo-

dynamics and Stiffness in Middle-Age Hypertensive Individuals," *Complementary Therapies in Clinical Practice* 30 (February 2018): 14–18, https://doi.org/10.1016/j.ctcp.2017.11.002.
9. Hiroyasu Satoh, "Acute Effects of Acupuncture Treatment with Baihui (GV20) on Human Arterial Stiffness and Wave Reflection," *Journal of Acupuncture and Meridian Studies* 2, no. 2 (June 2009): 130–34. https://doi.org/10.1016/S2005-2901(09)60045-5.
10. Ibid.
11. Gerhard Litscher, Lu Wang, Ingrid Gaischek, and Xin-Yan Gao, "Violet Laser Acupuncture: Part 4, Acute Effects on Human Arterial Stiffness and Wave Reflection," *Journal of Acupuncture and Meridian Studies* 4, no. 3 (September 2011): 168–74. https://doi.org/10.1016/j.jams.2011.09.004.
12. Shin Takayama et al., "Evaluation of the Effects of Acupuncture on Blood Flow in Humans with Ultrasound Color Doppler Imaging," *Evidence-Based Complementary and Alternative Medicine* 2012 (June 21, 2012): 1–8. https://doi.org/10.1155/2012/513638.
13. Ibid.

Chapter 31 Endnotes

1. Giovanni Maciocia, *The Foundations of Chinese Medicine: A Comprehensive Text for Acupuncturists and Herbalists*, 2nd ed. (Edinburgh: Churchill Livingstone, 2005), 383–396, 727.
2. Ibid.
3. Linlin Chen et al., "Inflammatory Responses and Inflammation-Associated Diseases in Organs," *Oncotarget* 9, no. 6 (December 14, 2017): 7204–7218, https://doi.org/10.18632/oncotarget.23208.
4. Amit Singh et al., "Aging and Inflammation," *Cold Spring Harbor Perspectives in Biology*, published online (December 5, 2023), https://doi.org/10.1101/cshperspect.a041197.
5. Ningcen Li et al. "The Anti-Inflammatory Actions and Mechanisms of Acupuncture from Acupoint to Target Organs via Neuro-Immune

Regulation." *Journal of Inflammation Research* 14 (December 21, 2021): 7191–7224. https://doi.org/10.2147/JIR.S341581.
6. Ji-Eun Oh and Seung-Nam Kim, "Anti-Inflammatory Effects of Acupuncture at ST36 Point: A Literature Review in Animal Studies," *Frontiers in Immunology* 12 (January 12, 2022): 813748, https://doi.org/10.3389/fimmu.2021.813748.
7. Jia Chen et al., "Efficacy of Acupuncture Combined with Active Exercise Training in Improving Pain and Function of Knee Osteoarthritis Individuals: A Systematic Review and Meta-Analysis," *Journal of Orthopaedic Surgery and Research* 18, no. 1 (2023): 728, DOI: 10.1186/s13018-023-04403-2

Chapter 32 Endnotes

1. Gardner, Hayley. "A Clinical and Philosophical Exploration of Jing." *Journal of Chinese Medicine*, October 10, 2024, https://www.jcm.co.uk/a-clinical-and-philosophical-exploration-of-jing/; Maciocia, Giovanni. *The Foundations of Chinese Medicine: A Comprehensive Text for Acupuncturists and Herbalists*. 2nd ed. London: Elsevier Churchill Livingstone, 2005, 44-45.
2. Maciocia, *The Foundations of Chinese Medicine*, 44-45.
3. Ibid.
4. Gardner, "A Clinical and Philosophical Exploration of Jing."
5. López-Otín, Carlos et al,. "The Hallmarks of Aging." *Cell* 153, no. 6 (2013): 1194–1217. https://doi.org/10.1016/j.cell.2013.05.039.
6. Ibid.
7. Saint-Pierre, Christian, and Julie Saint-Pierre. "Chinese Medical Perspectives on Longevity: Bridging Ancient Insights on Lifespan and Healthspan with Modern Research into IL-11." Unpublished manuscript.
8. Gardner, "A Clinical and Philosophical Exploration of Jing."
9. López-Otín et al., "The Hallmarks of Aging," 1194.,Gardner, "A Clinical and Philosophical Exploration of Jing."

10. Daniel Promislow et al., "Resilience Integrates Concepts in Aging Research," *iScience* 25, no. 5 (April 6, 2022): 104199. https://doi.org/10.1016/j.isci.2022.104199.
11. Dao-Fu Dai et al., "Mitochondrial Oxidative Stress in Aging and Healthspan," *Longevity & Healthspan* 3, no. 6 (May 1, 2014). https://doi.org/10.1186/2046-2395-3-6.
12. Haiyang Chen et al., "Targeting Mitochondrial Homeostasis: The Role of Acupuncture in Depression Treatment," *Neuropsychiatric Disease and Treatment* 19 (August 1, 2023): 1741–53. https://doi.org/10.2147/NDT.S421540.
13. Ibid.
14. Sarah Mockler et al., "Acupuncture Treatment Preserves Soleus Muscle Mass and Improves Mitochondrial Function in a Rat Model of Disuse Atrophy," *Integrative Medicine Research* 14, no. 3 (September 2025): 101178. https://doi.org/10.1016/j.imr.2025.101178.
15. Teng-I Huang and Ching-Liang Hsieh, "Effects of Acupuncture on Oxidative Stress Amelioration via Nrf2/ARE-Related Pathways in Alzheimer and Parkinson Diseases," *Evidence-Based Complementary and Alternative Medicine* (April 26, 2021): 6624976. https://doi.org/10.1155/2021/6624976.
16. Ibid.

Chapter 33 Endnotes

1. Dellara F. Terry et al., "Association of Longer Telomeres With Better Health in Centenarians," *Journals of Gerontology: Series A, Biological Sciences and Medical Sciences* 63, no. 8 (August 2008): 809–12, https://pubmed.ncbi.nlm.nih.gov/18772468; Angela R. Starkweather, Areej A. Alhaeeri, Alison Montpetit, Jenni Brumelle, Kristin Filler, Marty Montpetit, Lathika Mohanraj, Debra E. Lyon, and Colleen K. Jackson-Cook, "An Integrative Review of Factors Associated with Telomere Length and Implications for Biobehavioral Research," *Nursing Research* 63, no. 1 (January–February 2014): 36–50, https://doi.org/10.1097/

NNR.0000000000000009.
2. Ibid.
3. Giovanni Maciocia, *The Foundations of Chinese Medicine: A Comprehensive Text for Acupuncturists and Herbalists*, 2nd ed. (Edinburgh: Churchill Livingstone, 2005), 44–45.
4. Terry et al., "Association of Longer Telomeres With Better Health in Centenarians," *Journals of Gerontology: Series A* 63, no. 8 (2008): 809–12; Starkweather et al., "An Integrative Review of Factors Associated with Telomere Length," *Nursing Research* 63, no. 1 (2014): 36–50.
5. Maciocia, *The Foundations of Chinese Medicine*, 53.
6. Angela R. Starkweather et al., "An Integrative Review of Factors Associated with Telomere Length and Implications for Biobehavioral Research," *Nursing Research* 63, no. 1 (January–February 2014): 36–50, doi: 10.1097/NNR.0000000000000009.
7. Ibid.
8. Terry et al., "Association of Longer Telomeres With Better Health in Centenarians," *Journals of Gerontology: Series A* 63, no. 8 (2008): 809–12. doi: 10.1093/gerona/63.8.809
9. Dong Lin et al., "The Effect of Electroacupuncture versus Manual Acupuncture through the Expression of TrkB/NF-κB in the Subgranular Zone of the Dentate Gyrus of Telomerase-Deficient Mice," *Evidence Based Complementary and Alternative Medicine* 2018 (April 22, 2018): 1–9. https://doi.org/10.1155/2018/1013978.
10. Wei Wang et al., "Electroacupuncture Pretreatment Preserves Telomerase Reverse Transcriptase Function and Alleviates Postoperative Cognitive Dysfunction by Suppressing Oxidative Stress and Neuroinflammation in Aged Mice," *CNS Neuroscience & Therapeutics* 30, no. 2 (July 27, 2023): e14373. doi: 10.1111/cns.14373.
11. Ibid.
12. Maciocia, *The Foundations of Chinese Medicine*, 53.
13. Jun Wu and Lewis L. Lanier, "Natural Killer Cells and Cancer," *Advances in Cancer Research* 90 (2003): 127–156, https://doi.org/

10.1016/S0065-230X(03)90004-2.

14. Mattia E. Ligotti et al., "Sicilian Semi- and Supercentenarians: Age-Related NK Cell Immunophenotype and Longevity Trait Definition," *Translational Medicine UniSa* 25, no. 1 (October 17, 2023): 11–15, DOI: 10.37825/2239-9747.1041.

15. Michael Francis Johnston et al., "Acupuncture May Stimulate Anticancer Immunity via Activation of Natural Killer Cells," *Evidence-Based Complementary and Alternative Medicine* 2011 (March 10, 2011): 1–7. https://doi.org/10.1093/ecam/nep236

16. Ibid.

17. Meng Wang et al., "The Immunomodulatory Mechanisms for Acupuncture Practice," *Frontiers in Immunology* 14 (April 6, 2023): 1147718, doi: 10.3389/fimmu.2023.1147718.

18. Ibid.

Chapter 34 Endnotes

1. Unschuld, Paul U., Hermann Tessenow, and Zheng Jinsheng. *Huang Di Nei Jing Su Wen*. Vol. 1. Berkeley and Los Angeles, CA: University of California Press, 2011, 56.

2. Vincent Magnon, Frédéric Dutheil, and Guillaume T. Vallet, "Benefits from One Session of Deep and Slow Breathing on Vagal Tone and Anxiety in Young and Older Adults," *Scientific Reports* 11 (2021): 19267, https://doi.org/10.1038/s41598-021-98736-9; Dieu-Thuong Thi Trinh et al., "Heart Rate Variability during Auricular Acupressure at the Left Sympathetic Point on Healthy Volunteers: A Pilot Study," *Frontiers in Neuroscience* 17 (2023), https://doi.org/10.3389/fnins.2023.1116154; Davide Donelli et al., "Silence and Its Effects on the Autonomic Nervous System: A Systematic Review." in *Progress in Brain Research*, vol. 280 (2023): 103–144, doi.org/10.1016/bs.pbr.2023.06.002.

Chapter 35 Endnotes

1. Krystle Vermes, "Chinese Body Clock: About, Benefits, Research," *Healthline*, last modified March 17, 2020, https://www.healthline.com/health/chinese-body-clock.
2. Nicole P. Bowles et al., "The Circadian System Modulates the Cortisol Awakening Response in Humans," *Frontiers in Neuroscience* 16 (2022), https://doi.org/10.3389/fnins.2022.995452; Jessica Kimambo, "5 Science-Backed Morning Rituals to Maximize Daily Productivity," *Vocal Media*, accessed July 29, 2025, https://vocal.media/lifehack/5-science-backed-morning-rituals-to-maximize-daily-productivity.
3. Vermes, "Chinese Body Clock; Giovanni Maciocia, *Diagnosis in Chinese Medicine: A Comprehensive Guide* (Edinburgh: Churchill Livingstone, 2005), 195-197.
4. Tobias Stalder et al., "The Cortisol Awakening Response: Regulation and Functional Significance," *Endocrine Reviews* 46, no. 1 (2025): 43-59, https://doi.org/10.1210/endrev/bnae024.
5. Andrea Zaccaro et al., "How Breath-Control Can Change Your Life: A Systematic Review on Psycho-Physiological Correlates of Slow Breathing," *Frontiers in Human Neuroscience* 12 (2018), https://doi.org/10.3389/fnhum.2018.00353.
6. Sarah J. Hall et al., "The Acute Physiological Stress Response to an Emergency Alarm and Mobilization during the Day and at Night," *Noise & Health* 18, no. 82 (2016), DOI: 10.4103/1463-1741.181998
7. Konstantin V. Danilenko et al., "The Human Circadian Pacemaker Can See by the Dawn's Early Light," *Journal of Biological Rhythms* 15, no. 5 (2000): 437–46, https://doi.org/10.1177/074873000129001521; Angeliki Athanasatou et al., "Fluctuation of Water Intake and of Hydration Indices during the Day in a Sample of Healthy Greek Adults," *Nutrients* 11, no. 4 (2019): 793, DOI: 10.3390/nu11040793; Sidra Qayyum et al., "Association of Sleep Patterns and Water Intake with Cognitive Functions in Adults in an Urban Environment," *Pakistan Journal of Medical Sciences* 40, no. 4 (2024): 606–611, https://doi.org/10.12669/pjms.40.4.8268; Diane Freitas et al., "Glycemic Response, Satiety, Gastric Secretions and Emptying after Bread

Consumption with Water, Tea or Lemon Juice: A Randomized Crossover Intervention Using MRI," *European Journal of Nutrition* 61, no. 3 (2022): 1621–1636, https://doi.org/10.1007/s00394-021-02762-2.

8. Myeong Soo Lee, Hye-Sook Jang, and Sun-Rock Moon, "Effects of Qi-Therapy (External Qigong) on Autonomic Nervous System: A Randomized Placebo Controlled Pilot Trial," *Journal of International Society of Life Information Science* 22, no. 2 (2004): 314–316, https://doi.org/10.18936/islis.22.2_314; Albert Yeung et al., "Qigong and Tai-Chi for Mood Regulation," *Focus* 16, no. 1 (2018): 40–47, https://doi.org/10.1176/appi.focus.20170042; Jingyu Sun et al., "Effects of 3-Month Qigong Exercise on Heart Rate Variability and Respiration in Anxious College Students," *Scandinavian Journal of Medicine & Science in Sports* 34, no. 1 (2024): e14521, https://doi.org/10.1111/sms.14521.

9. Maciocia, *Diagnosis in Chinese Medicine*, 69-71.

Chapter 36 Endnotes

1. Mami Sakurai et al., "Conscious Slower Breathing Predominates Parasympathetic Activity and Provides a Relaxing Effect, in Healthy Japanese Adult Women," *Health* 15, no. 9 (2023): 852–868, https://doi.org/10.4236/health.2023.159064; Sophie Betka et al., "Breathing Control, Brain, and Bodily Self-Consciousness: Toward Immersive Digiceuticals to Alleviate Respiratory Suffering," *Biological Psychology* 174 (2022): 108329, https://doi.org/10.1016/j.biopsycho.2022.108329; Michael Christopher Melnychuk et al., "A Bridge between the Breath and the Brain: Synchronization of Respiration, a Pupillometric Marker of the Locus Coeruleus, and an EEG Marker of Attentional Control State," *PLOS Biology* 19, no. 10 (2021): e3001035, DOI: 10.3390/brainsci11101324; T.C. Koh, "Qigong—Chinese Breathing Exercise," *The American Journal of Chinese Medicine* 10, no. 1–4 (1982): 86–91, https://doi.org/10.1142/S0192415X82000142.

2. Stephen W. Porges, "Polyvagal Theory: A Science of Safety," *Frontiers in Integrative Neuroscience* 16 (2022), https://doi.org/10.3389/fnint.2022.871227.
3. Andrea Zaccaro et al., "How Breath-Control Can Change Your Life: A Systematic Review on Psycho-Physiological Correlates of Slow Breathing," *Frontiers in Human Neuroscience* 17 (2023), https://doi.org/10.3389/fnhum.2018.00353.
4. Ikuo Homma and Yuri Masaoka, "Breathing Rhythms and Emotions," *Experimental Physiology* 93, no. 9 (2008): 1011–1021, https://doi.org/10.1113/expphysiol.2008.042424.
5. Sakurai et al., "Conscious Slower Breathing Predominates Parasympathetic Activity."
6. Sophie Betka et al., "Breathing Control, Brain, and Bodily Self-Consciousness: Toward Immersive Digiceuticals to Alleviate Respiratory Suffering," *Biological Psychology* 174 (2022): 108329, https://doi.org/10.1016/j.biopsycho.2022.108329.
7. Porges, "Polyvagal Theory."
8. Mendo, Bruno, et al. "Can Yoga, Qigong, and Tai Chi Breathing Work Support the Psycho-Immune Homeostasis during and after the COVID-19 Pandemic? A Narrative Review." *Healthcare (Basel)* 10, no. 10 (2022): 1934. https://doi.org/10.3390/healthcare10101934; Tanya Coon "Qigong Breathing: Returning to the Rhythms of Nature," *Qigong Awareness*, accessed July 30, 2025, https://qigongawareness.com/blog/qigong-breathing-returning-to-the-rhythms-of-nature/.
9. Koh, "Qigong—Chinese Breathing Exercise."
10. Patrick R. Steffen et al., "Integrating Breathing Techniques Into Psychotherapy to Improve Heart Rate Variability: Which Approach Is Best?" *Frontiers in Psychology* 12 (2021), https://doi.org/10.3389/fpsyg.2021.624254.
11. Joshua Marchant et al., "Comparing the Effects of Square, 4-7-8, and 6 Breaths-per-Minute Breathing Conditions on Heart Rate Variability CO2 Levels, and Mood," *Applied Psychophysiology and Biofeedback* (2024), https://doi.org/10.1007/s10484-025-09688-z.

12. Gunjan Trivedi et al., "Humming (Simple Bhramari Pranayama) as a Stress Buster: A Holter-Based Study to Analyze Heart Rate Variability Parameters During Bhramari, Physical Activity, Emotional Stress, and Sleep," *Cureus* 15, no. 4 (2023): e37527, https://doi.org/10.7759/cureus.37527.
13. Bangalore G. Kalyani et al., "Neurohemodynamic Correlates of 'OM' Chanting: A Pilot Functional Magnetic Resonance Imaging Study," *International Journal of Yoga* 4, no. 1 (2011): 3–6, https://doi.org/10.4103/0973-6131.78171.
14. Jiayi Xia et al., "Effects of Conventional Speech Therapy with Liuzijue Qigong, a Traditional Chinese Method of Breath Training, in 70 Patients with Post-Stroke Spastic Dysarthria," *Medical Science Monitor* 29 (2023): e939451, DOI: 10.12659/MSM.939623.

Chapter 37 Endnotes

1. Eva Selhub, "Nutritional Psychiatry: Your Brain on Food," *Harvard Health Publishing*, last modified September 18, 2022, https://www.health.harvard.edu/blog/nutritional-psychiatry-your-brain-on-food-201511168626.
2. Paul Pitchford, *Healing with Whole Foods: Asian Traditions and Modern Nutrition*, 3rd ed. (Berkeley, CA: North Atlantic Books, 2002), 1-5.
3. Daniela Guarino et al., "The Role of the Autonomic Nervous System in the Pathophysiology of Obesity," *Frontiers in Physiology* 8 (September 14, 2017): 665, https://doi.org/10.3389/fphys.2017.00665.
4. Selhub, "Nutritional Psychiatry."
5. Gia Merlo, Gabrielle Bachtel, and Steven G. Sugden, "Gut Microbiota, Nutrition, and Mental Health," *Frontiers in Nutrition* 11 (2024), https://doi.org/10.3389/fnut.2024.1337889.
6. Junshi Chen, "Essential Role of Medicine and Food Homology in Health and Wellness," *Chinese Herbal Medicines* 15, no. 3 (May 25, 2023): 347–348. https://doi.org/10.1016/j.chmed.2023.05.001.
7. Christine E. Cherpak, "Mindful Eating: A Review of How the Stress-

Digestion-Mindfulness Triad May Modulate and Improve Gastrointestinal and Digestive Function," *Integrative Medicine (Encinitas)* 18, no. 4 (August 2019): 48–53. https://pubmed.ncbi.nlm.nih.gov/32549835/.
8. Pitchford, *Healing with Whole Foods*, 254, 339-346.
9. Ibid.

Chapter 38 Endnotes

1. Tomoko Ikeno and Lili Yan, "Chronic Light Exposure in the Middle of the Night Disturbs the Circadian System and Emotional Regulation." *Journal of Biological Rhythms* 31, no. 4 (2016): 352–364. https://doi.org/10.1177/0748730416642065; Junmei Wu, and Zhengyu Zhao. "Acupuncture in Circadian Rhythm Sleep-Wake Disorders and Its Potential Neurochemical Mechanisms." *Frontiers in Neuroscience* 18 (2024): 1346635. https://doi.org/10.3389/fnins.2024.1346635
2. Ikeno and Yan, "Chronic Light Exposure in the Middle of the Night."
3. Wu and Zhao, "Acupuncture in Circadian Rhythm Sleep-Wake Disorders," 1346635.
4. Ibid.
5. Ibid.
6. Peter Meerlo et al., "Restricted and Disrupted Sleep: Effects on Autonomic Function, Neuroendocrine Stress Systems and Stress Responsivity," *Sleep Medicine Reviews* 12, no. 3 (2008): 197–210, https://doi.org/10.1016/j.smrv.2007.07.007.
7. Giovanni Maciocia, *The Foundations of Chinese Medicine: A Comprehensive Text for Acupuncturists and Herbalists*, 2nd ed. (Edinburgh: Churchill Livingstone, 2005), 69-71.
8. Maciocia, *Foundations of Chinese Medicine*, 2nd ed., 335.
9. Maciocia, *Foundations of Chinese Medicine*, 2nd ed., 100.
10. Maciocia, *Foundations of Chinese Medicine*, 2nd ed., 335.
11. Ibid.
12. Vanessa Martins et al., "Effects of Light Exposure on Vagally-Mediated

NOTES

Heart Rate Variability: A Systematic Review," *Neuroscience and Biobehavioral Reviews* 176 (2025):
13. DOI: 10.1016/j.neubiorev.2025.106241; Laura Castro-Santos et al., "Sleep and Circadian Hygiene Practices Association with Sleep Quality among Brazilian Adults," *Sleep Med X* 6 (December 15, 2023): 100088, https://doi.org/10.1016/j.sleepx.2023.100088.

Chapter 39 Endnotes

1. Lauri Nummenmaa et al., "Bodily Maps of Emotions," *Proceedings of the National Academy of Sciences of the United States of America* 111, no. 2 (2014): 646–51, https://doi.org/10.1073/pnas.1321664111; Emily A. Butler, Frank H. Wilhelm, and James J. Gross, "Respiratory Sinus Arrhythmia, Emotion, and Emotion Regulation during Social Interaction," *Psychophysiology* 43, no. 6 (2006): 612–22, https://doi.org/10.1111/j.1469-8986.2006.00467.x.
2. Butler, Wilhelm, and Gross, "Respiratory Sinus Arrhythmia, Emotion Regulation"; Ya-Ting Lee, "Principle Study of Head Meridian Acupoint Massage to Stress Release via Grey Data Model Analysis," *Evidence-Based Complementary and Alternative Medicine* (2016): 4943204, https://doi.org/10.1155/2016/4943204.
3. Nummenmaa et al., "Bodily Maps of Emotions," 647.
4. Tiffany Field, "Touch for Socioemotional and Physical Well-Being: A Review," *Developmental Review* 30, no. 4 (2010): 367–83, https://doi.org/10.1016/j.dr.2011.01.001.
5. Ferenc Köteles et al., "Slow Stroking Evokes a More Pleasant Sensation but Similar Autonomic Nervous System Response than Rhythmic Touching," *Biological Psychology* 185 (2024): 108957, https://doi.org/10.1016/j.biopsycho.2024.108957.
6. Lee, "Head Meridian Acupoint Massage," 4943204.
7. Frédéric Flament, Aurélie Maudet, and Muriel Bayer-Vanmoen, "The Objective and Subjective Impact of a Daily Self-Massage on Visible Signs of Stress on the Skin and Emotional Well-Being," *International*

Journal of Cosmetic Science (2023), https://doi.org/10.1111/ics.12884.

8. "The History of Gua Sha," *Gua Sha Therapie*, accessed August 2, 2025, https://guashatherapie.nl/history/?lang=en; Mark Parzynski, "The History of Gua Sha: Ancient Origins to Modern Medicine," *AcuArtistry*, accessed August 2, 2025, https://www.acuartistry.com/acuarticles/the-history-of-gua-sha-ancient-origins-to-modern-medicine; The History of Gua Sha: Origins and Evolution," *Gua Sha Portugal*, accessed August 2, 2025, https://www.guasha.pt/en/the-history-of-gua-sha-origins-and-evolution/; Arya Nielsen, *Gua Sha: A Traditional Technique for Modern Practice*, foreword by Ted Kaptchuk (New York: Churchill Livingstone, 1995).
9. Parzynski, "The History of Gua Sha."
10. Ibid.
11. Ibid.
12. Ibid.
13. Arya Nielsen et al., "The Effect of Gua Sha Treatment on the Microcirculation of Surface Tissue: A Pilot Study in Healthy Subjects," *Explore* 3, no. 5 (2007): 456–66, https://doi.org/10.1016/j.explore.2007.06.001.
14. Nielsen et al., "Effect of Gua Sha," 2007.
15. Tingting Chen et al., "Gua Sha, a Press-Stroke Treatment of the Skin, Boosts the Immune Response to Intradermal Vaccination," *Cellular & Molecular Immunology* 13, no. 3 (2016): 391–93, DOI: 10.7717/peerj.2451
16. Sun-Hee Ahn et al., "Comparative Effects of Facial Roller and Gua Sha Massage on Facial Contour, Muscle Tone, and Skin Elasticity: Randomized Controlled Trial," *Journal of Cosmetic Dermatology* (2024), https://doi.org/10.1111/jocd.70236.

Appendix A. Epigraph Sources

Opening Epigraph

1. Ni, Maoshing. *The Yellow Emperor's Classic of Medicine: A New Translation of the Neijing Suwen with Commentary*. Boston: Shambhala, 1995, 1.

Part 1 - Foundations of Acupuncture and the Nervous System

1. Ni, Maoshing. *The Yellow Emperor's Classic of Medicine: A New Translation of the Neijing Suwen with Commentary*. Boston: Shambhala, 1995,17.
2. Huang Di. *Huang Di Nei Jing Su Wen*. Translated by Paul U. Unschuld and Hermann Tessenow. Vol. 1. Berkeley: University of California Press, 2011, 30.

Part II - When Survival Becomes the Pattern

1. Huang Di. *Huang Di Nei Jing Su Wen*. Translated by Paul U. Unschuld and Hermann Tessenow. Vol. 1. Berkeley: University of California Press, 2011, 30.
2. Hammer, Leon. *Dragon Rises, Red Bird Flies: Psychology and Chinese Medicine*. Revised edition. Seattle: Eastland Press, 2010, 59.

Part III - The Channels of Regulation

1. Unschuld, Paul U., trans. *Huang Di Nei Jing Ling Shu: The Ancient Classic on Needle Therapy*. Berkeley: University of California Press, 2016, 176.

Part IV - The Emotional Body

1. Huang Di. *Huang Di Nei Jing Su Wen*. Translated by Paul U. Unschuld and Hermann Tessenow. Vol. 1. Berkeley: University of California Press, 2011, 369.

Part V - Tracing the Currents of Balance

1. Huang Di. *Huang Di Nei Jing Su Wen*. Translated by Paul U. Unschuld and Hermann Tessenow. Vol. 1. Berkeley: University of California Press, 2011, 57.
2. Huang Di. *Huang Di Nei Jing Su Wen*. Translated by Paul U. Unschuld and Hermann Tessenow. Vol. 1. Berkeley: University of California Press, 2011, 53.

Part VI - From Regulation to Renewal

1. Huang Di. *Huang Di Nei Jing Su Wen*. Translated by Paul U. Unschuld and Hermann Tessenow. Vol. 1. Berkeley: University of California Press, 2011, 36.
2. Huang Di. *Huang Di Nei Jing Su Wen*. Translated by Paul U. Unschuld and Hermann Tessenow. Vol. 1. Berkeley: University of California Press, 2011, 41.

APPENDIX A. EPIGRAPH SOURCES

Part VII - Rhythms of Renewal

1. Ni, Maoshing. *The Yellow Emperor's Classic of Medicine: A New Translation of the Neijing Suwen with Commentary*. Boston: Shambhala, 1995, 1.

About the Author

Dr. Amanda Archuleta, D.A.O.M., L.Ac., is a nationally certified and New Mexico–licensed acupuncturist, herbalist, and educator. She earned her Doctorate of Acupuncture and Oriental Medicine from Five Branches University and completed her Master of Science in Oriental Medicine at Southwest Acupuncture College, with additional training at Heilongjiang University in Harbin, China.

Through her clinical practice, writing, and teaching, Dr. Archuleta explores the meeting place of modern health science and ancient healing traditions. Her work guides readers and patients alike back to balance, vitality, and spirit, weaving timeless wisdom with practical tools for well-being and longevity.

ABOUT THE AUTHOR

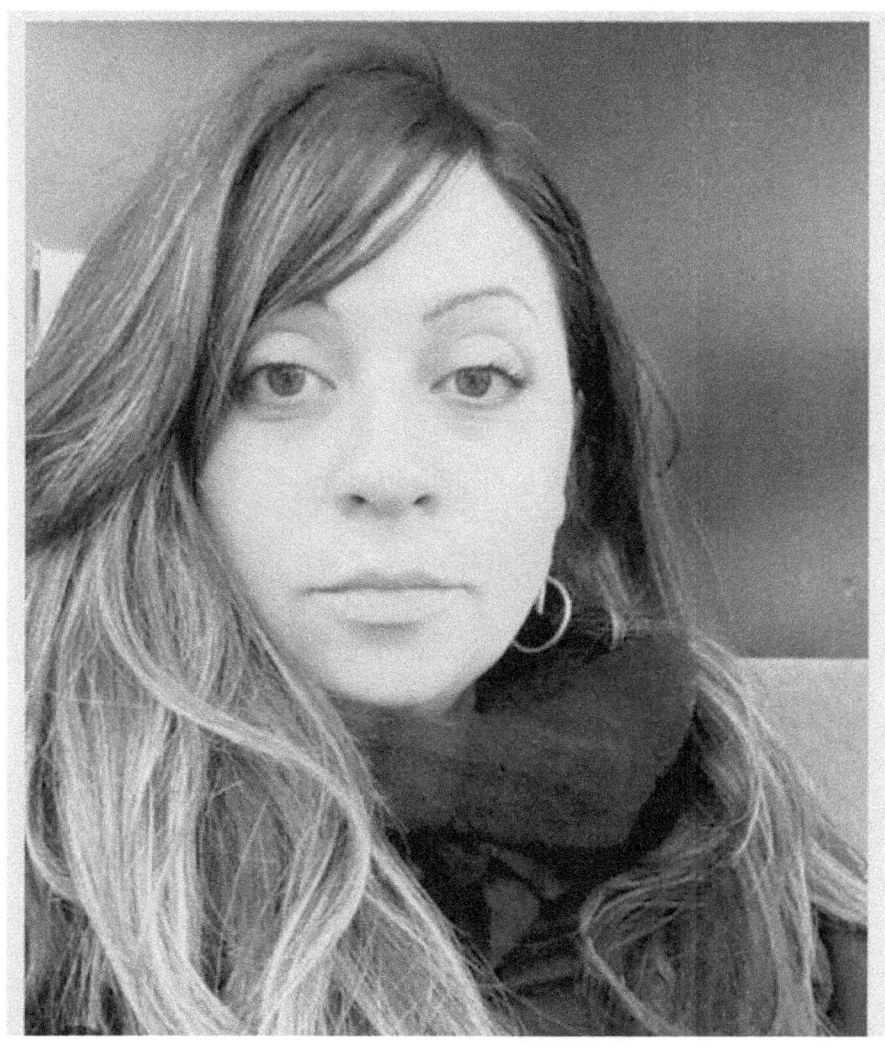

Stay Connected

Thank you for reading *Wired for Balance*. If you'd like to continue exploring these practices, you can join my free email community.

When you sign up, you'll receive:

- Selfcare ritual cards and guided meditations
- Seasonal wellness practices
- Updates on new journals, planners, and tools I'm creating

✧ Join here: ancient-vitality-tools.com

Share Your Experience

If you found this book helpful, I'd be so grateful if you left a review on the site where you purchased it. Your feedback helps others discover *Wired for Balance* and supports this work reaching more people.

www.ingramcontent.com/pod-product-compliance
Lightning Source LLC
Chambersburg PA
CBHW020452030426
42337CB00011B/86